CLINICAL

EKG

INTERPRETATION

&

Patient Management

Dedicated to: _____

_____
NIK NIKAM, MD, MHA

NIK NIKAM, MD, MHA

CLINICAL EKG INTERPRETATION

CLINICAL EKG INTERPRETATION

Copyright: S.G. (NIK) NIKAM, MD, MHA
All rights reserved ©2019

Editor: Navin Nikam, MD

Cover Graphics: NIK NIKAM, MD, MHA
Cataloging in Publication Date Jan. 2019

NIKAM, NIK
Clinical EKG Interpretation 2019
First eBook: 2019

Version 1.0

The information provided in this book is subject to this copyright notice. No part of this book may be copied, retransmitted, reported, duplicated, or used without the express written consent of the author, except by reviewers who may quote brief excerpts in connection with a review. United States laws and regulations are public domain and not subject to copyright. Any unauthorized copying, reproduction, translation, or distribution of any part of this material without permission by the author is prohibited and against the law.

Disclaimer and Terms of Use: The information provided here is for educational and entertainment purposes only. The information contained in this book is not a medical or professional advice.

Publication Date: March 10, 2019
ISBN: 9780976527558
EAN13: 978-0-9765275-5-8
Library of Congress Control Number: 2019901233

Language: English

NIK NIKAM, MD MHA
NNN Media
3130 GRANTS BLVD #17034
SUGAR LAND, TX 77496
drniknikam@gmail.com

Printed in the United States of America

CLINICAL
EKG
INTERPRETATION
&
Patient Management

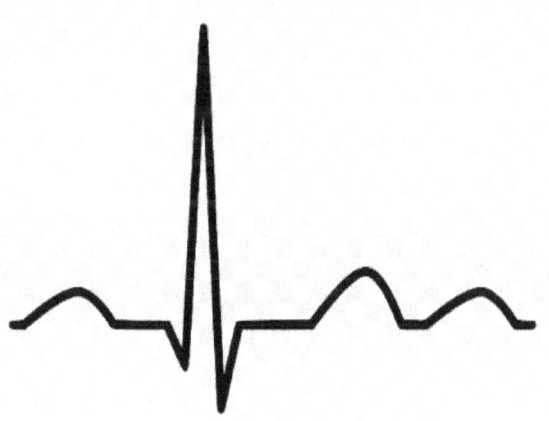

NIK NIKAM, MD, MHA

CLINICAL EKG INTERPRETATION

Publications by Nik Nikam, MD, MHA

Stressless Mind & Priceless Body (1995). Paperback.

Heart-Healthy Lifestyle (2010). Paperback and Kindle Editions.

RAMAYAN – An English Screenplay (2012). Paperback and Kindle Editions.

Cruise Crisis – An English Screenplay (2013). Kindle Edition.

Stressfree Lifestyle (2016). Paperback and Kindle Editions.

Cardiology Lecture Series:

https://www.youtube.com/channel/UCL1x8qabFk8zXn6XOHq8w1w

YOUTUBE: NIK NIKAM

Please visit our YouTube channel, "NIK NIKAM," and Subscribe to it.

It has more than 150 presentations under "Cardiology Lecture series," play list. It includes a comprehensive coverage of the cardiology section of the Internal Medicine Board Examination, the ACLS protocols, and ACLS EKG interpretations.

In fact, our presentation on ACLS-EKG interpretation has been watched by more than 250,000 people from all across the globe.

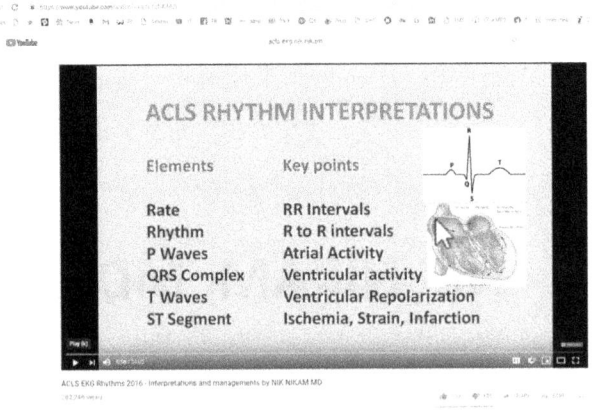

CLINICAL EKG INTERPRETATION

Author: Nik Nikam, MD, MHA

Dr. Nik Nikam has practiced cardiology in Houston and Sugar Land, Texas, for more than 38 years.

He had vast exposure to the medical field at the world-famous Texas Medical Center for more than three decades. His public-speaking skills and his interactions with a community of diverse people have created an everlasting reservoir of knowledge and experience.

He uses his experience in explaining the interpretation of the electrocardiogram from a clinical perspective to create a visual image of the heart in the patient's body. He explains how the heart reflects the electrocardiographic changes and how these changes may reflect the patient's overall prognosis

Dr. Nik has made hundreds of presentations on *Heart-Healthy Lifestyle*. He has published over 100 articles in many Houston-area newspapers and across the United States.

He is a Distinguished Toastmaster, speaker, writer, auctioneer, and a talk show host. His YouTube channel, "NIK NIKAM NETWORK – NNN," has more than 140 videos covering important cardiology topics, including ACLS protocols.

He loves to deliver an engaging educational presentation sprinkled with a unique sense of humor.

For speaking engagements, you can contact Dr. Nik at:

Nik Nikam, MD, MHA
3130 Grants Blvd., #17034
Sugar Land, TX 77496
281-745-4161

CLINICAL EKG INTERPRETATION

Inspirations come from different angles

When I attended my first EKG conference in Clearwater Florida, Dr. Marriott was the only featured presenter. That was in the year 1980. Even to this day, his words and art of uncovering the hidden mystery have inspired and mesmerized me. Even his book on treadmill testing was very educational. His method of teaching and describing events in cardiology in time, dimension, and space had a lasting impression on my cardiology journey.

While I was researching for this book, I came across an online EKG interpretation by Dr. Ary Goldberger, which I found to be the most practical. It provided an in-depth look at an electrocardiogram and making a clinical diagnosis based only on the salient features on an electrocardiogram that only a master can see and perceive.

There are authors, there are researchers, and then there are true masters of communication who can build a new generation of responsible professionals.

Another inspiration for me to write this book came from a YouTube video series I did on ACLS protocols. Just one 35-minute video on ACLS-EKG interpretation was watched by more than 250,000 people from all across the globe.

Many times, heartfelt inspirations have come when I have made presentations to students, nurses, and residents. As you read this book, if you come across an interesting electrocardiogram, please share a screen copy of the same along with some background information. We will be happy to respond to you and proudly add that to our collection of EKGs that can benefit future students.

Nik Nikam, MD
drniknikam@gmail.com

CLINICAL EKG INTERPRETATION

Mission:

The mission of the Clinical EKG Interpretation book is to help you:

- Recognize common EKG patterns you come across in your daily practice.

- Correlate them with underlying anatomical and pathological changes in the cardiovascular system.

- Apply the EKG knowledge in clinical decision making in the management of patients at the bedside.

- Anticipate future events based on the current electrocardiographic and clinical presentations.

- Pass your board examination EKG sections.

- Get a better understanding of ACLS EKG arrhythmias.

- Feel confident that you can, "Do it!"

We need your help:

As we continue to provide basic, clinical, patient-focused, EKG interpretations, we invite your input, tracings, and suggestions for the next edition so we can surely provide the readers maximum return on their time and effort.

Also, please take a moment to comment on the Amazon website about your impressions of this book and how we can improve it in the future.

CLINICAL EKG INTERPRETATION

Table of Contents—Summary

Chapter	01	Introduction	01
Chapter	02	Electrical Axis	31
Chapter	03	Conduction Disturbances	37
Chapter	04	Bundle Branch Blocks	49
Chapter	05	Chamber Enlargements	67
Chapter	06	Sinus Node Dysfunction	83
Chapter	07	Bradycardias	91
Chapter	08	Supraventricular Arrhythmias	101
Chapter	09	Ventricular Arrhythmias	141
Chapter	10	Ischemia and Infarction	163
Chapter	11	ST Segment Abnormalities	183
Chapter	12	T Wave Abnormalities	193
Chapter	13	Pacemaker Rhythms	203
Chapter	14	Miscellaneous Conditions	215
Chapter	15	Cardiac Monitoring	245
Chapter	16	Multiple-Choice Questions 1-100	247
Chapter	17	Interpretation Quiz: 1-50 Tracings	282
Chapter		References	310

CLINICAL EKG INTERPRETATION

Table of Contents

Chapter 1 Introduction   01

- Introduction
- Lead Placement
- Rate, Rhythm, and Normal EKG
- Coronary Anatomy and EKG Correlation
- Heart Structure and EKG Changes
- Action Potential and EKG Correlation
- The Electrical System of the Heart
- Basic Measurements

Chapter 2 Electrical Axis   31

- Normal
- Left Axis
- Right Axis
- Indeterminate Axis

Chapter 3 Conduction Disturbances   37

- 1st-degree AV Block
- 2nd-degree AV Block: Type-1 and Type-II
- Incomplete Heart Block (ICHB)
- Complete Heart Block (CHB)
- Preexcitation
- LGL Syndrome

Chapter 4 Bundle Branch Blocks   49

- RBBB
- LBBB
- LAHB
- Fascicular Block
- IVCD
- Wide QRS Complexes
- Brugada Syndrome

Chapter 5 Chamber Enlargements   67

- Left Atrial Enlargement
- Right Atrial Enlargement
- Biatrial Enlargement
- Right Ventricular Hypertrophy
- Left Ventricular Hypertrophy
- Biventricular Hypertrophy

Chapter 6 Sinus Node Dysfunction   83

- Sinus Arrhythmia
- Sinus Exit Block
- Sinus Pauses
- Sinoatrial Block
- Sick Sinus Syndrome
- Hyperdynamic Circulation

Chapter 7 Bradycardias   91

- Sinus Bradycardia
- Slow Junctional Rhythm
- Ventricular Rhythm
- Idioventricular Rhythm
- Agonal Rhythm
- Asystole
- Lead Displacement

Chapter 8 Supraventricular Arrhythmias   101

- Sinus Tachycardia
- Paroxysmal Supraventricular Tachycardia (PSVT)
- Junctional Rhythm
- PACs
- Blocked Atrial Beats
- Atrial Bigeminy
- Atrial Fibrillation
- Atrial Flutter
- Multifocal Atrial Tachycardia
- Junctional Tachycardia

Chapter 9 Ventricular Arrhythmias   141

- PVCs
- Ventricular Bigeminy
- Ventricular Tachycardia
- Ventricular Flutter

- Ventricular Fibrillation
- Idioventricular Rhythm
- Agonal Rhythm

Chapter 10 Ischemia and Infarction   163

- Acute Myocardial Infarction
  - ASMI
  - ALMI
  - IMI
  - Posterior MI
  - Right Ventricular MI
- Ventricular Ischemia
- Subendocardial Ischemia
- Giant Negative T Waves
- Nonspecific T Wave Changes
- Nonspecific ST-T Changes

Chapter 11 ST Segment Abnormalities   183

ST Elevation

- Normal Variation
- Early Repolarization
- ST Segment Elevation with LBBB
- ST Segment Elevation with Acute MI
- ST Segment Elevation with Pericarditis
- J Point Elevation
- Left Ventricular Aneurysm

ST Depression

- Horizontal ST Depression
- Downsloping ST Depression
- Upsloping ST Depression
- Nonspecific ST-T Changes
    - Reciprocal ST Depression in Acute MI
    - Subendocardial Ischemia v. Infarction

Chapter 12 T Wave Abnormalities — 193

- Normal T Wave Variations
- T Wave Changes with BBBs
- Ventricular Ischemia
- Cerebrovascular Accidents
- Tall Peaked T Waves

Chapter 13 Pacemaker Rhythms — 203

- Ventricular Pacing
- AV Sequential Pacing
- Atrial Sensing and Ventricular Pacing
- Atrial Pacing and Ventricular Pacing

Chapter 14 Miscellaneous Conditions — 215

- Low Voltage
- Electrical Alternans
- Hypokalemia
- Hyperkalemia
- Hypocalcemia
- Hypomagnesemia

- Hypothermia
- Cardiac Transplant

Chapter 15 Cardiac Monitoring   245

EKG Multiple-Choice Questions 1-100   247

EKG Interpretation Quiz: 1-50 Tracings   282

References   310

Sermon before we start this journey!

John, a farmer, takes his preacher on a tractor to show his fields. As he drives around the field, the preacher is impressed with acres and acres of beautifully cultivated land.

The preacher looks at John and says, "John, you and the good Lord have made it here together."

John replies, "Yes, brother, you should have seen it when your good Lord had it by himself!"

***

Hopefully, you, also, can cultivate some good EKG skills from this book. That's going to depend on you, the John.

CLINICAL EKG INTERPRETATION

Chapter 1 Introduction

- Introduction
- Lead Placement
- Rate, Rhythm, and Normal EKG
- Coronary Anatomy and EKG Correlation
- Heart Structure and EKG Changes
- Action Potential and EKG Correlation
- The Electrical System of the Heart
- Basic Measurements

INTRODUCTION

An electrocardiogram (EKG) is an important, simple test done at the bedside. It can provide a great volume of information about the status of the current electrical system of the heart, shed some light on how the heart has performed over decades and what type of transformations it has undergone over the years, and provide some important and unique diagnostic clues, as well as provide information about what to expect in the future.

It has stood the test of time and continues to be an important diagnostic tool at hospitals and medical offices. Yet, it may be intimidating even to an experienced cardiologist as the complexity of some tracings can challenge their intellectual acumen in the medical field.

As the name indicates—*Clinical EKG Interpretation*—this book provides clinical tips for students, nurses, technologists, physicians, paramedical professionals, and others on how to recognize some important findings that can shed light on the underlying heart condition and how it provides vital signals such as a STEMI, arrhythmias, or high-grade heart blocks that need immediate medical attention.

Use this as a reference—in your office, on the field, or in a hospital setting—to familiarize yourself with the pattern recognition until it becomes second nature. After that, every time you see an EKG you can appreciate what is not apparent beyond the obvious. Note that doing an electrocardiogram differs from knowing what is on the electrocardiogram that adds to your knowledge about a patient's overall condition and how it helps you to plan your patient's management

The electrocardiogram represents the electrical activity of the heart. It reflects the rhythmic pattern of depolarization and repolarization of the atria and the ventricles and indirectly the contraction and relaxation of the same chambers. It also helps to pinpoint the site of origin of the electrical impulse, the manner in which it is propagated, and how it terminates. Thus, it not only helps us in identifying the normal heart function, but it also uncovers a plethora of electrical conduction disturbances, cardiac enlargements, acute cardiac events such as ischemia or infarction, tachycardia or bradyarrhythmias, electrolyte and metabolic effects on the heart, certain congenital heart diseases, and many others that will be covered in the following chapters. It is an accurate measure of the duration of the ventricular contraction, the conduction delays at the Atrioventricular node, and ventricular relaxation.

ELECTRICAL SYSTEM OF THE HEART

It is amazing how a human heart weighing only 300 grams has such a complex electrical system yet it can last a lifetime and, in some cases, span more than a century. No man-made electrical grid can stand that test of time and evolve over challenging circumstances while learning from the experiences.

1. INTRODUCTION

Sinus Node: The Sinus node is located at the junction of the right atrium and the superior vena cava (Fig: 01.01). It gives rise to three internodal branches that traverse the right atrium and a Bachman's bundle that reaches the left atrium. The sinus node has the potential to spontaneous depolarization; as a result, it acts at the pacemaker cell, initiating the electrical impulse. This characteristic feature is called the "Automaticity."

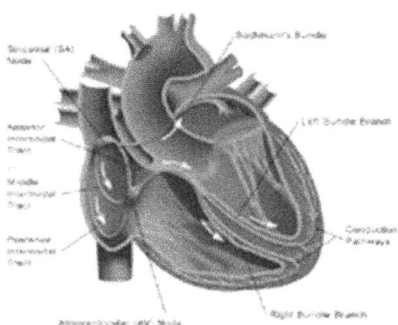

Fig: 01.01 Electrical system of the heart

It is also influenced by the autonomic nervous system. The adrenergic stimulation increases the heart rate while acetylcholine released by vagal nerve stimulation slows the heart rate. The sinus node activates from 60 to 100 times per minute.

Intra-Atrial Fibers: These are specialized conducting cells radiating from the sinus node and supply both atria. They conduct the sinus impulse to the atrial cells which in turn are activated, resulting in an action potential at the atrial level. All the atrial cells contract at the same time, squeezing the chamber, reducing the cavity size, and pushing the blood into the ventricles.

AV Node: The AV node (Atrioventricular) is located at the junction of the Tricuspid valve near the isthmus. The main purpose of the AV node is to delay the impulse so the atria can completely fill the ventricles before the ventricles begin to contract.

Bundle of His: It arises from the AV node and traverses a short distance before it divides into the right and left bundle branches.

CLINICAL EKG INTERPRETATION

Right Bundle Branch: The right bundle arises from the bundle of His, travels through the interventricular septum, turns around the apex, and supplies the right ventricular free wall.

Left Bundle Branch: The left bundle arises from the bundle of His, travels through the interventricular septum, and divides into the anterior fascicle and the posterior fascicle. The main fascicle turns around the apex and supplies the left ventricular free wall. It also gives rise to a small septal branch that activates the interventricular septum.

Purkinje Fibers: The Purkinje fibers arise from the bundle branches and provide a rich network of fibers that connects the myocardial cells at the subendocardial level. From there, the impulses are transmitted to the rest of the myocardium through the cells and the interstitial tissues. So, the Purkinje fibers activate the endocardial layer of cells and from there the impulse travels to the rest of the myocardium, reaching the epicardium.

All or None Phenomenon: The heart muscle's response to an electrical impulse differs from that of a skeletal muscle. When the atrial myocardium receives an electrical impulse, all the atrial cells contract simultaneously, shrink the atrial size, and squeeze the blood into the ventricles. Similarly, the right and the left ventricles respond to the electrical impulses from the Purkinje fibers, contract simultaneously, and squeeze blood into the great vessels.

Accessory Pathways: Wolf Parkinson White Syndrome (WPW): This condition is characterized by accessory pathways from the atria to the ventricles, which transmit the impulse from the atria to the ventricles earlier than the impulse going through the AV node (Fig: 01.02). Often, these accessory pathways are located in the lateral atrial wall. This early activation, known as the Delta waves, leads to the initial slurred upstroke of the QRS complexes. As the impulse from the AV node catches up with the delta wave, it conducts rapidly through the bundle branches and the Purkinje fibers leading to the terminal normal QRS complex. These accessory pathways having differential conductance can facilitate a reentry tachycardias which are the hallmark of WPW.

1. INTRODUCTION

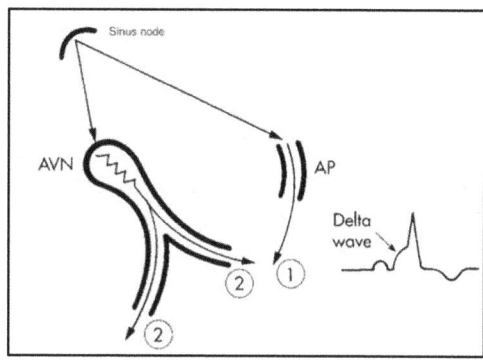

Fig:01.02. Accessory pathway

Similarly, other accessory pathways circling the tricuspid annulus may also lead to atrial flutter with rapid ventricular responses. The impulse conduction can be clockwise or counterclockwise, creating a different type of atrial flutter, which will be covered in detail in the following chapters (Fig: 01.02B).

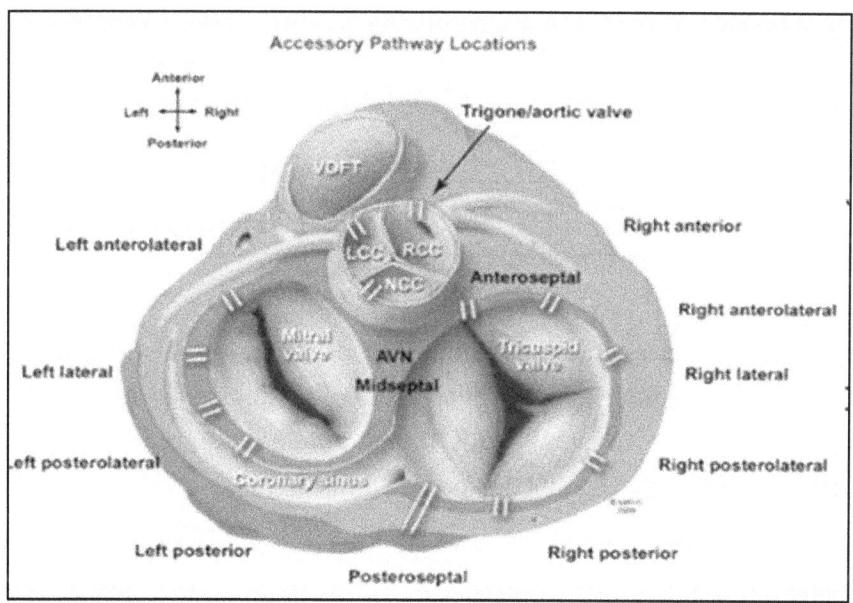

Fig: 01.02B. Accessory pathways located along the tricuspid valve and along the left atrial free wall.

Accessory pathways around the pulmonary veins are presumed to set off microcircuits in the atria, leading to atrial fibrillation. These microcircuits can arise anywhere in the atria in atrial fibrillation.

ACTION POTENTIAL

As you recall from physiological studies, the resting cardiac cell has a negative potential of -90 mV (voltage). It is called the repolarized state. When the cardiac muscle receives an electrical signal or an impulse, an action potential is generated. An action potential has five distinct phases: 0, 1, 2, 3, and 4. All the changes in the action potential are related to the movement of sodium (Na⁺), potassium (K⁺), calcium (Ca⁺), and other elements across the cardiac cell membrane (Fig: 01.03).

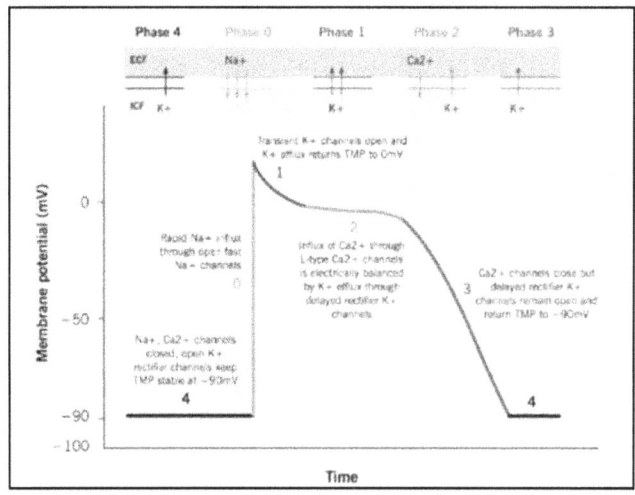

Fig: 01.03. Action potential

Phase 4: It represents the resting membrane potential of -90 mV. At rest, the intracellular space is negatively charged and the interstitial space is positively charged. The main ions found outside the cell are sodium and chloride, while inside the cell it is potassium.

Phase 0: Refers to the acute depolarization of the cardiac cell that is brought on by a sudden influx of the sodium and calcium from the extracellular space into the intracellular space. That shifts the membrane potential to +30 to 50 mV. Thus, during the depolarization phase, there is a sudden shift inside the cell to a positive charge brought primarily by the influx of sodium ions (Na⁺) into the cells through the rapid channels. This is followed by the mechanical atrial or ventricular contraction.

1. INTRODUCTION

Immediately following the rapid depolarization of the cardiac cell, the positive charge inside the cardiac cell is maintained by phases 1 and 2. This is followed by rapid repolarization represented by phase 3.

Phase 1: This is characterized by the movement of the intracellular potassium (K^+) to the extracellular space. The positive charge inside the cardiac cell dips a little before it begins to plateau.

Phase 2: There is a movement of calcium (Ca^+) into the cell, while the potassium (K^+) continues to leak into the extracellular space. This plateau maintains the action potential in a state of positive charge.

Phase 3. At this stage, the calcium (Ca^+) channels close and the potassium (K^+) channels pump the potassium (K^+) outside the cells, resulting in a gradual decline in the positive action potential inside the cell. It also represents the repolarization of the cardiac cell toward the resting membrane potential of -80 mV. This is represented on the surface electrocardiogram by the T waves of ventricular repolarization before the electrical activity returns to the baseline.

Phase 4: Once the action potential reaches the resting membrane potential of -90 mV, it remains in that state until it receives the next electrical signal.

Below is a chart showing the concentration of various ions in the intracellular and extracellular space (Fig: 01.03B).

Element	Ion	Extracellular	Intracellular	Ratio
Sodium	Na^+	135 - 145	10	14:1
Potassium	K^+	3.5 - 5.0	155	1:30
Chloride	Cl^-	95 - 110	10 - 20	4:1
Calcium	Ca^{2+}	2	10^{-4}	$2 \times 10^4 : 1$

Fig: 01.03B. Intracellular and extracellular ion concentrations

CLINICAL EKG INTERPRETATION

Spontaneous Depolarization: Unlike the myocardial cells, the pacemaker cells, such as the sinus node, the AV node, and the Bundle of His, have spontaneous depolarization properties, of which there is a gradual depolarization of the resting membrane potential (Fig: 01.04). When it reaches a certain threshold, the rapid depolarization begins and sets off a new action potential.

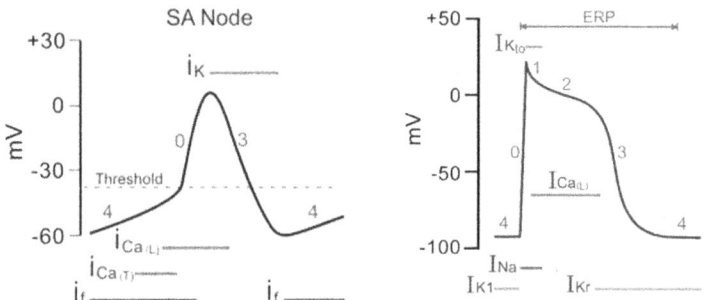

Fig: 01.04. Notice the slow spontaneous depolarization in the sinus node cell as opposed to the myocardial cell which has a steady resting membrane potential.

However, the rate at which each pacemaker cell or a cardiac cell spontaneously depolarizes determines the dominant impulse generator that controls the heart rate. When a top-rate pacemaker cell fails, the next cell that has an inherent rate greater than the rest takes over.

Site	Rate
Sinus node	60-100
AV node	40-60
Idioventricular	30-40

The entire mechanical cardiac function is based on the movements of these ions powered by the ATP energy molecules. Hence, changes in the serum potassium and calcium levels not only can influence the myocardial function but also can provide vital diagnostic information on the surface electrocardiogram.

1. INTRODUCTION

NORMAL CARDIAC CYCLE

An entire cardiac cycle consists of atrial activation, the AV nodal delay, the ventricular activation, diastasis, the ventricular relaxation, and the beginning of the next cardiac cycle (Fig: 01.05).

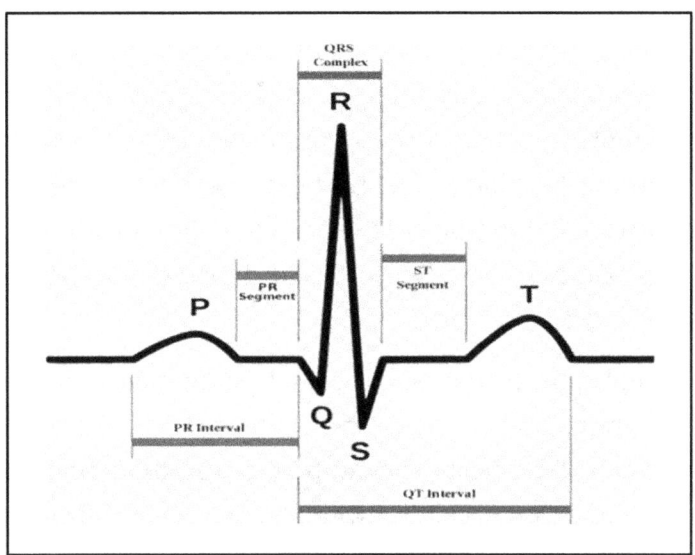

Fig: 01.05. Normal cardiac cycle

P Waves: It results from activation of the atrial muscles. It represents the depolarization of the atrial cells. It is a positive deflection varying from 100 to 120 ms. The electrical depolarization of the atria is followed by the mechanical contraction of the atria pumping the blood into the ventricles.

Note that the contraction of the atria extends beyond the P wave duration. Normally, we may not see an atrial repolarization wave as we would with the ventricular repolarization, because of the very low amplitude generated by atrial repolarization.

It helps us to identify the site of origin of the atrial impulse, such as from the sinus node where the P waves are positive in lead I, or from an ectopic focus such as a low atrial site where the P waves will be inverted in lead I.

Sometimes, in patients with chronic lung disease the origin of the atrial impulse can be from multiple sites [Multifocal Atrial Tachycardia (MAT)].

CLINICAL EKG INTERPRETATION

The P waves may also show evidence of right, left, or biatrial enlargements, which will be covered later. Rarely, we may see a negative deflection immediately following the P wave which may represent atrial infarction.

PR Interval: The PR interval is measured from the beginning of the P wave to the beginning of the QRS complex. An extremely high level of engineering has gone into building this interval as it provides time for the atria to completely empty the blood into the ventricles before the ventricles begin to contract. Without this delay, if all four chambers act at the same time there will be no forward blood flow. Praise the Lord! The normal PR interval is less than 200 ms. Occasionally, we may see depression of the PR interval in patients with acute pericarditis.

QRS Complex: As its name indicates, it is the most complex wave on the electrocardiogram, as it reflects the composite electrical activity of both ventricles. It actually reflects the ventricular (both) depolarization, and the mechanical contraction occurs between 40 and 60 ms after the beginning of the QRS complex. These time intervals are very important to understand as there are several concepts in the diagnosis and management of cardiac conditions.

The **Initial Q** wave is a negative deflection of the impulse moving backward in the interventricular septum. This is related to the septal activation. It is seen in leads I, aVL, and the lateral chest leads.

The tall **R wave** results from the activation of both ventricles moving forward and to the left axillary area. Hence, it produces a positive wave in the chest leads, except for lead V1 where it is negative, as V1 is located on the right side of the chest.

That is followed by an **S wave**. The S wave represents the movement of impulse away from the electrode. The point where the S wave ends and the ST segment begins is called the J point, an important pivotal point that is altered in a variety of conditions such as acute myocardial ischemia, cardiac enlargement, bundle branch blocks, and others.

1. INTRODUCTION

The QRS complex duration can help us in differentiating bundle branch blocks (BBB), Intra-ventricular conduction delays, or ventricular arrhythmias.

QRS Nomenclature: Whenever an electrical impulse travels toward a positive electrode it produces a positive deflection. When the electrical impulse is moving away from the monitoring electrode, it records a negative deflection.

There is a positive deflection in V1 due to the initial septal activation from the left to the right. As the rest of the impulse travels toward the left side, it records the dominant negative deflection thus producing a rose pattern in V1. On the other hand, the V6 electrode records an initial tiny Q wave, followed by a dominant R wave. The R wave is followed by an S wave representing the impulse moving away from the electrode.

Depending on the initial, middle, and terminal deflections, the QRS complexes can be labeled as follows. This is especially true in the presence of bundle branch blocks and chamber enlargements (Fig: 01.06).

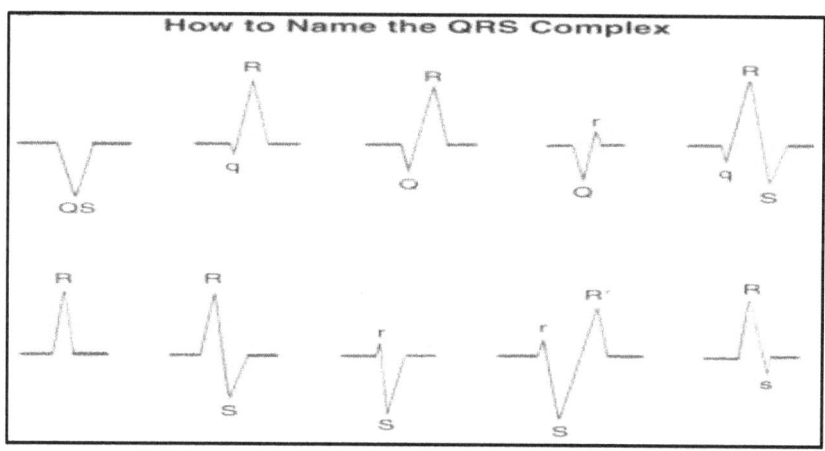

Fig: 01.06. Various QRS morphologies

Based upon the morphology of the normal and abnormal QRS complexes, we can identify ventricular hypertrophy, abnormal ventricular activation, old myocardial infarctions (MI), and bundle branch blocks (BBB), among others.

J Point: The terminal segment of the QRS complex reaches the baseline and continues as the ST segment. The J point is altered in a variety of conditions such as acute myocardial ischemia, myocardial infarction, or pericarditis, where it is usually elevated. It may also be elevated in the anterior leads in the presence of left bundle branch block. The 'J' point may be depressed along with the ST segments in the presence of ventricular dilatation or hypertrophy, which signals the strain pattern.

ST Segment: This segment marks the continued mechanical ventricular ejection phase and is usually isoelectric to the baseline. The variation in ST segment may signal acute myocardial infarction, normal variations, pericarditis, ventricular arrhythmias, subendocardial ischemia, and others. The duration of ST segment does not bear much significance in the diagnosis of heart conditions.

T Waves: They represent the ventricular repolarization. They have a smooth upslope, a rounded top, and a fairly steep decline before they reach the baseline. The T wave has a gradual upslope and a steeper downslope. Variations in T-wave morphology provide clues to a variety of conditions ranging from electrolyte abnormalities to myocardial infarction. They are also involved in chamber enlargements. Peaked T waves may signal hyperkalemia while flat T waves may be seen in patients with hypothyroidism. Even though the duration of the T wave may not be greatly significant, the QT interval has great importance.

QT Interval: It is the distance from the beginning of the QRS complex to the end of the T wave. It represents the electrical and mechanical contraction of the left ventricle or the systolic phase of the cardiac cycle. So, the ventricular contraction involves both the QRS and T-wave durations.

The QT interval must be corrected to the heart rate (QTc). The normal QTC for men is 440 ms; for women it is 450 ms. QTc interval >440 ms in men or >450 ms in women is associated with a tendency for ventricular arrhythmias. In fact, many antiarrhythmic drugs tend to prolong the QT interval and some of them may need to be titrated based on the QTc intervals.

U Waves: Occasionally, we may see a positive deflection following the T wave. This represents the U wave. It is presumed to represent the papillary muscle repolarization. It also may be seen in patients with hypokalemia and hypothyroidism.

1. INTRODUCTION

Prominent U waves may be seen in patients with cerebrovascular accidents or those who are taking drugs like Quinidine, sotalol, or phenothiazines.

TP Interval: Even though most people don't give much weight to the TP interval, it is the interval during which the slow ventricular filling occurs as the ventricular pressure begins to fall. It is also the elastic period that is most affected by the heart rate. When the heart rate accelerates, the TP interval shortens.

Normal Variations: The T waves can be inverted in V2 in young female patients. They may also be seen in V3. These are sometimes called Juvenile T waves. These findings are seen in 10% of young females. Occasionally, the T waves in III and aVF may be flat or inverted.

Varying RR Intervals: We may see minor variations in RR intervals in sinus arrhythmia and during labored respirations.

ELECTRICAL VS. MECHANICAL ACTIVATION OF THE HEART

The main purpose of the electrical impulse is to activate the myocardium and initiate a contraction and relaxation to pump the blood forward. As you can see in the diagram, following the P wave there is atrial activation as reflected in the pressure tracing. Similarly, following the QRS complex there is a steep rise in the left ventricular pressure. There is approximately a 40 to 60 ms delay between the electrical and mechanical activation of the heart. Following the T wave, which represents the ventricular repolarization, there is a slow ventricular filling phase (Fig: 01. 07).

CLINICAL EKG INTERPRETATION

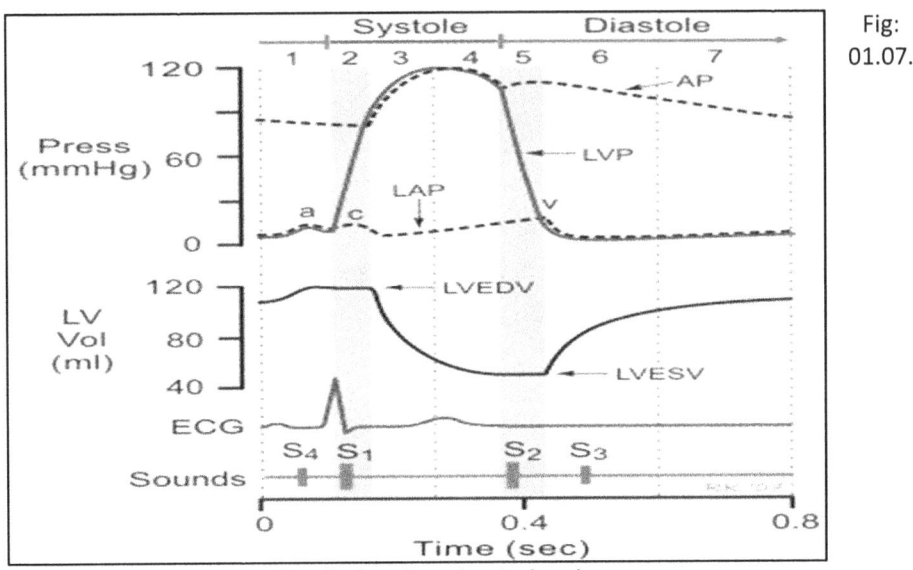

Electrical and mechanical cycle

EKG PAPER, VOLTAGE, AND TIME INTERVALS

An electrocardiogram (EKG) represents the composite electrical activity of the heart over time. It consists of a series of heartbeats recorded on EKG graph paper.

The EKG paper has a series of 1 mm squares in the horizontal and vertical directions (Fig: 01.08). After every five blocks, there is a dark line in both the horizontal and vertical axes to help us better visualize the graph.

Vertical Axis: Each vertical square represents 0.1 mV. So, 10 mm represents 1 mV.

Calibration: At the beginning of each tracing, you will see a vertical deflection of 10 mm followed by a short horizontal line and a sudden downward deflection. This represents the voltage calibrated to 1 mV/10 boxes. Occasionally, when the EKG QRS voltage is very high, the EKG paper may be calibrated to ½ standard (1 mV/5 boxes).

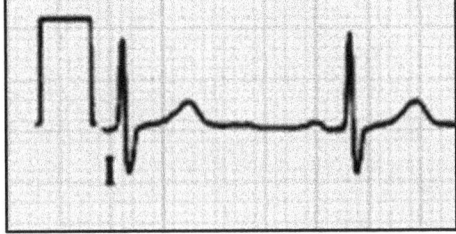

1. INTRODUCTION

Horizontal Axis: The paper speed is 25 mm/sec or 25 small boxes/sec in the horizontal axis. Each horizontal box represents 40 ms and aids us in measuring various time intervals. It also represents five big boxes.

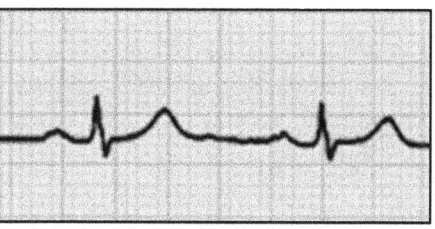

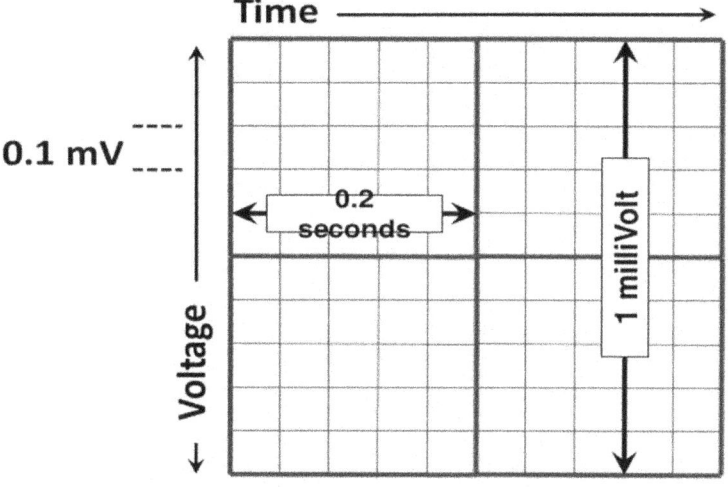

Fig: 01.08. EKG graph paper and small boxes

Six Seconds Markers: At the top of the EKG paper there are vertical lines that are 30 squares, or 6 seconds, apart (Fig: 01.08B). These are useful to measure the heart rate when the RR intervals vary from beat to beat. We can measure the number of R waves in 6 seconds and multiply them by 10 to get an approximate heart rate per minute. On rhythm strips, you may see 3-second markers.

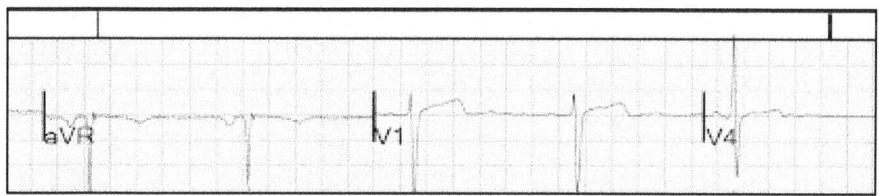

Fig: 01.08B. Six-second markers at the top of the graph

CLINICAL EKG INTERPRETATION

HEART RATE

Rule of 300: Count the number of big boxes between the RR intervals. Divide 300 by the number of big boxes and that will get you the heart rate. This is only useful if the rate is regular and you can see the R waves matching the lines.

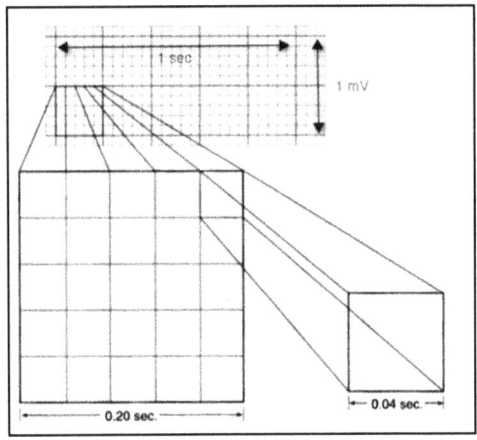

Fig: 01.09. Time covered by each small box

Count the number of large boxes (groups of five small boxes) and use the table below to familiarize yourself with the heart rate (Fig: 01.09). Next, create a mental vision of this table until it becomes second nature for you to determine the heart rate based on the number of large boxes between the RR spike (Fig: 01.10).

Boxes	Math	HR
5	300/5	60 bpm
4	300/4	75 bpm
3	300/3	100 bpm
2	300/2	150 bpm
1	300/1	300 bpm

Fig: 01.10. Heart rate chart

1. INTRODUCTION

Here is a practical way of looking at RR peaks and determining the number of large boxes. If the RR peaks fall on the exact number of boxes, we can use this table.

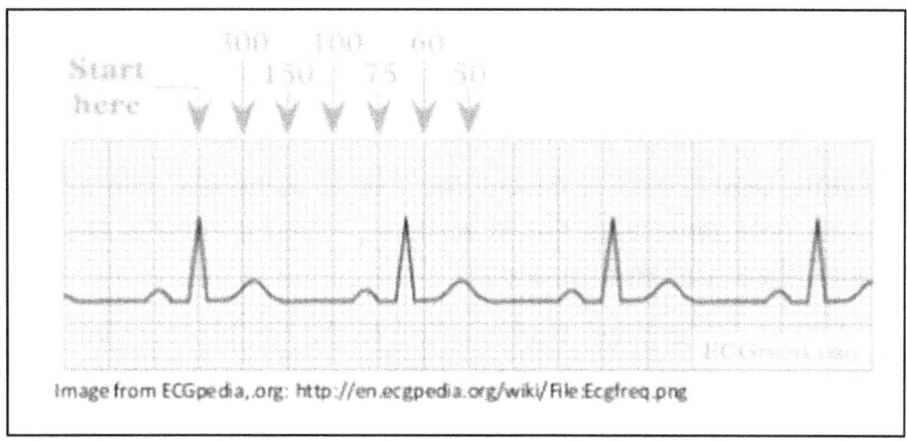

Fig: 01.11. Heart rate calculation based on the number of large boxes

If the RR interval falls midway between 4 and 3, the heart rate is between 75 and 100, which is more like 87 bpm. Similarly, if the RR interval is between 3 and 2, the approximate heart rate is 125 bpm (Fig: 01.11).

Rhythm Strips: On top of most EKG rhythm strips there are vertical lines that represent the 3-second markers. Measure the number of RR intervals in a 6-second strip and multiply that by 10 and you will get an approximate HR. This is useful when the RR intervals are irregular as in atrial fib, atrial flutter, or multifocal atrial tachycardia.

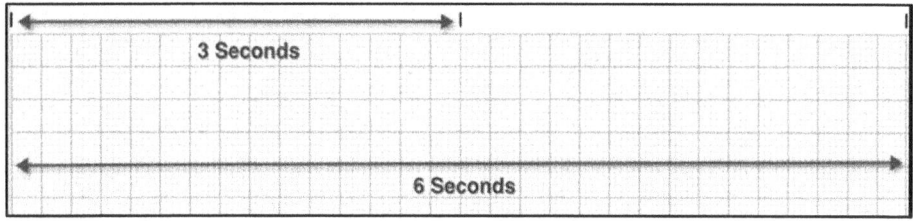

Fig: 01.12. Heart rate based on a 6-second rule

CLINICAL EKG INTERPRETATION

LEADS AND CONNECTIONS

An EKG represents the heart's electrical activity from various angles and locations. It has three Limb Leads, namely leads I, II, and III. There are three augmented limb leads, namely aVR, aVL, and aVF. There are six precordial leads that record the electrical activity at various locations directly over the chest overlying the heart.

Limb Leads: They represent the frontal plane EKG (Fig: 01.13). The positive pole represents the direction in which it records the electrical activity. There are leads I, II, and III.

As the impulse moves from the right to the left, lead I records a positive deflection.

Similarly, an impulse moving from top to bottom will record a positive deflection in leads II, III, and aVF.

Most of the time the impulse moves from the right to left side so the aVR records a negative deflection.

Augmented Leads: In the augmented leads such as aVR, aVL, and aVF, the last letter represents the positive electrode and the other two form the negative electrode. For example, in aVR the right arm represents the positive electrode and the left arm and left leg form the negative electrode. These are also called the unipolar leads.

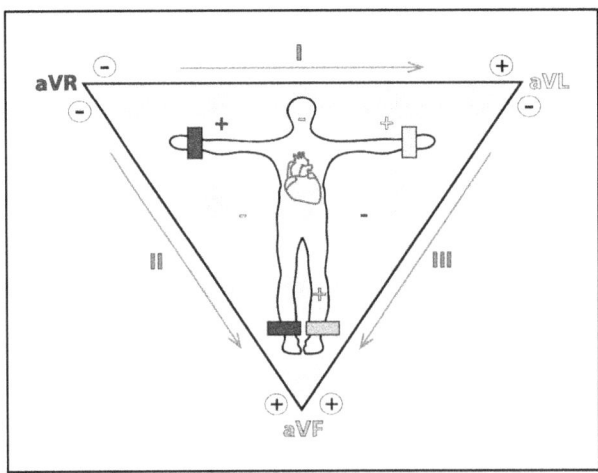

Fig: 01.13. Limb leads and augmented leads configuration

1. INTRODUCTION

Chest Leads or Precordial Leads: Leads V1 to V6 have the positive electrodes at the tip of their leads. They record the electrical activity in close proximity to the chest leads (Fig: 01.14).

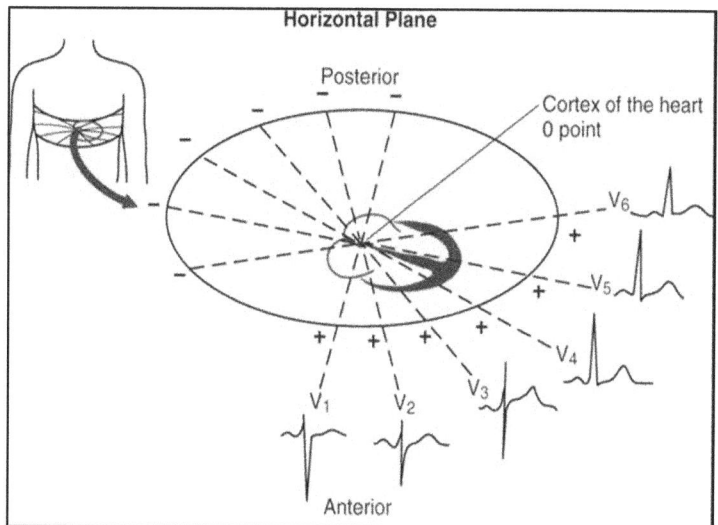

Fig: 01.14. The chest leads orientation

They also record the electrical activity of the heart in the horizontal plane as the chest leads move from the right side of the chest to the left axillary line. The electrical activity of the right and left ventricles is reflected here.

The heart's electrical activity remains the same. But, recording from each lead can be different as the positive electrode moves with reference to the electrical impulse. When the depolarization wave moves toward an electrode, it records a positive deflection. When it moves away from the electrode, it records a negative deflection. The T waves follow similar patterns.

LEADS AND THE MYOCARDIAL AREA REPRESENTATIONS

- Leads I and aVL, represents the electrical activity from the high anterior wall or the high lateral wall of the left ventricle (the area supplied by the diagonal branches).

CLINICAL EKG INTERPRETATION

- Leads II, III, and aVF represent the electrical activity from the inferior wall of the left ventricle, the area supplied by the right coronary artery and occasionally by circumflex branch.

- The precordial leads V1 and V2 represent the electrical activity from the interventricular septum, the area supplied by the septal branches.

- The precordial leads V3 and V4 represent the electrical activity from the anterior wall of the left ventricle, the area supplied by the LAD.

- The precordial leads V5 and V6 represent the electrical activity from the lateral wall of the left ventricle, the area supplied by circumflex marginals.

SUMMARY OF LEADS AND THEIR CONNECTIONS

LEAD	POSITIVE	NEGATIVE
I	LT. arm	RT. arm
II	LT. leg	RT. arm
III	LT. leg	LT. arm
aVR	RT. arm	LT. arm + RT. leg
aVL	LT. arm	RT. arm + LT. leg
aVF	LT. leg	RT. arm + LT.
V1	Right 4th ICS (intercostal space)	Central Terminal
V2	Left 4th ICS	Central Terminal
V3	Between V2 and V_4	Central Terminal
V4	Left midclavicular line, 5th ICS	Central terminal
V5	Left anterior axillary line,	Central terminal
V6	Left mid axillary line, 5th ICS	Central terminal

1. INTRODUCTION

NORMAL EKG PATTERN

A 12-lead electrocardiogram consists of three limb leads (I, II, and III), three augmented leads (aVR, aVL, and aVF), and six precordial leads (V1 to V6) (Fig: 01.15).

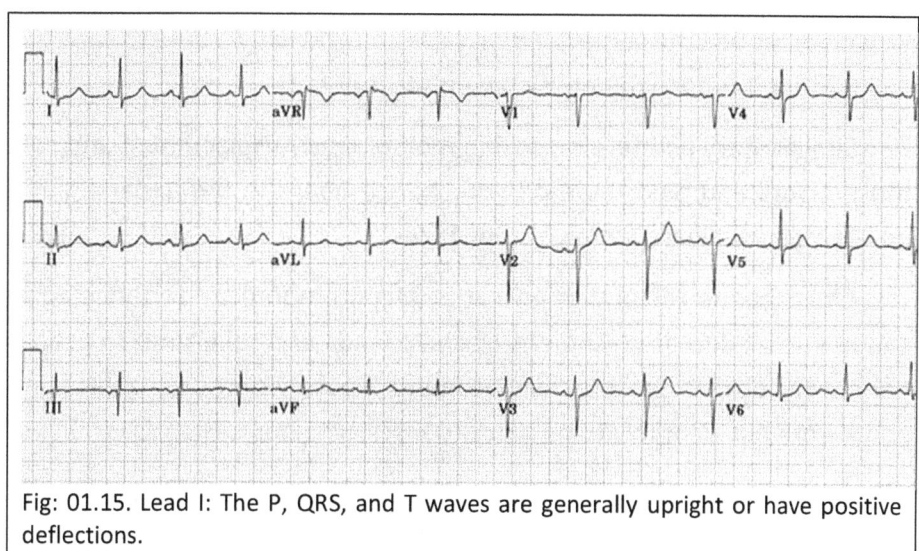

Fig: 01.15. Lead I: The P, QRS, and T waves are generally upright or have positive deflections.

The Recording of an Electrocardiogram: Recording of electrocardiogram as a routine as it may seem, needs extra precaution to make sure the leads are placed in the proper places, the leads stick to the skin well, and there is no patient movement during the recording. If you see a 60-cycle interference, try to hook up the machine to a different electrical outlet to see if you can get rid of the 60-cycle electrical disturbances.

Check that the name and demographics match with the patient.

If the room is cold, cover the patient adequately to avoid muscle tremors.

You should be able to recognize common patterns such as rapid heartbeats, V. Tach, or Acute MI, which deserve immediate attention and action. If you see these findings on the EKG, immediately alert the nurse and the attending physician.

CLINICAL EKG INTERPRETATION

Limb Leads Misplacement: Proper lead placement is an essential foundation for a good electrocardiogram. It reflects your knowledge and diligence in taking excellent electrocardiograms.

Make sure the limb leads are properly matched to the extremities. Practice this on one of your co-workers when you have time and deliberately interchange the right and left arm leads and see what changes you notice. When you notice the same in a real situation you will be able to spot the error and correct it before the physician points it out.

Similarly, try a different combination or lead misplacement and collect all those errors and post them on your notice board in the department so the newcomers can learn from your mistakes.

Chest Leads Misplacement: It is of paramount importance to have a sound knowledge of placement of chest leads and take time to prepare the patient for proper chest leads placement. There won't be trophies given for good work but people will be quick to highlight your mistakes.

Learn to correctly count the intercostal spaces. In obese patients, the heart is situated more horizontally and higher-up in the chest cavity. In a really thin and tall patient, the heart is more vertically situated and you may need to place the leads lower down on those patients.

One of the common mistakes is the placement of all the chest leads in the 2nd or 3rd intercostal spaces, which will create a QS complex in all the chest leads. This happens more often when dealing with a female patient with large breasts. Take the extra time to place the leads underneath the breast if necessary to obtain a proper electrocardiogram.

Repeat the electrocardiogram in various lead positions until you get a good tracing as your job depends on that.

1. INTRODUCTION

Poor EKG Technique Red Flags:

- ➢ Muscle tremors
- ➢ 60-cycle artifacts
- ➢ Wandering baselines
- ➢ Loss of R waves in all the precordial leads
- ➢ Negative deflections in lead I or all positive deflections in aVR
- ➢ R wave flying off the graph paper (reduce the calibration to ½)
- ➢ Blaming the patient?
- ➢ Emergency? Come back and get a good tracing,
- ➢ EKG machine? See if a different tech can reproduce the mistake.

Proper Leads Placement: Follow the guidelines listed below for proper leads placement before recording an electrocardiogram. The diagram shows the limb leads connections (Fig: 01.16).

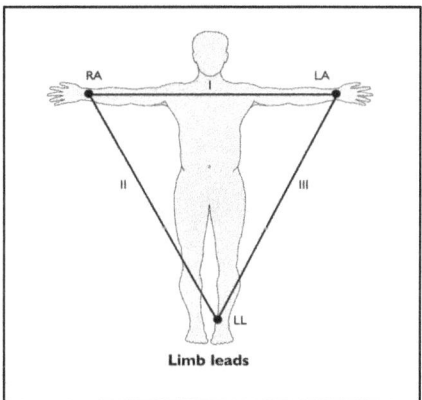

Fig: 01.16. Limb leads placement

Make sure you place the limb leads, namely RA, LA, RL, and LL, on the designated locations.

- **RA:** Right shoulder
- **LA:** Left shoulder
- **RL:** Right leg or lower part of the abdomen on the right side
- **LL:** Right leg or lower part of the abdomen on the left side

CLINICAL EKG INTERPRETATION

Horizontal Plane Chest Leads Placement: Memorize the proper placement of the chest leads (Fig: 01.17).

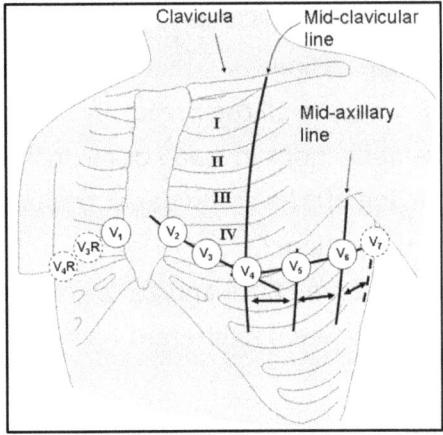

Fig: 01.17. The chest leads placement

Lead V1: 4th intercostal space to the right of the sternum.

Lead V2: 4th intercostal space to the left of the sternum

Lead V3: V2 and V4

Lead V4: 5th ICS in the mid-clavicular space

Lead V5: 5th ICS along the anterior axillary line

Lead V6: 5th ICS along the mid-axillary line

The right-side chest leads are placed along the same guidelines, on the right side of the chest. Mostly, you may record V1, V3R, and V4R.

If you suspect posterior infarction, leads V7, V8 and V9 can be placed along the left posterior chest in the 5th ICS.

1. INTRODUCTION

AUTONOMIC SYSTEM EFFECTS ON CARDIOVASCULAR SYSTEM

ADRENERGIC SYSTEM

The adrenergic system is controlled by the cardiopulmonary center in the brain. Through the spinal cord, it sends out impulses to the preganglionic nerve center (Fig: 01.18). The post-ganglionic fibers innervate the various organs where they exert their actions on the cardiovascular, muscular, and visceral systems.

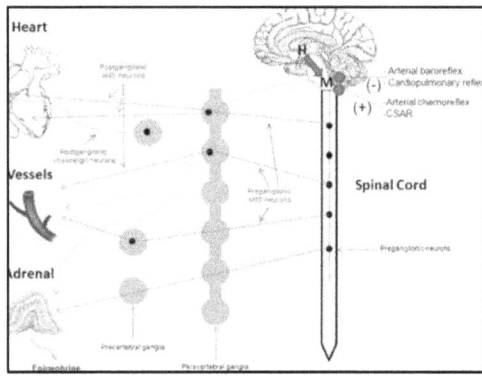

Fig: 01.18. Adrenergic system

The adrenergic system exerts a variety of responses on the cardiovascular system. All these responses are geared to prepare the body for a fight-or-flight response. The norepinephrine is the main hormone responsible for many of the cardiovascular effects as a result of sympathetic nervous system stimulation.

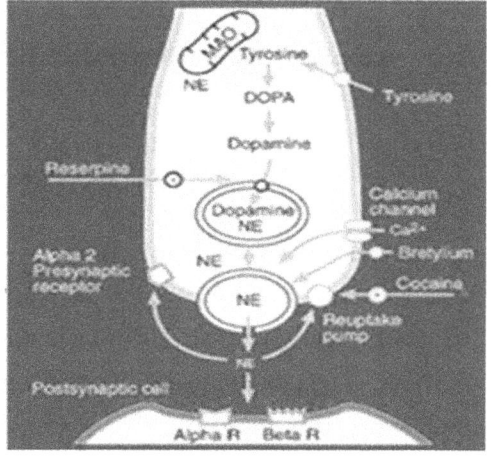

The adrenergic system transmits its signals to a disk-like terminal called the bouton (button in French) located on the cardiac and vascular smooth muscle cells. This releases the norepinephrine, which activates the adrenergic receptors, which bring about the changes mentioned above.

In the heart, it activates the Beta$_1$ adrenergic receptors, stimulating the SA node, increasing the heart rate, contractility, improving AV conduction, and conduction through the atrial and ventricular muscles, and increasing contractility. It also increases the myocardial irritability which can lead to ectopic beats. Epinephrine is secreted by the adrenal glands, which exert even more potent stimulation of the heat's Beta$_1$ receptors.

Adrenergic Cardiovascular Responses

- **Accelerate Heart Rate (Chronotropic Response)**
- **Increase Cardiac Contractility (Inotropic Response)**
- **Accelerate Cardiac Relaxation (Lusitropy)**
- **Enhance AV Conduction (Dromotropic Response)**
- **Decrease Venous Capacitance**
- **Constrict Cutaneous Vessels**

PARASYMPATHETIC SYSTEM

The parasympathetic system exerts the opposite effects of the sympathetic system on the cardiovascular system, thus maintaining a balance to meet varying demands on the cardiovascular system from moment to moment. The parasympathetic system acts through the Vagus nerve, which innervates the heart, aorta, and vascular system. The activation of the parasympathetic system releases the acetylcholine at the cholinergic nerve

1. INTRODUCTION

terminals located on the myocardial cells and the smooth muscle cells on the vascular bed.

It inhibits the sinus node, thus slowing the heart rate or in some cases causing a temporary long sinus pause. It also slows the conduction through the AV node and the conduction systems, decreases myocardial contraction, and dilates the peripheral blood vessel, increases the vascular capacitance, and drops the blood pressure.

This is commonly known as the vasovagal or vasodepressor response, where people experience dizziness, weakness, and near syncope. Occasionally, it may lead to syncope. Once the effects of this sudden cholinergic rush dissipate, the cardiovascular function slowly returns to the baseline.

In addition, the parasympathetic activation may also indirectly inhibit the sympathetic ganglia that innervate the same organs. A combination of a slow heart rate and profound vasodilation is a perfect set-up for "drop attacks" following activation of the parasympathetic system.

*****

COMEDY RELIEF!

Dr. Nik: "Ma'am, do you drink coffee?"

Patient: "Yes!"

Dr. Nik: "How many cups?"

Patient: "Five cups before sunrise."

Dr. Nik: "Ma'am, do you realize coffee is a slow poison?"

Patient: "Must be Dr. Nik! I am 83 and it's still trying to get my heart!"

*****

CLINICAL EKG INTERPRETATION

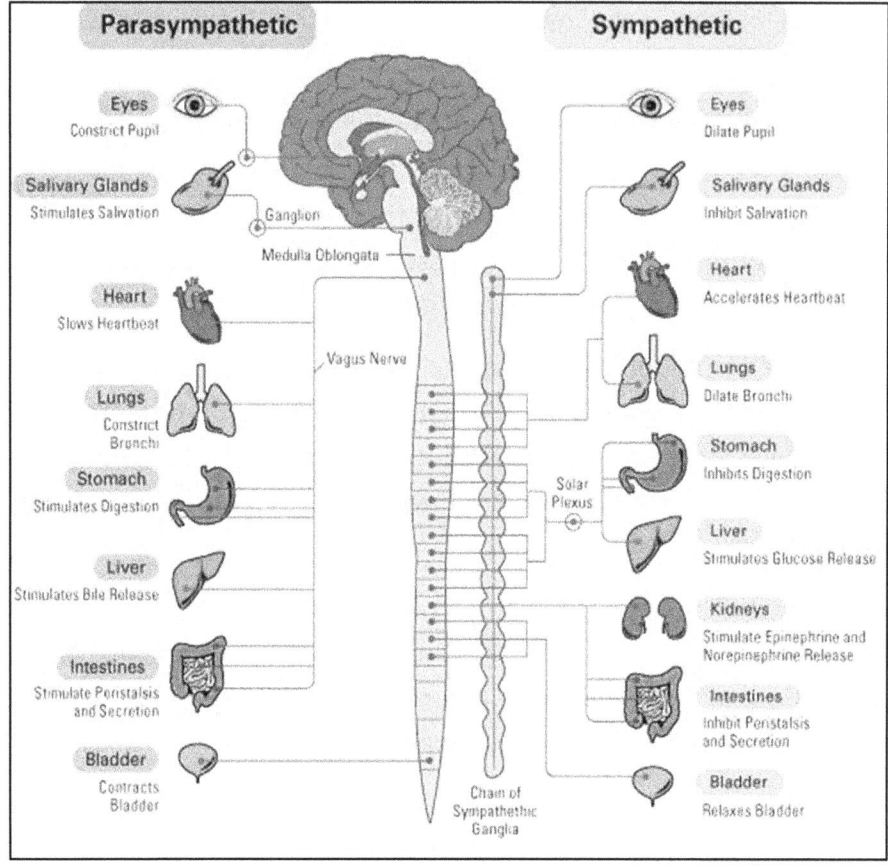

Fig: 01.19. Autonomic nervous system

Neuro-Cardiogenic Syncope: This commonly happens in elderly patients who experience dizziness and near syncope upon prolonged standing. Normally, this is compensated by sympathetic stimulation, which causes an increase in heart rate and blood pressure. However, in some elderly patients there are inadequate heart rate and vasoconstrictive responses. Hence, a partially filled ventricular contraction stimulates an undesirable parasympathetic response. This further slows the heart rate and drops the blood pressure, thus reducing the cerebral blood flow leading to syncope.

Prevention is the best cure here by avoiding prolonged standing. Exercising the leg muscles periodically to pump the blood back to the circulation may also help.

1. **INTRODUCTION**

QUIZ

Label the various waves and intervals.

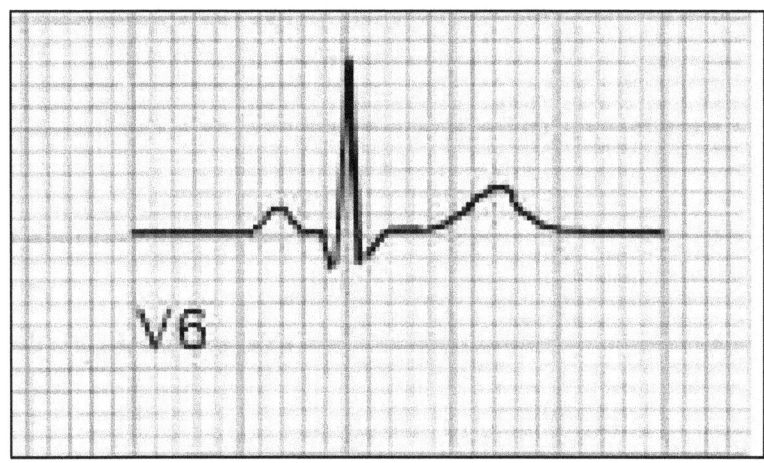

Which waves are negative?

___

Which waves are positive?

___

What is the R wave amplitude?

___

Which is the QT interval?

___

Action Potential

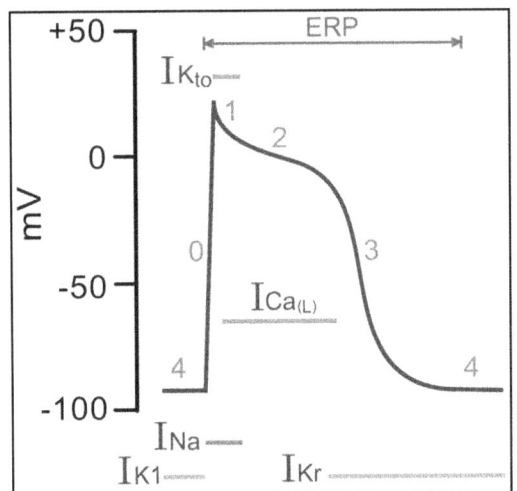

The resting membrane potential is _____ mV.

Describe:

Phase 0 _____

Phase 1 _____

Phase 2 _____

Phase 3 _____

Phase 4 _____

Chapter 2 Electrical Axis

- Normal
- Left Axis
- Right Axis
- Indeterminate Axis

The electrical axis of the heart is a representation of the direction in which the electrical activation of the heart happens during a cardiac cycle and not necessarily the way the heart is situated in the mediastinum (Fig: 02.01). Nonetheless, the electrical axis of the heart provides important clues to the underlying status electric grid and chamber enlargements, among others.

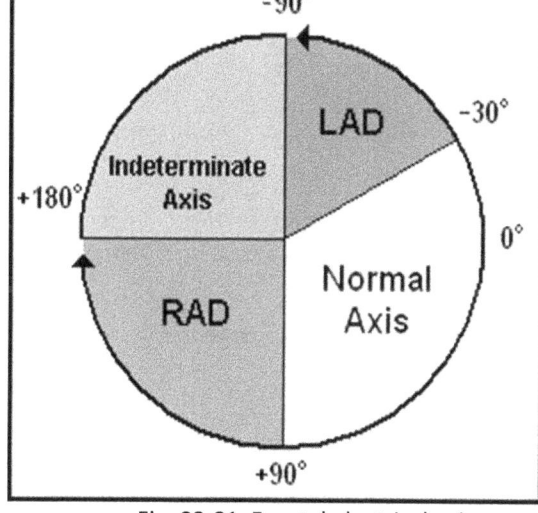

Fig: 02.01. Frontal electrical axis

CLINICAL EKG INTERPRETATION

The normal electrical axis of the heart ranges from -30° to +90°. It is considered a right axis (RAD) when the axis is between 90° and 180°. The right axis deviation may be seen in patients with right ventricular hypertrophy, corpulmonale, acute pulmonary embolism, and congenital heart diseases.

When the axis is between -30° and -45° it is considered a leftward axis and when the axis is between -45° and -90° it is called the Left Axis Deviation (LAD). The LAD deviation may be related to the left anterior hemiblock.

HOW TO DETERMINE THE ELECTRICAL AXIS

There are two main ways to determine the electrical axis.

Equiphasic Method: Here you look at a lead that has equal positive and negative deflections or a net zero deflection. Then, the axis should be 90° to that lead (Fig: 02.02).

So, in lead aVF, which represents the 90° position, if the negative and positive deflections are equal, the axis should be perpendicular to that. In other words, the axis should be 0°.

Lead II, which represents 60°, is equiphasic and the axis is –30°.

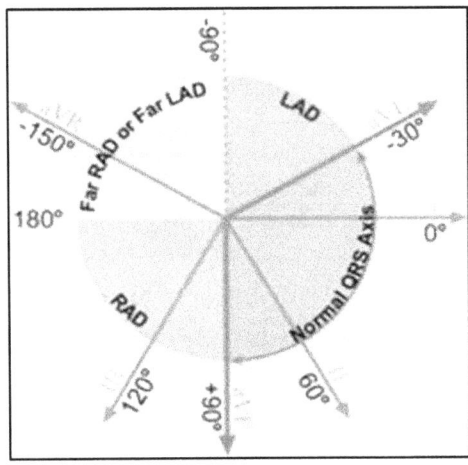

Fig: 02.02. Frontal electrical axis

CHAPTER 2. ELECTICAL AXIS

Left Axis Deviation: If the negative deflection in lead II is more than the positive deflection, the axis will be more than -30°. This will lead to left axis deviation. Left axis deviation is often seen in patients with left ventricular hypertrophy, and we should look for other features of left ventricular hypertrophy. The left axis deviation also can occur in the presence of left anterior hemiblock, which may reflect on the status of the electrical system in the heart (Fig: 02.03).

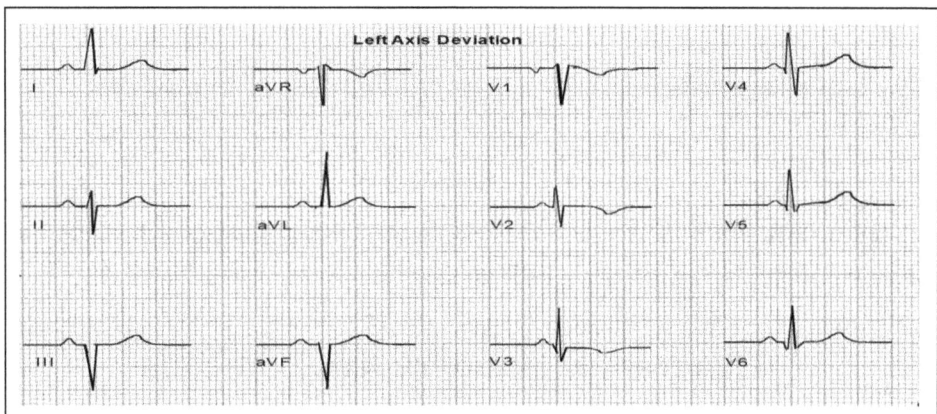

Fig: 02.03. Sinus rhythm. Left axis deviation (-45°), left atrial enlargement, and T wave changes. Tiny R waves are noted in III and aVF

Right Axis Deviation: If the negative deflection in lead I is greater than the positive deflection along with a positive deflection in aVF, it represents a right axis beyond +90°. If lead II is equiphasic and the lead aVR is positive, then the axis will be on the right side, resulting in a right axis deviation. Along with right axis deviation, we may also look for any right atrial and/or right ventricular hypertrophy which may support the diagnosis of a right axis deviation (Fig: 02.04).

CLINICAL EKG INTERPRETATION

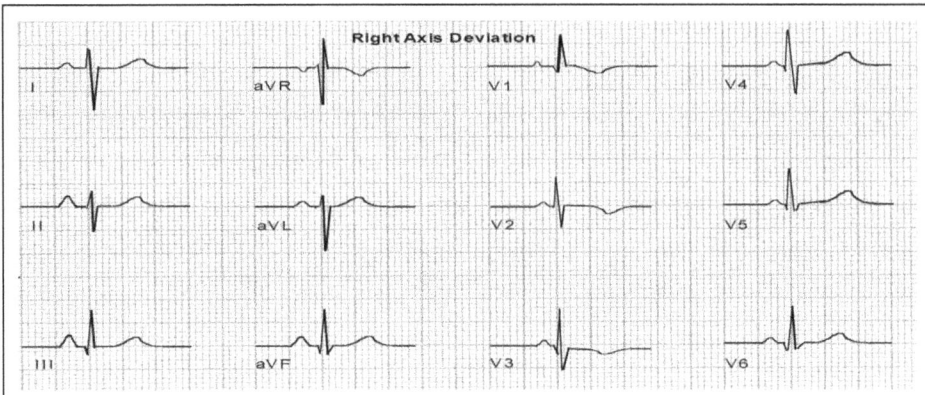

Fig: 02.04. Sinus rhythm. Right axis deviation, right atrial enlargement, and right ventricular hypertrophy.

Quadrant Method: By just looking at the QRS deflections in leads I and aVF, we can approximate the axis (Fig: 02.05).

Quadrant Method for Axis Detection

- **If leads I and aVF are positive the electrical axis is normal.**

- **If lead I is negative and aVF is positive we have a right axis deviation**

- **If lead II is negative and aVF is negative, we have a left axis deviation.**

		Lead aVF	
		Positive	Negative
Lead I	Positive	Normal Axis	LAD
	Negative	RAD	Indeterminate Axis

Fig: 02.05. Frontal electrical axis

CHAPTER 2. ELECTRICAL AXIS

Indeterminate Axis: Sometimes, we may see an equiphasic RS or an SR pattern in all the limb leads and it may be impossible to determine the axis. Occasionally, we may see QS complexes in multiple limb leads, like QS in I, III, aVF, and aVL (Fig: 02.06).

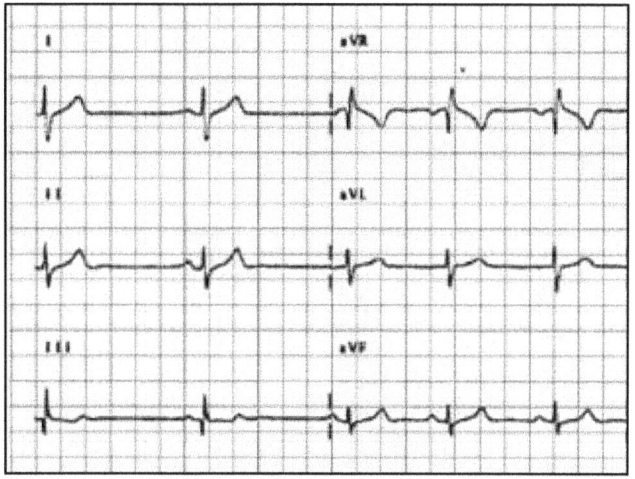

Fig: 02.06. RS Pattern seen in all the limb leads

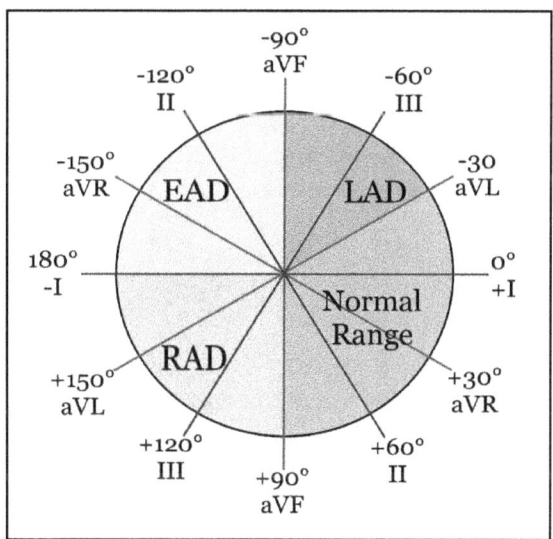

Fig: 02.07. Frontal electrical axis

CLINICAL EKG INTERPRETATION

QUIZ

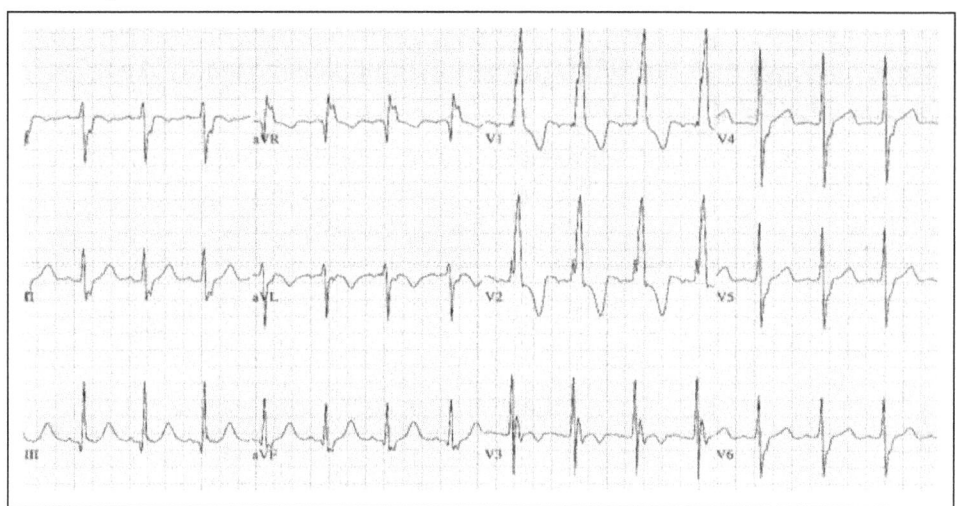

What is your diagnosis?

_____

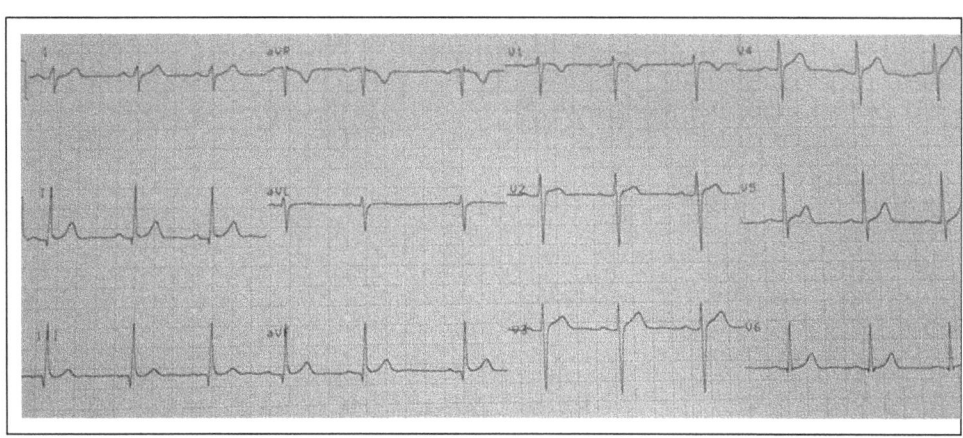

What is your diagnosis?

_____

Chapter 3 Conduction Disturbances

- 1st-degree AV Block
- 2nd-degree AV Block: Type 1 and Type II
- Incomplete Heart Block (ICHB)
- Complete Heart Block (CHB)
- Preexcitation
- LGL Syndrome

Conduction disturbances could be located anywhere along the heart's electrical grid. Many conduction disturbances are pathological and signify important underlying heart diseases.

THE 1ST-DEGREE AV BLOCK

The 1st-degree AV block refers to the prolongation of the PR interval. It is the interval from the beginning of the P wave to the beginning of the Q wave. The normal PR interval is less than 200 ms. It is an important interval as it involves impulse conduction through the intra atrial specialized conduction fibers and the AV nodal tissue itself (Fig: 03.01).

Diseases involving the AV node could suggest disease elsewhere down the specialized conduction system now or in the future. In the example below, the PR interval is 280 ms, which suggest a significant delay in the electrical impulse conduction from the sinus node to the ventricles.

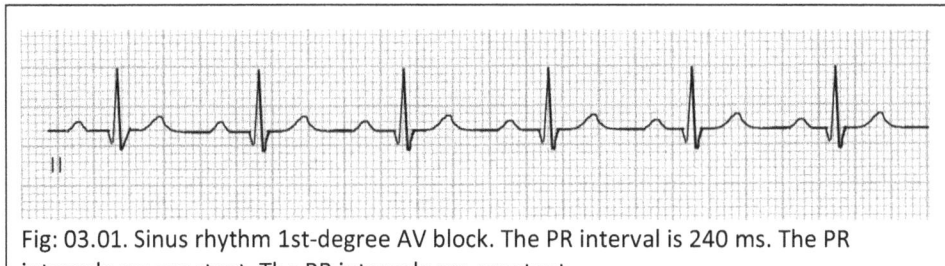

Fig: 03.01. Sinus rhythm 1st-degree AV block. The PR interval is 240 ms. The PR intervals are constant. The RR intervals are constant.

The PR interval is an important interval as it determines the optimal cardiac function. This is especially true in patients with advanced heart failure, where the optimal ventricular filling is essential to improve the forward stroke volume. Hence, in patients who have heart failure and advanced pacemakers, we often adjust the PR interval to optimize the cardiac output.

THE 2ND-DEGREE AV BLOCK

It refers to a condition where some sinus impulses fail to conduct to the ventricles. In the 1st-degree AV block, just the PR interval is prolonged but all the impulses eventually reach the ventricles. However, with 2nd-degree AV block the ventricular conduction is variable.

Based on the ventricular conduction, the second AV block is divided into two groups:

- Mobitz Type I or Wenckebach
- Mobitz Type II AV block

Wenckebach AV Block (Type I): This is commonly seen in a patient with inferior myocardial infarction.

There is a progressive prolongation of the PR interval until one of the P waves fails to conduct to the ventricles, creating a pause, and then the cycle repeats. Each cycle can have 3 or more beats before the impulse fails to reach the ventricles (Fig: 03.02).

This also leads to a cycle of one QRS dropped every 3-4 beats (3:2 or 4:3 conduction). You will also see a grouping of the QRS complexes before there is a pause, which should be a clue to the presence of Wenckebach.

3. CONDUCTION DISTURBENCES

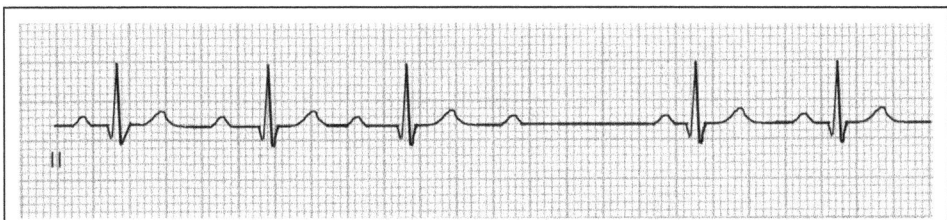

Fig: 03.02. Sinus rhythm Wenckebach Type I 2nd-degree AV block. Note the progressive prolongation of the PR interval, shortening of the RR intervals, and shorter PR after the pause compared to the PR before the pause.

AV Wenckebach in an acute inferior MI is often related to high vagal tone or nodal ischemia. The block is at the AV nodal level and transient. It is usually seen with occlusion of a dominant right coronary artery that also supplies the AV node and possibly the posterior wall.

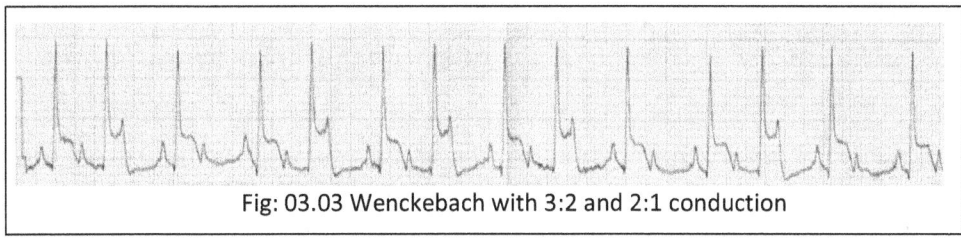

Fig: 03.03 Wenckebach with 3:2 and 2:1 conduction

Wenckebach occurring in the presence of acute MI is self-limiting. It doesn't need a temporary or permanent pacemaker. As the MI progresses, these changes resolve in a week's period.

Quiz: Describe what you see:

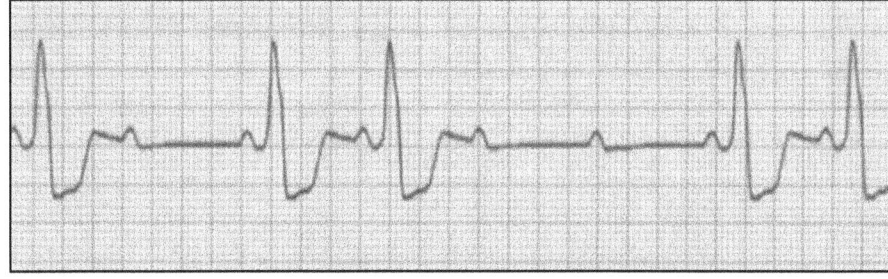

Features of Wenckebach

- The PP intervals remain the same as the sinus node is not affected.

- The PR intervals progressively increase as the rhythm progresses.

- The RR intervals become shorter and shorter, which may alter the refractory period of the ventricle and may account for some impulses not being able to conduct into the ventricle.

- After the pause, the regular sinus rhythm may continue or another episode of the dysrhythmia may appear.

- It generally doesn't cause any significant hemodynamic changes.

- In many cases, it is self-limiting and may improve with time in the case of myocardial infarction.

- Rarely, it may progress to more advanced forms of AV block.

3. CONDUCTION DISTURBENCES

Mobitz Type II AV Block: This rhythm is characterized by a periodic dropping of the QRS complexes. The PR intervals remain constant. However, more than one P wave may fail to conduct to the ventricles. The RR intervals may vary (Fig: 03.04).

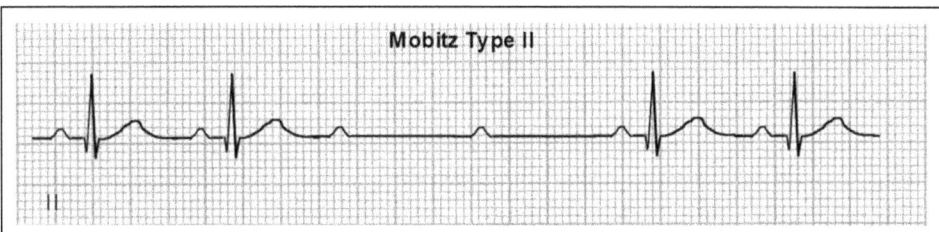

Fig: 03.04. Sinus rhythm Mobitz II 2nd-degree AV block. Note the normal PR intervals and two dropped P waves.

When every other P wave fails to conduct, it may be difficult to differentiate it from Mobitz Type I block. One important clue is the PR interval in the Mobitz Type II remains the same whereas in Mobitz Type I the PR interval following the pause will be shorter than the previous PR interval.

Mobitz Type II AV block is more serious than Mobitz Type I block. Very often, this block involves the infranodal tissue. This conduction disturbance can rapidly progress to complete heart block; these patients eventually will need a permanent pacemaker.

When several P waves are dropped, it is called a high-grade AV block. This is more serious than the other types of blocks as it can quickly progress to complete heart block (CHB).

COMPLETE HEART BLOCK (CHB

This is a more serious condition, where none of the sinus impulses can reach the ventricles. As a result, the atria will be beating at the sinus rate, while the ventricles may be beating at a much slower rate. The ventricular impulses could be arising from the ventricular myocardium at a rate ranging from 40 to 45 beats per minute (Fig: 03.05).

A complete heart block can occur in the presence of acute inferior myocardial infarction, which is transient and resolves within two weeks. It is related to the damage to the AV node, which is supplied by the right coronary artery.

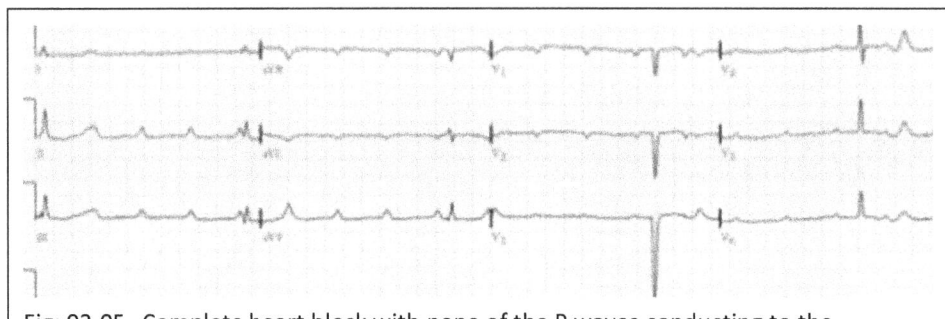

Fig: 03.05. Complete heart block with none of the P waves conducting to the ventricles. The QRS complexes are narrow, suggesting a His bundle origin

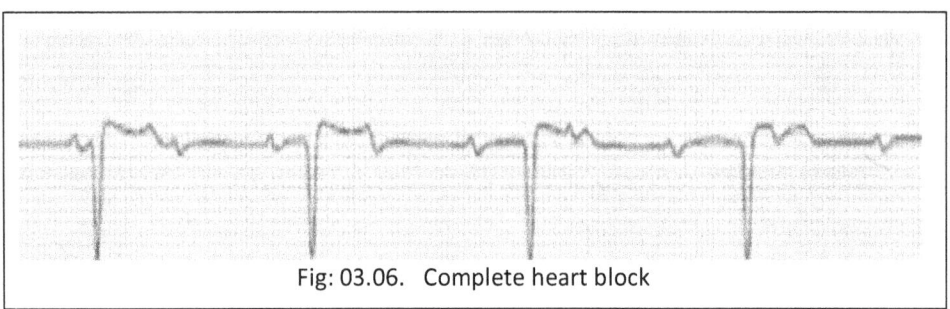

Fig: 03.06. Complete heart block

The above tracing is an example of a complete heart block. The narrow QRS complex may suggest a ventricular rhythm arising from the junction or one of the bundle branches (Fig: 03.06).

- The PP intervals are regular
- The RR intervals are regular
- There is no relationship between the P and the QRS complexes.

The QRS complex could be narrow (from the junction or bundle) or wide (ventricular escape rhythm).

3. CONDUCTION DISTURBENCES

The complete heart block seen in anterior myocardial infarction is related to damage involving the distal conducting system and is usually permanent. This may necessitate the need for a permanent pacemaker.

Patients with complete heart block can have the weakness, dizziness, fatigue, shortness of breath. It also may cause hypotension. Since there is severe disease involving the AV node, atropine may not be useful in speeding the ventricular rate. In addition, the AV dissociation and loss of atrial contribution can account for the low cardiac output.

Atropine may be useful if the QRS is narrow, suggesting a nodal rhythm. It blocks the vagal nerve release of acetylcholine and thus speeds up the heart rate. Idioventricular rhythm doesn't respond to atropine.

Complete heart block (CHB) related to beta-blocker overdose may respond to glucagon, while the CHB due to calcium channel blocker responds to calcium chloride, and the CHB resulting from digitalis toxicity may respond to Digoxin immune Fab.

The treatment options for complete heart block will include:
- Transcutaneous pacemaker
- Temporary transvenous pacemaker
- Ultimately, all these patients will need a permanent pacemaker.

As most patients with advanced conduction disease may also have advanced cardiac diseases, they would benefit from an AV sequential pacemaker to synchronize the atrial and ventricular functions in optimizing their cardiac output. In patients with advanced heart failure using an additional pacer wire in the coronary sinus to active both ventricles simultaneously may be necessary to improve their cardiac output and symptoms (Fig: 03.07). This will be covered in the chapter on pacemakers.

CLINICAL EKG INTERPRETATION

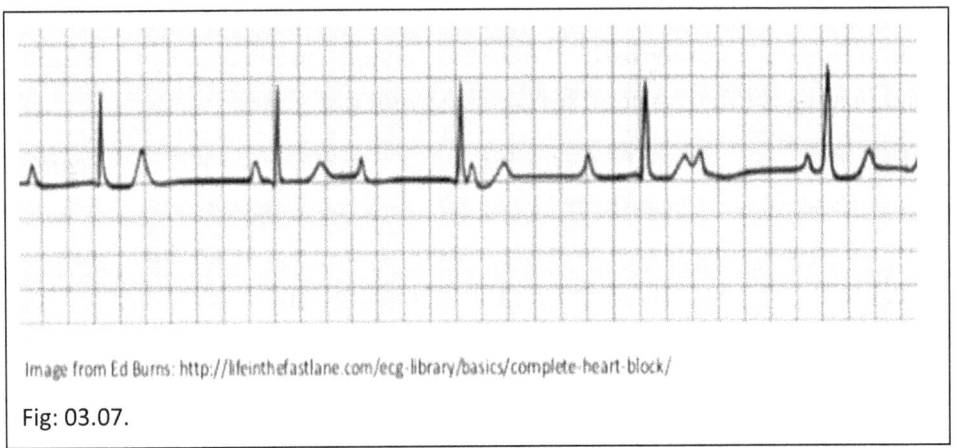

Fig: 03.07.

EKG QUIZ

EKG 3.1

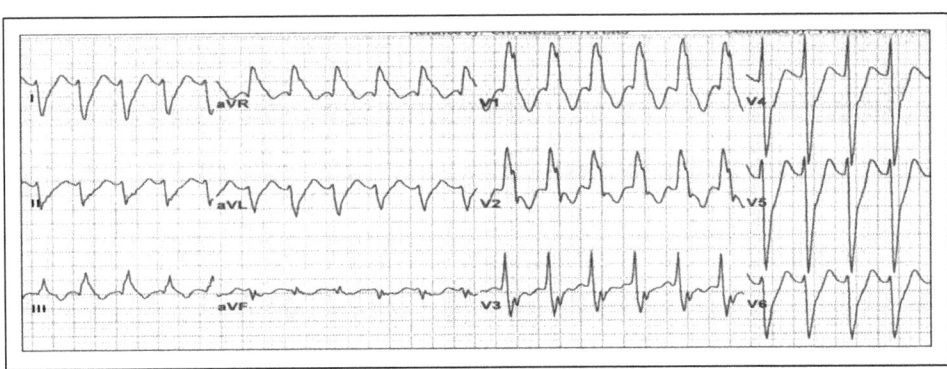

EKG 3.2

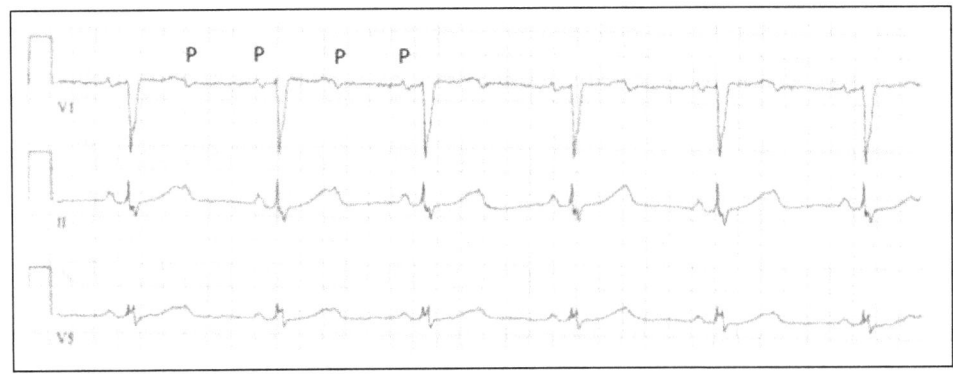

3. CONDUCTION DISTURBANCES

EKG 3.3

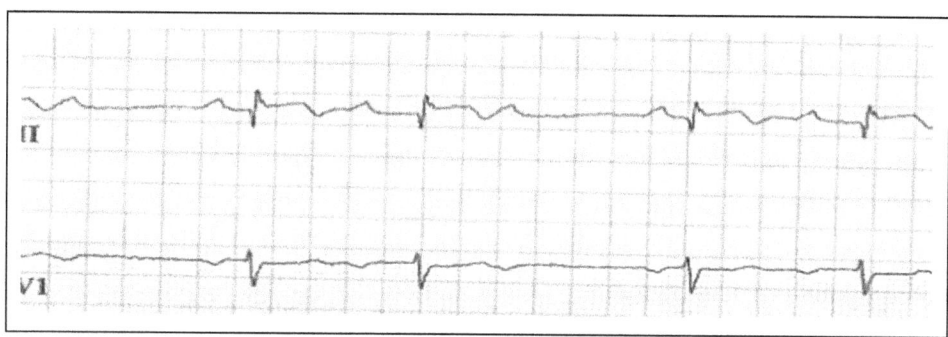

EKG 3.4

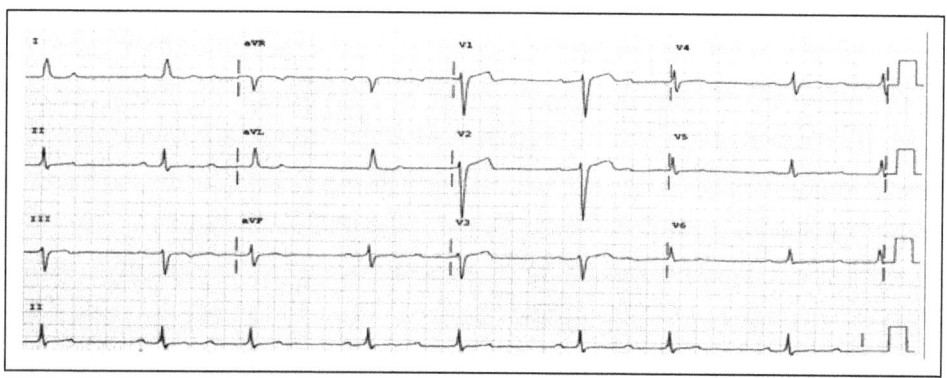

EKG 3.5

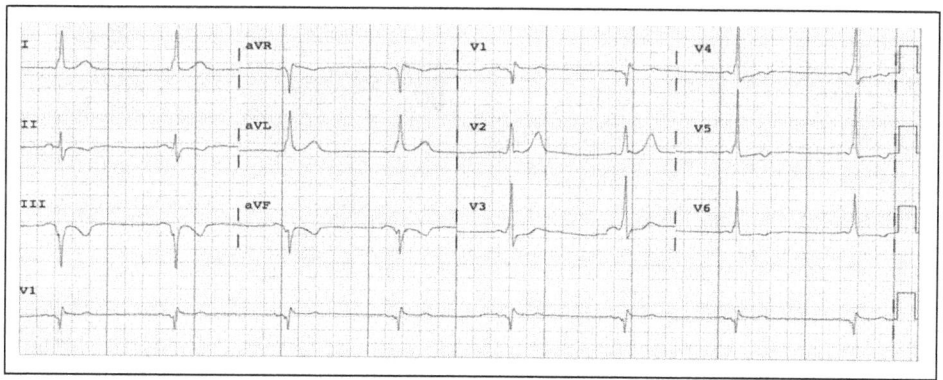

CLINICAL EKG INTERPRETATION

EKG 3.6

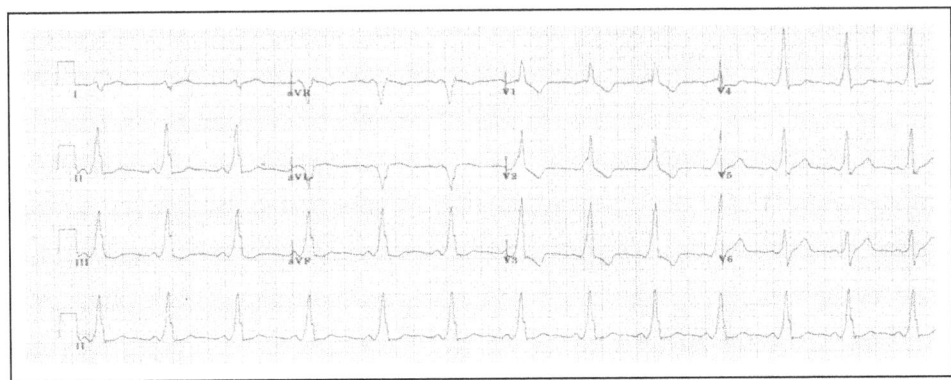

EKG 3.7

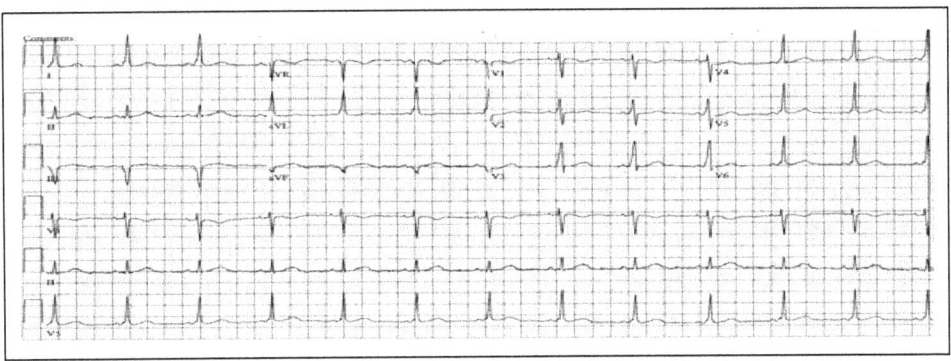

EKG 3.8

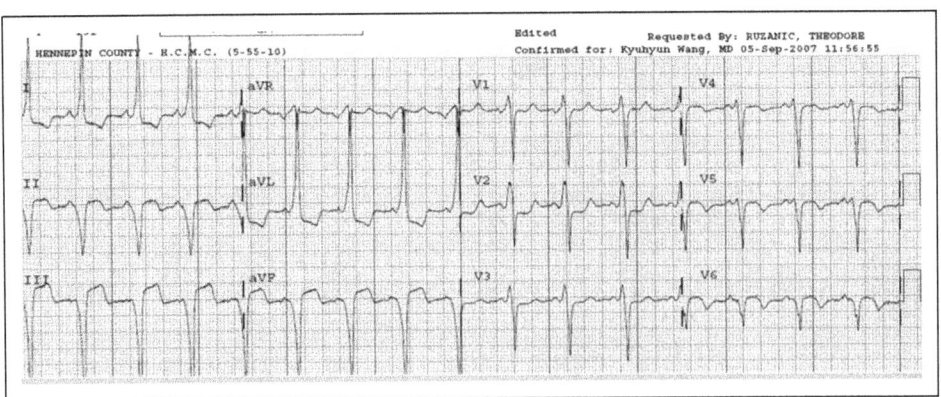

3. CONDUCTION DISTURBENCES

EKG 3.9

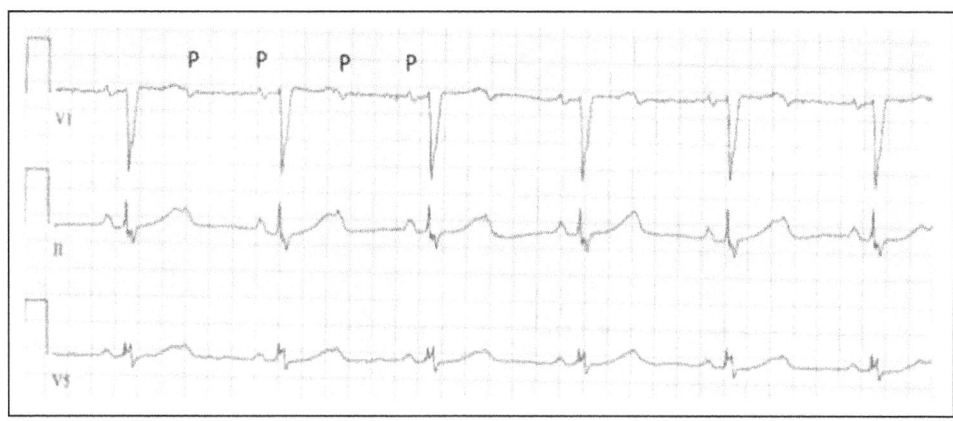

Contact the author for interpretations.

CLINICAL EKG INTERPRETATION

COMEDY TIME

Roll'em up?

As soon as I walked into a patient's room, the patient said, "Hi Dr. Nik, could you please give me a prescription for some cigarettes. This young nurse says I can't smoke in the hospital!"

"You must be out of your mind. You had heart surgery two days ago, and you want me to write a prescription for cigarettes?"

"In that case, I need a second opinion."

The nurse said, "You already had two opinions. The doctor's and mine."

"Yes, you are out of your quota!" I said.

"Come on Dr. Nik. I'm very nervous, jittery, can't you see. I've been smoking all my life!"

"I can understand that. I can order some Nicorette gum. I could lose my license for writing a prescription for cigarettes, did you know?"

"In that case, I'm going' to role'em up all your bills and start smoking'em!"

The young nurse, standing next me said, "Oh ho! You will be smoking'em for a long, long time, perhaps until you come back for your next heart surgery!"

ACLS QUIZ:

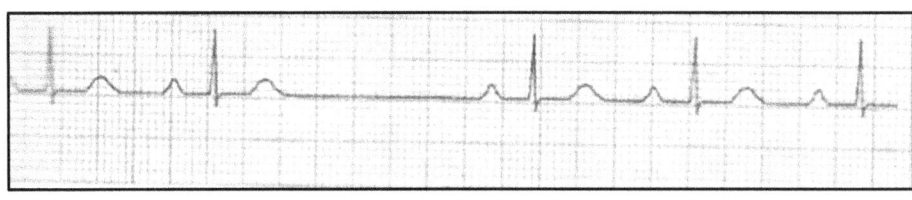

What do you see? _____

Chapter 4 Bundle Branch Blocks

- LBBB
- RBBB
- LAHB
- Fascicular Block
- IVCD
- Wide QRS Complexes
- Brugada Syndrome

In this chapter, we will look at various types of conduction disturbances in the electrical grid of the heart and their significance. Most of the conduction disturbances are abnormal and some may have a grave prognosis, while others may have no clinical significance.

Sometimes, these conduction disturbances may not only mimic myocardial infarction, but may also mask myocardial infarctions in other cases. We will explore the pattern recognition of such conduction disturbances while emphasizing their clinical significance in the patients' diagnoses and overall prognosis.

These conduction disturbances reflect the underlying pathology involving the conduction system and also may shed light on what to expect in the future. It will also aid us in avoiding certain drugs that can make the conduction disturbances worse.

CLINICAL EKG INTERPRETATION

LEFT BUNDLE BRANCH BLOCK (LBBB)

A Left Bundle Branch Block or LBBB as it is commonly called is always pathological. It signifies an underlying heart disease that needs more attention. It should trigger your mind to question the etiology of LBBB.

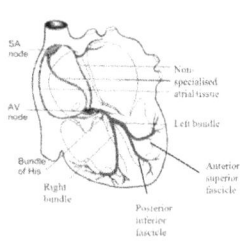

The Left Bundle Branch arises from the Bundle of His and it divides into the left anterior and the left posterior fascicles. The anterior fascicle is smaller and shorter compared to the posterior fascicle which wraps around the apex and supplies the lateral and posterior walls. Depending on where the left bundle is blocked, the EKG morphology may be different. If the anterior fascicle is also blocked, the EKG may show left axis deviation and left anterior hemiblock, besides traditional LBBB changes.

Complete LBBB: It results from the interference of the impulse propagation in the left bundle. The cardinal EKG findings of an LBBB are the widening of the QRS complexes in most leads. The QRS duration may exceed 120 ms. The QRS complexes are biphasic or notched in the lateral leads, while you may notice deep S waves in the anterior leads V1, V2, and V3 (Fig: 04.01).

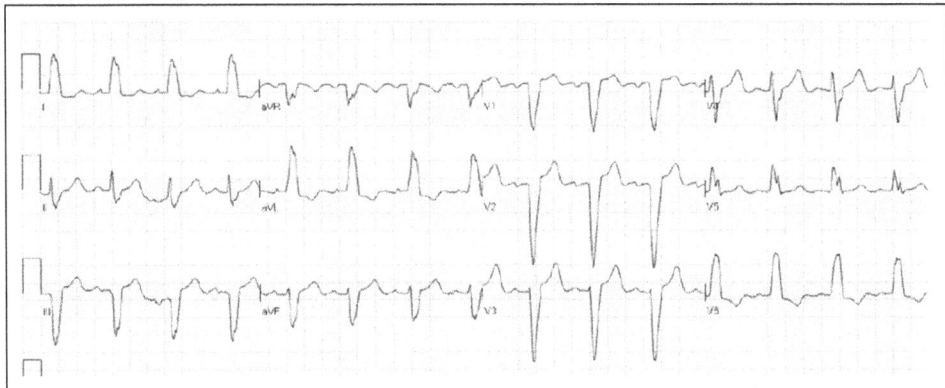

Fig: 04.01. Wide QRS in I, aVL, v5, v6. ST-T changes. Deep S waves in the anterior leads. Left axis deviation (-30°), not enough to call left anterior hemiblock. Also, note a 2 mm St elevation in leads V1, V2, and V3, which are common findings in LBBB.

CHAPTER 4. BUNDLE BRANCH BLOCKS

> **Complete LBBB Features:**
>
> - Wide QRS Complex in the lead I, aVL, and Lateral Chest Leads with a Notch at the Top.
>
> - The QRS Duration Can be >140 ms.
>
> - There Are Discordant ST-T changes.
>
> - Tiny r waves in the Anterior Leads with Deep S waves.
>
> - Peaked R waves in the Lateral Leads >60 ms.
>
> - A Notch in the R Wave in Lateral Chest Leads Resembling an "M."

More than 90% of the time the LBBB is due to underlying heart diseases such as hypertension, myocardial infarction, myocarditis, valvular heart disease, or congestive heart failure.

There is a slight delay in the activation of the left ventricle compared to the right due to the LBBB. It may not make a big difference in a patient with normal left ventricular function. However, in patients with heart failure, especially with a QRS complex >120 ms, the asynchrony could compromise already depressed left ventricular output. In such patients, Cardiac Resynchronization Therapy or (CRT) can play a significant role in improving the forward cardiac flow and a patient's symptoms. It is very important to read the EKG beyond what is clear to the naked eyes.

The Left bundle branch block can also produce septal wall motion abnormalities on the Echocardiogram and produce false-positive results on the nuclear stress test. The EKG findings on a stress test may be useless in patients with left bundle branch block.

CLINICAL EKG INTERPRETATION

Development of new-onset LBBB in an anterior myocardial infarction signals a grave prognosis. As you recall, the anterior myocardial infarction is caused by occlusion of the left anterior descending artery. A new LBBB may signal more proximal occlusion of the left anterior descending branch resulting in a septal infarction, damage to the left bundle branch, besides extensive anterolateral myocardial damage.

The Left bundle branch block may also mask left ventricular hypertrophy (LVH). The left atrial abnormality, increased precordial voltage, and QSR prolongation of >150 ms may suggest LVH.

The discordant ST-T changes associated with left bundle branch block can mimic subendocardial ischemia or infarction. You need to compare these changes with the previous EKGs and correlate them with other clinical presentations of acute coronary syndrome.

Occasionally, the LBBB can be rate-related. This is due to an increased refractory period of the conducting system during rapid ventricular rates.

It is difficult to diagnose acute myocardial infarction in the presence of a complete LBBB. In a given clinical setting, look for concordant ST changes in the anterior or inferior leads that could be a clue for acute ischemia or infarction. The ST-T changes are discordant to the QRS complex direction in LBBB. If you see concordant ST-T changes with chest pain or shortness of breath, they could be clues for underlying ischemia. Serial evolving electrocardiographic changes could also aid in the diagnosis of myocardial infarction in patients with LBBB.

Differential diagnoses should include hyperkalemia with wide QRS complexes, drug toxicity from Flecainide, or pre-excitation.

DIAGNOSIS OF MI IN PATIENTS WITH LBBB

The diagnosis of acute myocardial infarction in patients with LBBB becomes complicated as some may have ST elevation as a manifestation of LBBB. However, it is important to correlate with the patient's presentation, previous EKGs, and associated findings such as elevated cardiac enzymes that may provide hidden clues to the diagnosis of acute myocardial infarction in LBBB.

CHAPTER 4. BUNDLE BRANCH BLOCKS

Sgarbossa et al. in 1916 described certain EKG criteria that can support the diagnosis of acute myocardial infarction in LBBB.

Sgarbossa Criteria for MI detection in LBBB

- ST Elevation >1 mm and in the Same Direction (Concordant) with the QRS Complex = 5 points

- ST Depression >1 mm in leads V1, V2 or V3 = 3 Points

- ST Elevation > 5 mm and in the Opposite Direction (Discordant) with the QRS = 2 Points

It requires a score of 3 points to diagnose an acute MI.
It essentially requires either criteria 1 or criteria 2.
Criteria #3 is under debate as to its usefulness.

RIGHT BUNDLE BRANCH BLOCK

The right bundle branch block (RBBB) is more common than the left bundle branch block. It results from interruption of the electrical impulse transmission through the right bundle branch. As a result, the impulse travels through the normal left bundle and then activates the right ventricle through the spread of the impulse via the muscle fibers. So, it produces the classic rsR' pattern in V1 and a slurred deep S wave in V6 (Fig: 04.02).

It can occur with no structural heart disease. It is commonly found in patients with right ventricular hypertrophy, atrial septal defect, pulmonary hypertension, pulmonary embolism, Brugada syndrome, rheumatic heart disease, myocarditis, or cardiomyopathy.

CLINICAL EKG INTERPRETATION

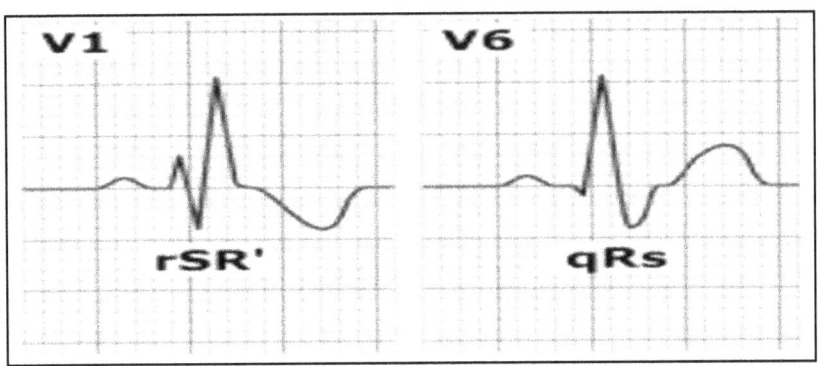

Fig: 04.02. rSR' in V1 and qRs in V6. Discordant ST-T changes in V1.

Right Bundle Branch Block - RBBB

- There is an rSR' in V1

- Right Axis Deviation (RAD)

- Slurred Terminal S Waves in Anterolateral Leads

- QRS Complex >120 ms

- ST-T Changes Discordant to the QRS Complexes

- No change in the Electric Axis of the Heart

- If the QRS Duration is Between 110-120 ms = IRBBB

CHAPTER 4. BUNDLE BRANCH BLOCKS

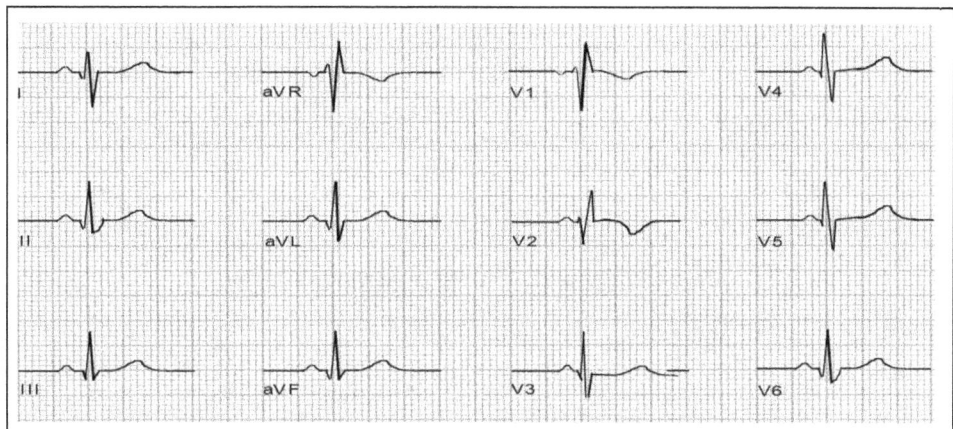

Fig: 04.03. Sinus rhythm with an rSR' in V1, V2, and discordant ST-T changes in the right precordial leads

In most cases, the right bundle branch block does not impact cardiovascular outcomes.

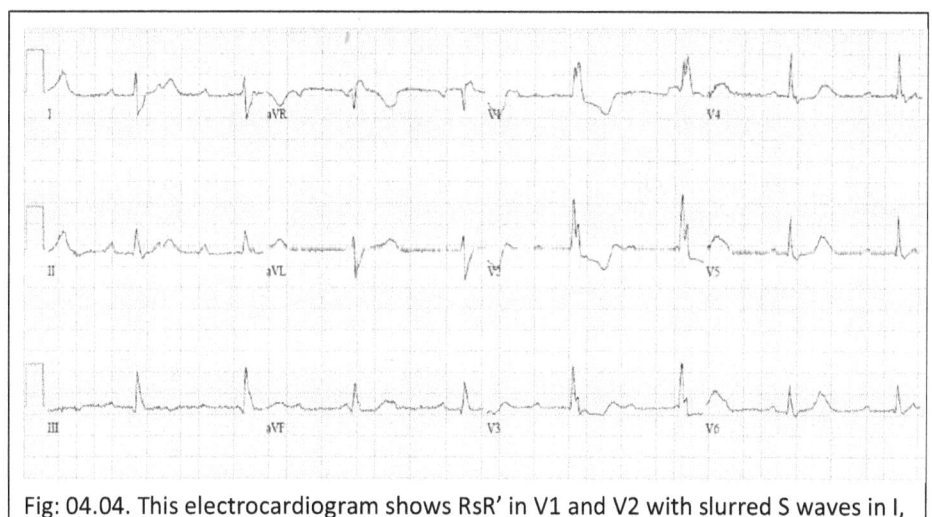

Fig: 04.04. This electrocardiogram shows RsR' in V1 and V2 with slurred S waves in I, aVL, V4-V6.

You notice the discordant ST-T changes in leads that display an rSr' pattern (Fig: 04.03). New development of a right bundle branch block with myocardial infarction may suggest the proximal left anterior descending artery involvement. RBBB associated with a left anterior fascicular block may progress to complete heart block with a grave prognosis.

CLINICAL EKG INTERPRETATION

Since the right bundle branch block doesn't involve the initial 40 ms of the QRS complex, it doesn't mask an acute myocardial infarction change.

A normal variation is an rSr' in V1 and V2, with a tiny r wave of less than 2 mm and a QRS duration of 100 to 110 ms may be mistaken for incomplete RBBB.

Here are some variations of QRS complexes in the anterior leads in patients with RBBB.

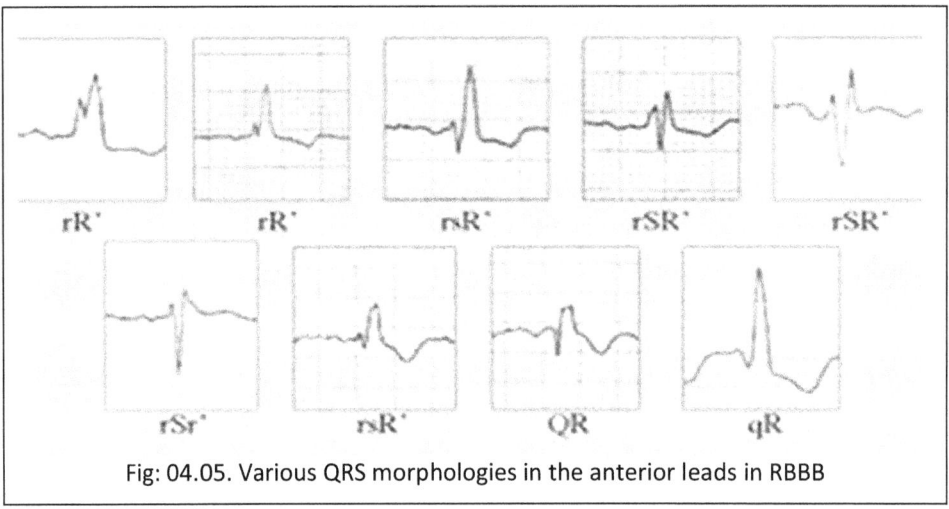

Fig: 04.05. Various QRS morphologies in the anterior leads in RBBB

More examples of RBBB:

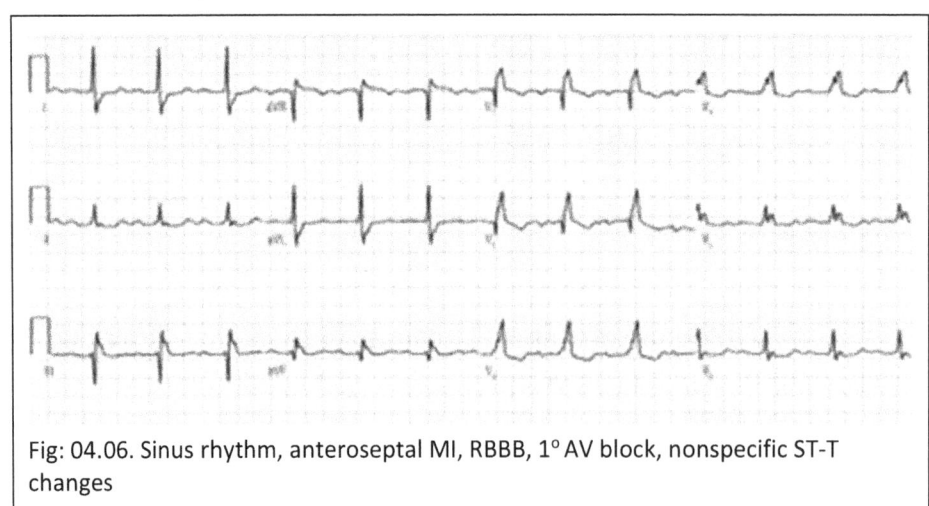

Fig: 04.06. Sinus rhythm, anteroseptal MI, RBBB, 1° AV block, nonspecific ST-T changes

CHAPTER 4. BUNDLE BRANCH BLOCKS

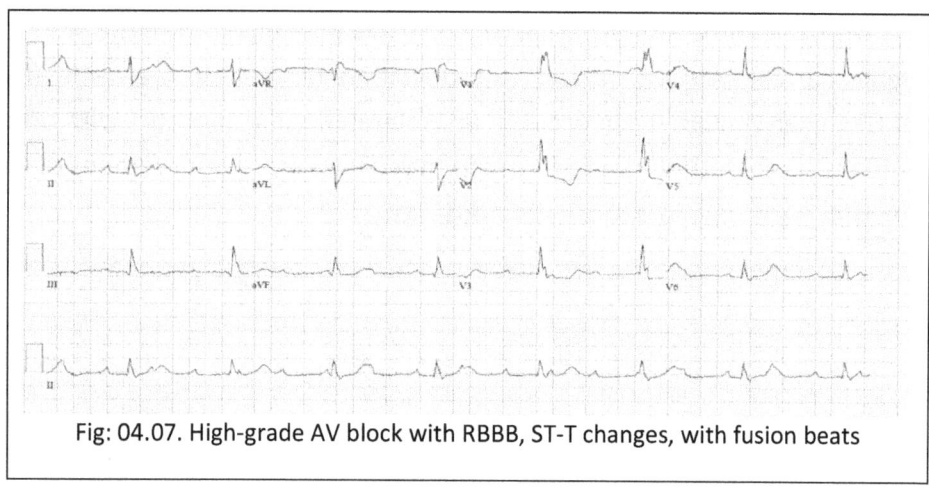

Fig: 04.07. High-grade AV block with RBBB, ST-T changes, with fusion beats

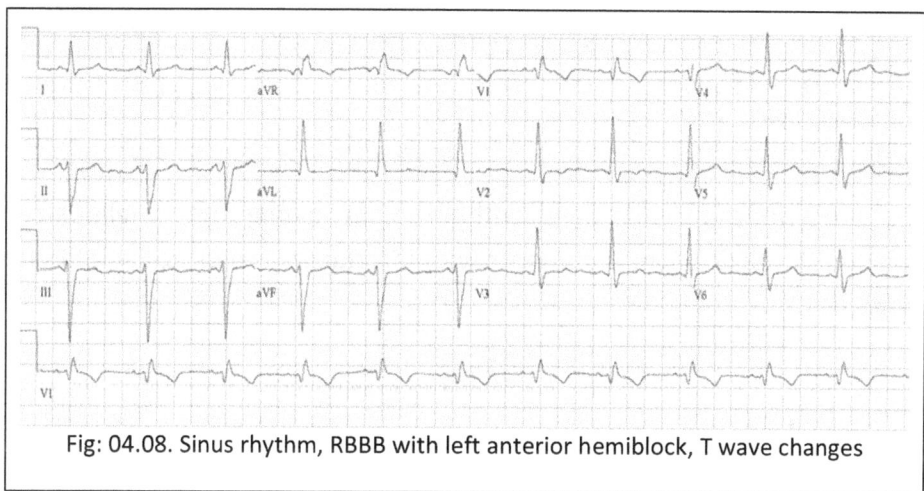

Fig: 04.08. Sinus rhythm, RBBB with left anterior hemiblock, T wave changes

LEFT ANTERIOR FASCICULAR BLOCK (LAFB):

The left anterior fascicle activates the superior septum, the left ventricular anterior wall, and the anterior papillary muscle. When the left anterior fascicle of the left bundle is blocked, the impulse travels through the posterior fascicle and then activates the rest of the ventricular myocardium through the Purkinje system. This leads to the left superior orientation of the electrical axis of the heart. However, it doesn't affect the mechanical function of the left ventricle as long as the posterior fascicle carries the bulk of the electrical impulse.

CLINICAL EKG INTERPRETATION

The left anterior fascicular block (LAFB) manifests on the surface electrocardiogram with a left axis deviation of greater than -45° (Fig: 04.09). Even though it can occur as an isolated finding, it occurs with other findings such as RBBB or LBBB, which may signal more involvement of the electrical system and a more ominous sign.

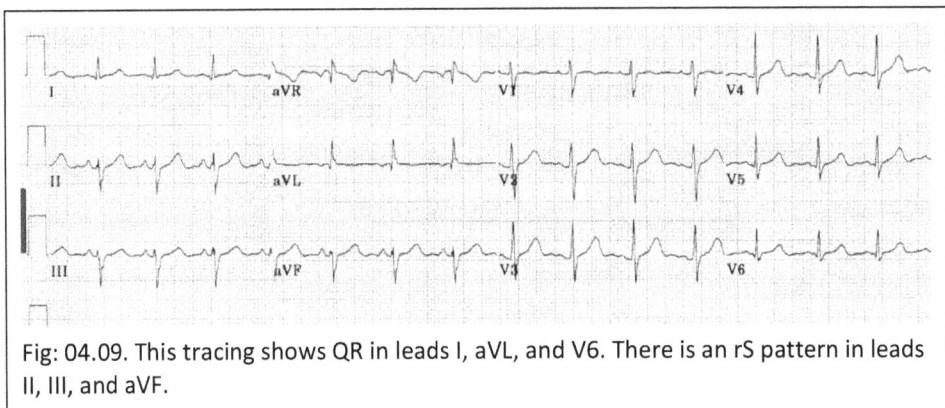

Fig: 04.09. This tracing shows QR in leads I, aVL, and V6. There is an rS pattern in leads II, III, and aVF.

LAFB doesn't signify significant pathology, owing to its smaller size. It may mask the Q waves in patients with inferior wall myocardial infarction (Fig: 04.10).

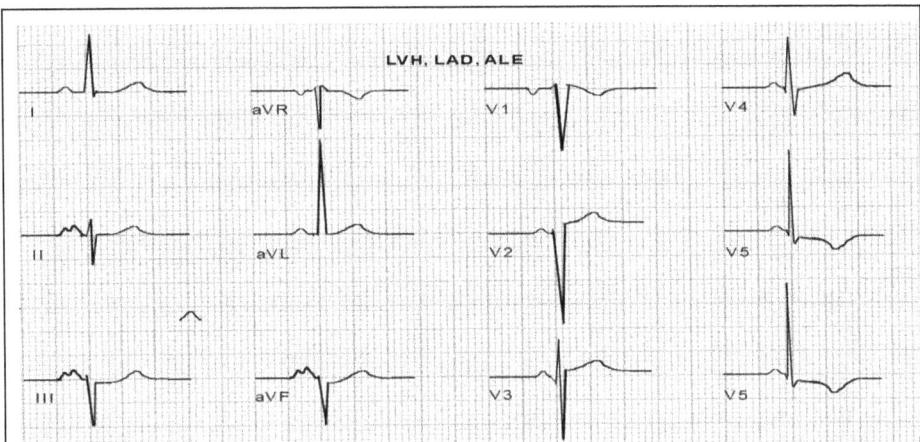

Fig: 04.10. This electrocardiogram shows Left axis deviation, left atrial enlargement, and left ventricular hypertrophy with strain pattern. Note the tall and double-peaked P waves in leads II, III, and aVF.

CHAPTER 4. BUNDLE BRANCH BLOCKS

Left Anterior Fascicular Block (LAFB) Features

- QRS Duration of <120 ms
- More Negative Deflection in lead II
- Time to Peak R Wave in aVL >45 ms
- Leads II, III, and aVF Show rS Patterns
- Leads I, aVL, V5, and V6 Show qR Patterns

LEFT POSTERIOR FASCICULAR BLOCK

It is very rare. Often, it occurs in combination with RBBB. The LPHB electrocardiographic features include:

Left Posterior Fascicular Block Features

➢ The QRS Axis of 120^0 (RAD)

➢ The QRS Width is <120 ms

➢ rS Pattern in I and aVL

➢ qR Complexes in II, III, and aVF

➢ Exclude Other Causes of RAD: RVH, PE, COPD, Lateral MI

CLINICAL EKG INTERPRETATION

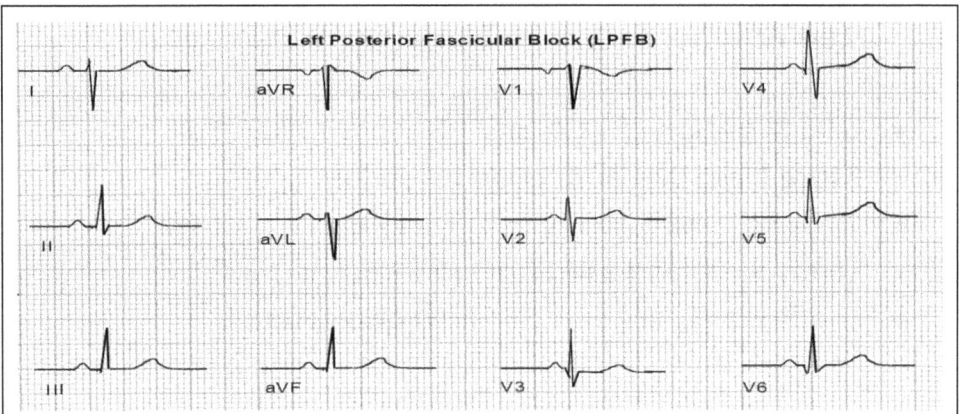

Fig: 04.11 This electrocardiogram reveals rS complexes in leads I, aVL, and the QRS duration is <120 ms, and qR in III.

BRUGADA SYNDROME

The diagnostic feature is an rSr' in the anterior chest leads mimicking a RBBB (Fig: 04.11). There is also 'J' point and ST elevation in the anterior leads. These patients are prone to ventricular tachyarrhythmias. The QRS duration is between 100 and 110 ms. The T waves can vary in their direction.

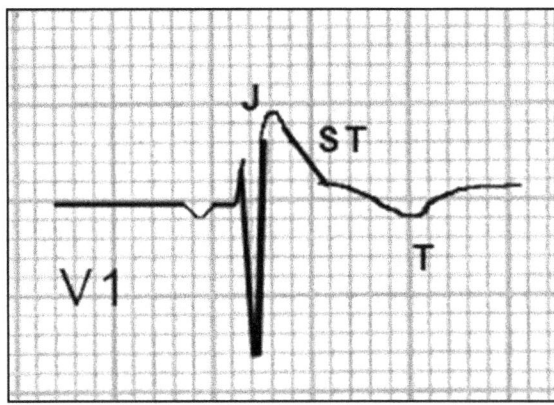

Fig: 04.11. An rSr' pattern with ST elevation and slurring in V1

There are three main types of this syndrome and all of them can be seen in a single individual from time to time. Calcium channel blockers given intravenously can unmask hidden ST-T changes (Fig: 04.12).

CHAPTER 4. BUNDLE BRANCH BLOCKS

Brugada Syndrome	Type I	Type II	Type III
J Wave Amplitude	≥2 mm	≥2 mm	≥2 mm
ST-T Segment	Curved	Saddleback	Saddleback
ST Segment	Gradual Slope	Elevated	Elevated
T Waves	Negative	Lifted 1 mm	Lifted 1 mm

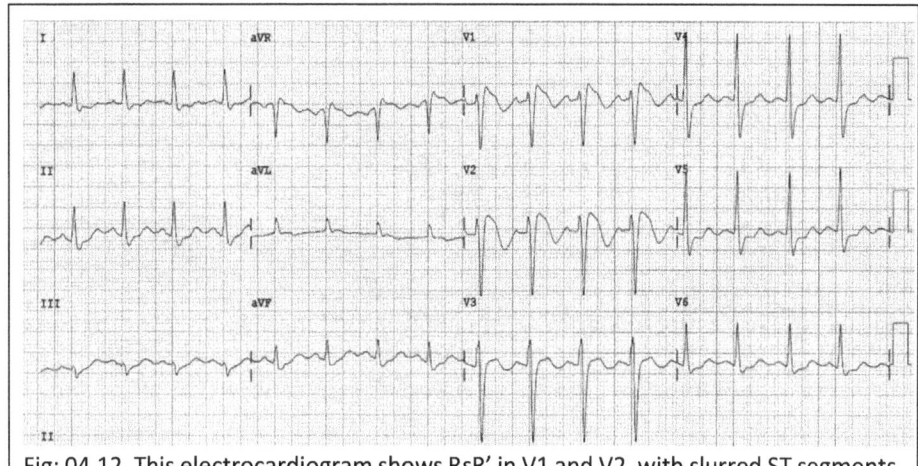
Fig: 04.12. This electrocardiogram shows RsR' in V1 and V2, with slurred ST segments.

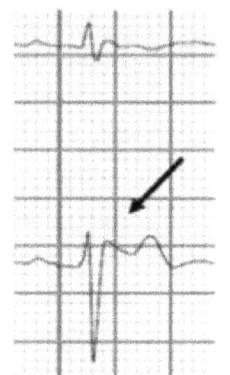
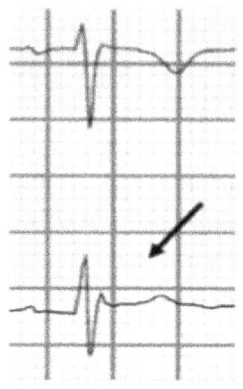

Type 1:
Coved type
ST-segment
elevation

Type 2:
saddle-back type
ST-segment
elevation

Type 3:
Saddle-back type
"ST-segment
elevation"

BIFASCICULAR BLOCK

A Bifascicular block can result from a block involving more than one site. It can be a combination of:

RBBB+Left anterior fascicular block LAFB (Fig: 04.13)

RBBB+Left posterior fascicular block LPFB

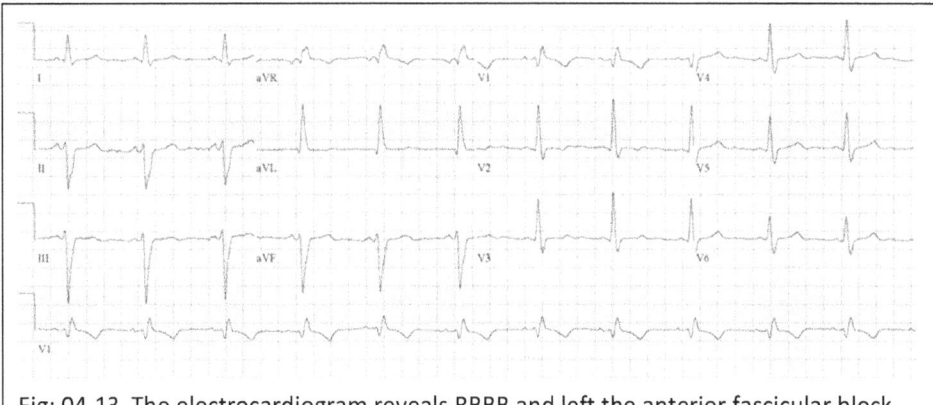

Fig: 04.13. The electrocardiogram reveals RBBB and left the anterior fascicular block (LAFB).

TRIFASCICULAR BLOCK

Even though we have only two bundle branches, sometimes we can see involvement in more than two branches. Take for example an electrocardiogram with an RBBB and left anterior hemiblock that also had prolongation of the PR interval. In this case, there is pathology involving the right bundle, the left anterior fascicle, and the AV node. This signifies a more extensive involvement of the conduction system in general. These patients are at high risk of developing high-grade AV block or even complete heart block. It will be challenging to use any drugs that affect the AV conduction or heart rate as the patient may develop complete heart block.

INTRA-VENTRICULAR CONDUCTION DELAY (IVCD)

You often see this interpretation when the QRS duration is greater than 120 ms and it doesn't fit the usual RBBB or the LBBB pattern.

CHAPTER 4. BUNDLE BRANCH BLOCKS

PRE–EXCITATION SYNDROME (WPW)

It is characterized by a slurred upstroke of the R waves because of an accessory pathway between the atria and the ventricles. The initial conduction of the impulse through the bypass tract in Wolff-Parkinson-White syndrome (WPW), results in an earlier activation of ventricles than the normal impulse, accounting for the slurred upstroke or the delta waves.

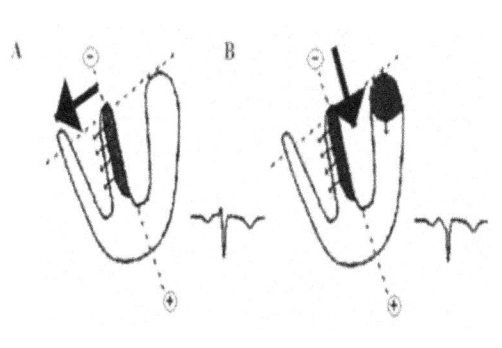

Classic WPW Features

➤ **Short PR Interval**

➤ **The Typical Slurring of the R wave Resulting in the Delta Wave**

➤ **Wide QRS Complex of >120 ms**

The QRS morphology is a fusion beat (Fig: 04.14). It's a combination of conduction through the accessory pathway causing the initial slurred delta wave. As the normal AV nodal conduction arrives, it rapidly activates the ventricles through the bundle branch system, resulting in a terminal steep R wave. This variation is QRS morphology can mimic infarctions, BBB, hypertrophy, or myocardial ischemia.

CLINICAL EKG INTERPRETATION

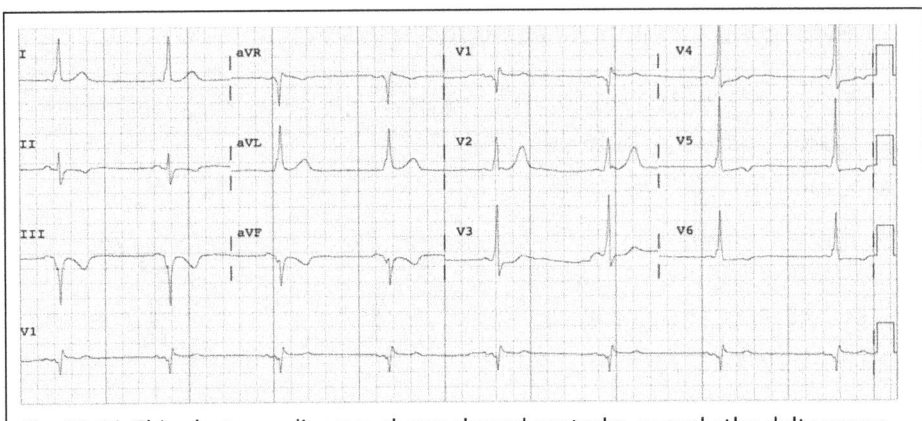

Fig: 04.14. This electrocardiogram shows slurred upstroke, namely the delta waves in multiple leads. There are nonspecific ST-T changes.

The bypass tracts from the left atrium may connect to the AV node, the His bundle, or fascicular tracts. Up to 45% to 60% of the accessory pathways are on the left atrial free wall. A pre–excitation pattern with a PR interval of >120 ms indicates a left atrial free-wall pathway.

There are two types of WPW.

Type A has R waves in V1 (left-sided pathways). They have positive delta waves, short PR interval, wide QRS complexes, and reciprocal ST-T changes (Fig: 04.15).

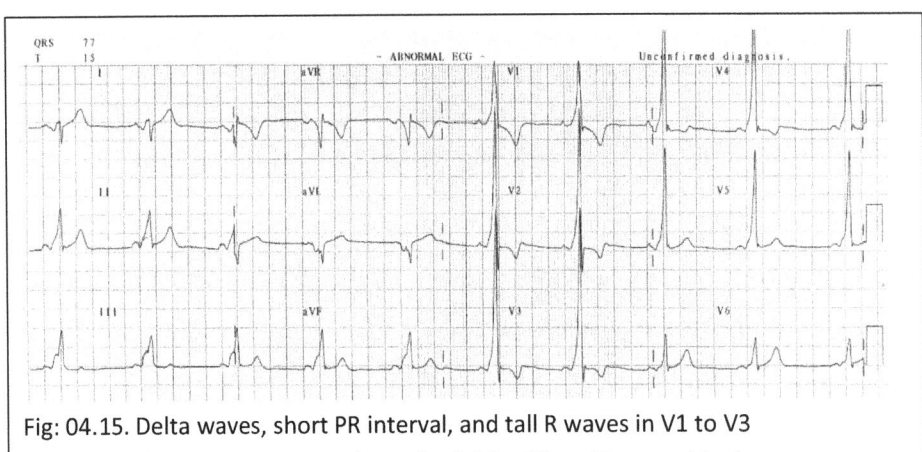

Fig: 04.15. Delta waves, short PR interval, and tall R waves in V1 to V3
Ref: https://www.resus.com.au/2016/02/13/wolff-parkinson-white/

CHAPTER 4. BUNDLE BRANCH BLOCKS

WPW Type B has QS complex in V1 (right-sided pathways). They have negative delta waves in leads II, III, and aVF, short PR interval, QS complex in V1, and wide QRS complexes (Fig: 04.16). The negative dealt waves in the inferior wall can cause a pseudo-infarction pattern. Also, notice the ST-T changes in the opposite direction.

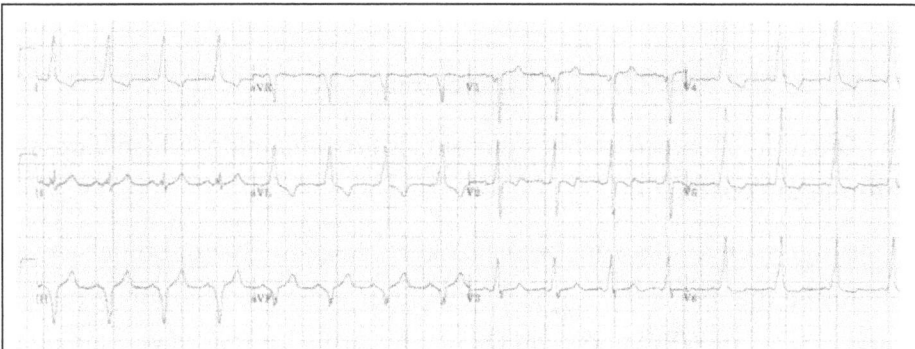

Fig: 04.16. WPW with QS complexes in V1, negative delta waves in leads II, III, and aVF, short PR interval, and wide QRS complexes. Notice the pseudo-infarction pattern in the inferior leads.

Coexisting conditions such as acute MI or LVH may alter the QRS morphology.

Since the accessory pathway and the normal AV nodal tissue have different conduction velocities, it can set off an Atrioventricular reentry tachycardia (AVRT).

Patients with antidromic tachycardia have a shorter refractory period.

The most common symptoms of WPW syndrome are palpitation, chest pain, shortness of breath, and dizziness. Syncope may signal very rapid ventricular rates. Often, patients with WPW pattern are asymptomatic and the WPW patterns are discovered on a routine electrocardiogram.

The onset of tachycardia is sudden. Caffeine, stress, menstrual periods, or pregnancy can precipitate a tachyarrhythmia.

CLINICAL EKG INTERPRETATION

In WPW, a negative in wave leads III and aVF along with tall R waves in the V1 to V3 may suggest left posterior bypass tracks. This pattern may simulate Inferoposterior MI. WPW may also simulate RVH, LVH, and bundle branch blocks. The key is to identify the delta waves and short PR intervals in any leads.

Treatment of WPW with Tachycardia

The drug of choice in these patients is Procainamide, which blocks the anterograde conduction.

Drugs such as Digoxin, beta-blockers, calcium channel blockers, and Adenosine that block the AV node should be used with caution in patients with a history of WPW and wide QRS tachycardia for fear of worsening the tachycardia. This is especially true in a patient with WPW and atrial flutter or fibrillation.

The disappearance of the delta wave during an exercise test in patients with WPW syndrome identifies patients who are at low risk for sudden arrhythmic death.

The most common indication for an electrophysiological study is a decision to perform catheter ablation. All competitive athletes, pilots, and bus drivers with WPW should undergo these studies.

ACLS QUIZ:

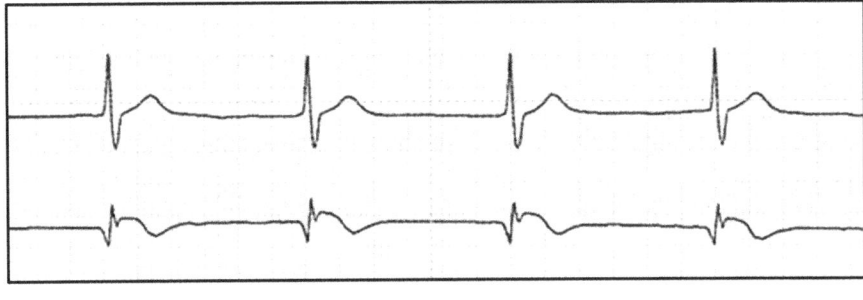

How many points can you see? _____

Chapter 5 Cardiac Enlargement

- Left Atrial Enlargement
- Right Atrial Enlargement
- Biatrial Enlargement
- Left Ventricular Hypertrophy (LVH)
- Right Ventricular Hypertrophy (RVH)
- Biventricular Hypertrophy
- Hypertrophic Cardiomyopathy (HCM)

There are two mechanisms by which the heart responds to pressure or volume changes chronically. When there is volume overload in conditions such as mitral regurgitation, aortic regurgitation, or tricuspid regurgitation, the heart responds by dilatation. The sarcomeres duplicate in sequence.

When there is pressure overload in situations such as aortic stenosis, hypertension, or pulmonary hypertension, the heart responds by concentric hypertrophy. Here, the sarcomeres respond by parallel duplication, thus increasing the thickness. In either case, the electrocardiographic changes are almost similar.

In the case of atria, we commonly refer to them as enlargement, where as in case of ventricles, we call hypertrophy even if the underlying changes are dilatation.

The position of the heart in the chest may also influence the P waves. For example, in dextrocardia the P waves may be inverted in leads I and aVL.

CLINICAL EKG INTERPRETATION

RIGHT ATRIAL ENLARGEMENT

The right atrial enlargement is most often seen in patients with either right ventricular pressure or volume overload. It is rare to see an isolated right atrial enlargement unless we are dealing with tricuspid stenosis. The right atrial enlargement occurs in association with right ventricular enlargement or hypertrophy. The most common causes of this combination of findings are chronic lung disease or primary pulmonary hypertension. Both pressure and volume changes lead to dilatation of the right atrium.

The right atrial enlargement is reflected best in the inferior leads II, III, and aVF. Normally, the P waves in these leads are monophasic and less than 2.5 mm and less than 120 ms in duration. In case of isolated right atrial enlargement, the P waves in these leads may appear peaked. The voltage can be more than 2.5 mm but not greater than 120 ms in duration. More often, we may see a biphasic P wave in these leads.

In the electrocardiogram below (Fig: 05.01), there are peaked P waves in leads II, III, and aVF. In addition, they're all tall R waves in V1 and V2. There is also a right axis deviation and increased voltage in leads V1 and V2 suggestive of right ventricular hypertrophy. The composite picture is that of right ventricular hypertrophy with strain (ST-T changes in V1-V2) along with right atrial enlargement.

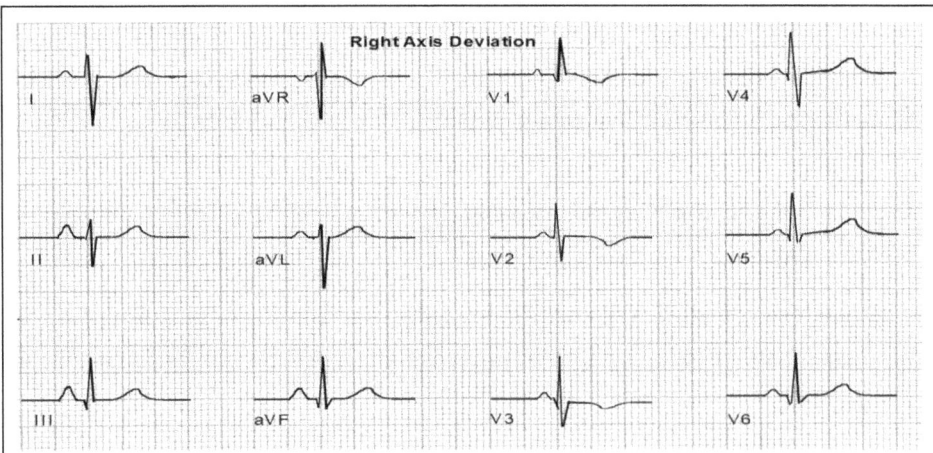

Fig: 05.01. This electrocardiogram shows right axis deviation, right atrial enlargement, and right ventricular hypertrophy. Note the tall and peaked P waves in leads II, III, and aVF. There are nonspecific ST-T changes.

CHAPTER 5. CARDIAC ENLARGEMENT

When we analyze an EKG, we need to keep in mind that nothing happens in isolation. When you see changes suggesting right atrial enlargement always look for other supporting findings that can confirm the diagnosis.

Isolated right atrial overload can be associated with a negative P wave in V1 which appears narrow (pseudo LAA). The picture may also be related to the right atrium beneath the V1 position. Leads II, III, and aVF should show a narrow-peaked P waves.

LEFT ATRIAL ENLARGEMENT

The correct terminology is left atrial abnormality as it only refers to the electrical activity of the left atrium and not the actual structural changes. The hallmark of left atrial enlargement is seen in V1, where the negative deflection of the P wave is greater than 40 ms and deeper than at least 1 mm. In other words, if the P wave in V1 occupies more than one smaller square, and if the P wave is more than 120 ms, it represents left atrial enlargement. In addition, we can appreciate biphasic P waves in leads II, III, and aVF. The second wave represents the left atrial activity (Fig: 05.02).

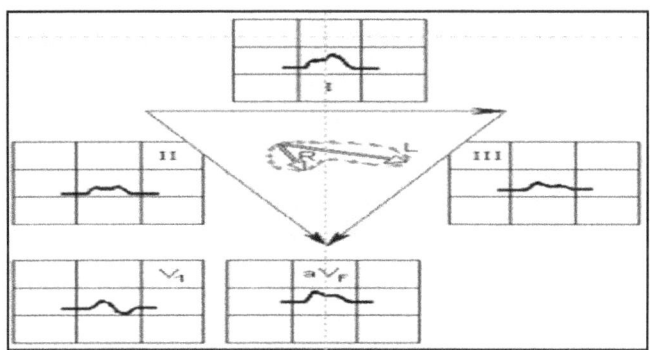

Fig: 05.02. This tracing shows left atrial enlargement. Biphasic P waves in II, III, aVF and negative P wave in V1.

CLINICAL EKG INTERPRETATION

Left atrial enlargement rarely occurs in isolation. Most often, it occurs in conjunction with changes that reflect left ventricular hypertrophy as characterized by a deep S waves in the anterior chest leads, tall R wave in leads I, aVL, and lateral chest leads. We need to consider these combinations as a group which will help us better appreciate the effect of pressure or volume overload on the entire heart, not just a single chamber. Sometimes atrial fibrillation may make it difficult to appreciate left atrial enlargement. However, atrial fibrillation is considered an indirect marker for left atrial enlargement.

In the following electrocardiogram, we can appreciate several findings. There is a prominent negative deflection in V1 covering more than one box (Fig: 05.03). In addition, there are other features of left ventricular hypertrophy as evidenced by Deep S waves in the anterior chest lead, tall R waves in the Lateral chest leads, along with ST-T changes in the lateral chest leads suggestive secondary change to left ventricular hypertrophy. Thus, look at an entire electrocardiogram, in the context of a patient's clinical findings, which will add more value to each part of the puzzle while arriving at a logical clinical diagnosis.

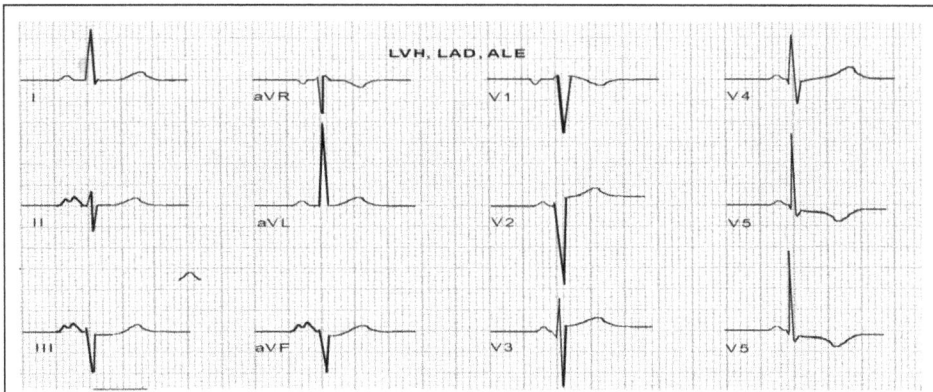

Fig: 05.03. This electrocardiogram shows left axis deviation, left atrial enlargement, and left ventricular hypertrophy with a strain pattern. Note the tall and double peaked P waves in leads II, III, and aVF.

CHAPTER 5. CARDIAC ENLARGEMENT

BIATRIAL ENLARGEMENT

It is not uncommon to see biatrial enlargement in patients with far advanced heart disease involving the left side of the heart, in conditions such as cardiomyopathy, advanced heart failure with pulmonary hypertension, and others (Fig: 05.04). When you come across bilateral enlargement think of global involvement of the heart and a poor outcome. It is amazing how a simple beside electrocardiogram can shed so much light on the underlying pathology.

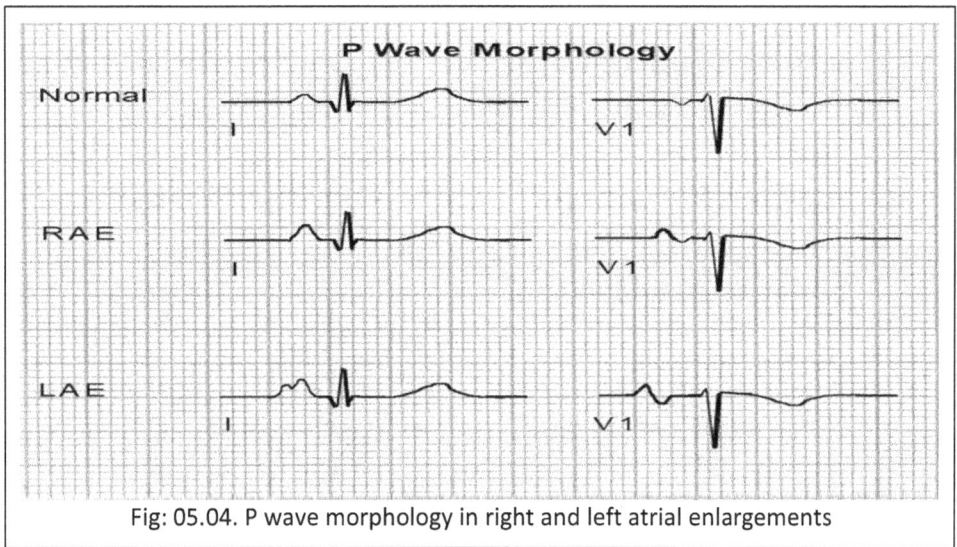

Fig: 05.04. P wave morphology in right and left atrial enlargements

Biatrial enlargement may be seen in mitral stenosis. The P duration may be greater than 120 ms. The P waves may appear notched in leads I, II, and aVF. The P waves in V1 will be biphasic with the terminal negative deflection occupying more than one box.

There is also evidence for a right axis deviation and prominent R waves in the right precordial leads suggestive of RVH.

Differential Diagnosis of Varying P Wave Morphology

➤ Atrial fibrillation: The P waves are just undulating narrow waves to almost a flat line in some leads.

➤ Atrial flutter: It has distinct P waves which have a sawtooth appearance in at least one or more deals.

➤ Wondering pacemaker: The rhythm is slower and the change in P wave morphology is more gradual.

➤ AV nodal reentrant tachycardia: The P waves, if visible, could be seen after the QRS complex and they are generally inverted.

➤ Multifocal tachycardia: It has a rapid, irregular rate with P waves arising from multiple foci, thus having distinct P waves but with varying morphology

CHAPTER 5. CARDIAC ENLARGEMENT

RIGHT VENTRICULAR HYPERTROPHY

Right ventricular hypertrophy (RVH) should alert you to possible etiologies such as chronic obstructive lung disease, pulmonary hypertension, pulmonic stenosis, among others.

Electrocardiographic features of RVH

RVH Criteria (Fig: 05.05)

Presence of Right Atrial Enlargement

Prominent Rs Pattern in V1 and V2.

Discordant ST-T Changes in Leads V1, V2, V3

The RS Pattern in Leads V1 to V5.

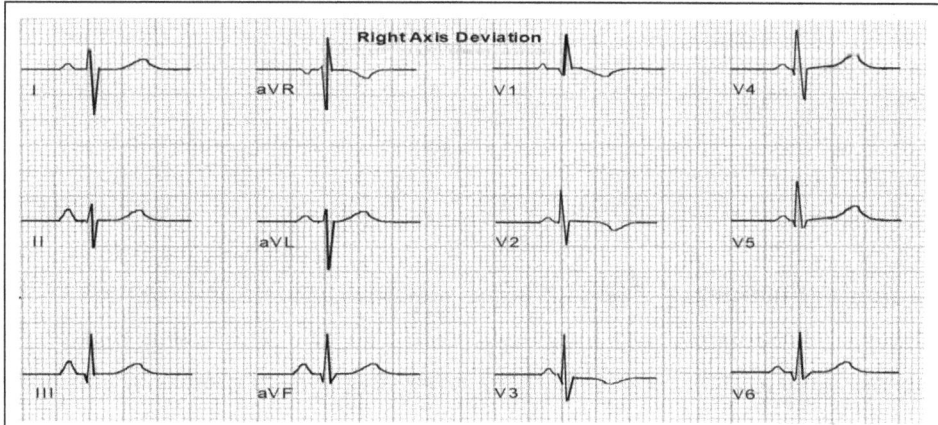

Fig: 05.05. This electrocardiogram shows right axis deviation, right atrial enlargement, and right ventricular hypertrophy. Note the tall and peaked P waves in II, III, and aVF. There are nonspecific ST-T changes.

CLINICAL EKG INTERPRETATION

Whenever you come across RVH and right axis deviation think about what is causing these EKG changes. It will help us to fine-tune the clinical diagnosis and treatment plans.

Chronic Corpulmonale

Chronic obstructive pulmonary disease may be characterized by peaked P wave (P pulmonale) in II, III, aVF, right axis deviation, low voltage, RVH, poor R wave progression across the chest leads (Fig: 05.06). Note the narrow negative P in V1 may represent a right atrial enlargement and no Left atrial enlargement. These patients may also have hypertension or coronary artery disease which may produce changes in the left chest leads that can confound the picture.

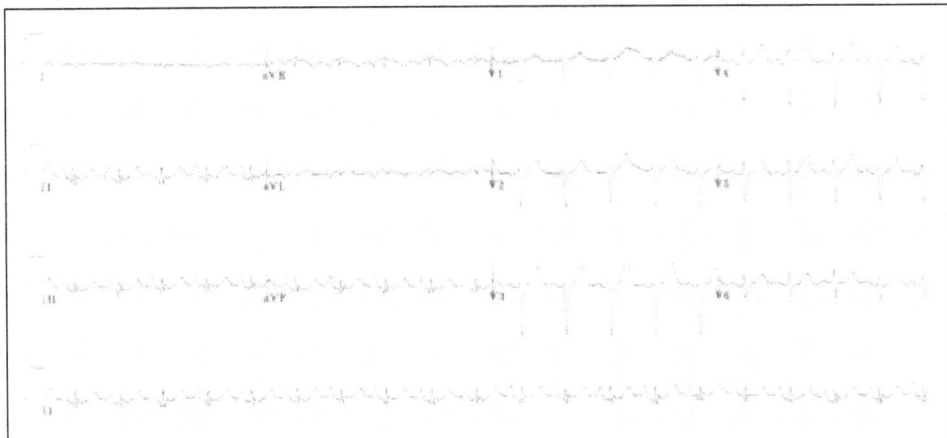

Fig: 05.06. This electrocardiogram shows sinus rhythm, low voltage, loss of R waves in the chest leads.

Acute Pulmonary Embolus: The electrocardiographic features of a pulmonary embolus include sinus tachycardia S1, Q3, and T3 (Fig: 05.07). This is second only to D Dimer in sensitivity in the diagnosis of pulmonary embolus. It may also show evidence of peaked P waves in II, III, aVF. There may be prominent r wave in V1 and V2 suggestive of right ventricular dilatation along with right ventricular strain pattern. When a middle-aged patient present with chest pain, shortness of breath, weakness, and palpitation, the most Definitive test, will be a chest CT with a PE protocol.

CHAPTER 5. CARDIAC ENLARGEMENT

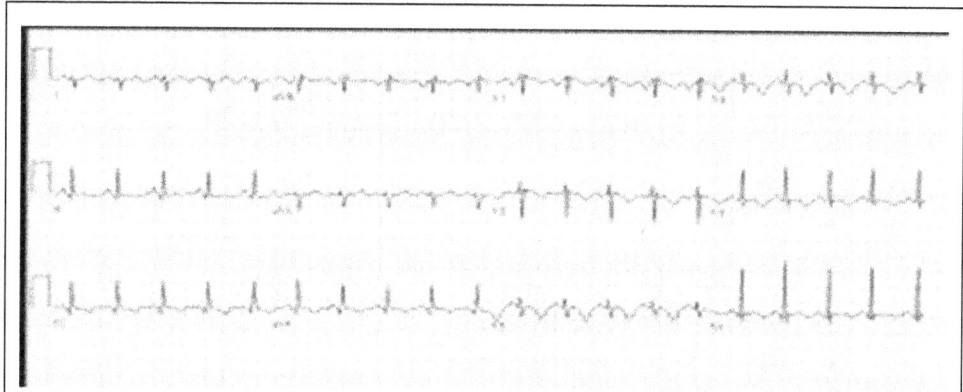

Fig: 05.06. This electrocardiogram shows sinus tachycardia, right axis deviation, S1, Q3, T3 pattern, and incomplete RBBB.

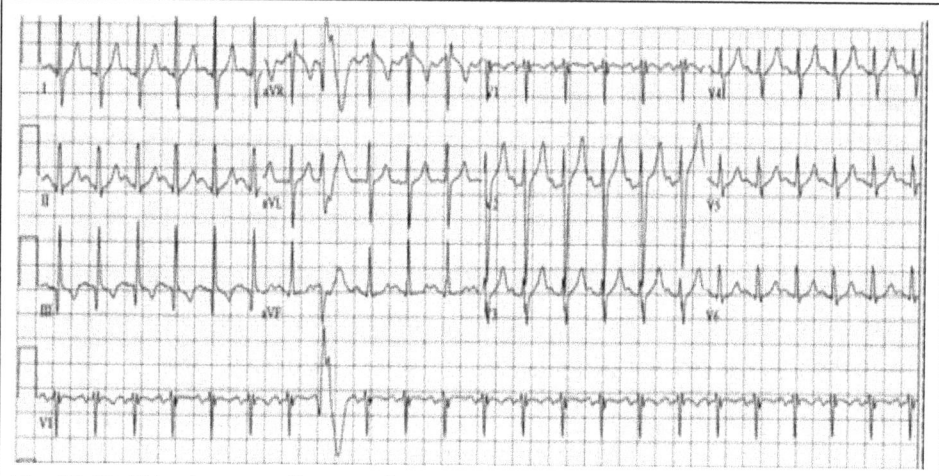

Fig: 05.08. This electrocardiogram shows sinus tachycardia, right axis deviation, S1, Q3, T3 pattern, and incomplete RBBB, which is characteristic of acute pulmonary embolus.

Tall R waves can be seen in a variety of conditions unrelated to the right ventricular hypertrophy.

TALL R WAVES IN THE ANTERIOR LEADS V1, V2

Tall R waves in the Anterior Leads V1, V2
- RBBB
- RVH
- Posterior Myocardial Infarction
- Thin Athletic Build
- Acute Pulmonary Embolus
- Primary Pulmonary Hypertension
- Juvenile Pattern
- WPW Syndrome

Similarly, you can see a poor R wave progression across the chest leads. Normally, you see an rS pattern in V1 with a tiny 'r' wave. In V2 the QRS pattern is rS and in V3 the QRS pattern is RS. From V4 to V6 you expect to see prominent R waves with tiny S waves. However, there a number of conditions where you may not see this normal r wave progression. You should be able to differentiate between the technical errors and pathological conditions that cause poor R wave progression across the chest LEADS.

LOSS OF R WAVES, RS, OR QS IN THE ANTERIOR LEADS

Loss of R waves, rS, or QS in the Anterior Leads
- Anteroseptal Myocardial Infarction
- LBBB
- Pacemaker Rhythm
- WPW Syndrome
- LVH
- COPD
- Low Chest Lead Placement
- Dextrocardia

CHAPTER 5. CARDIAC ENLARGEMENT

LEFT VENTRICULAR HYPERTROPHY:

The left ventricular hypertrophy occurs commonly in association with hypertension, heart failure, aortic stenosis, cardiomyopathy among others. The dominant features of LVH on the electrocardiogram include (Fig: 05.09):

- High voltage in the lateral chest leads
- Left atrial enlargement,
- Discordant ST-T changes in I, aVL, V5, and V6
- Biphasic P waves in the inferior leads.

The higher voltage in the chest leads alone may not be indicative of LVH as we can see similar findings in a patient with thin chest walls and in athletes.

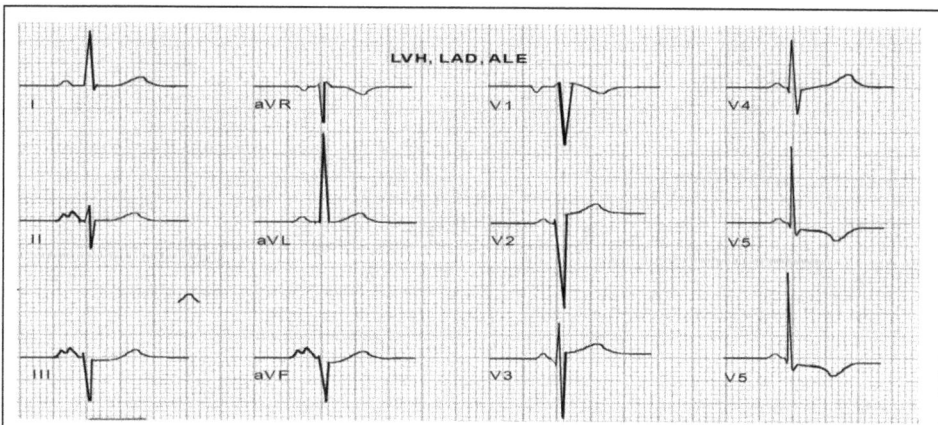

Fig: 05.09. This electrocardiogram shows Left axis deviation, left atrial enlargement, and left ventricular hypertrophy with strain pattern. Note the tall and double peaked P waves in II, III, and aVF.

Some patients may have left axis deviation and left anterior hemiblock. In fact, the presence of LVH should alert you to future complications such as the development of LBBB or Intraventricular conduction delay.

CLINICAL EKG INTERPRETATION

LVH CRITERIA FROM VARIOUS AUTHORS

Romhilt-Estes LVH criteria	
LVH Criteria	Points
R or S in any Limb Leads ≥ 2mV or 20 mm in Height	3
Or S in Lead V1 or V2 > ≥ 2mV or 20 mm in Height	
Or R in Lead V5 or V6 > 3mV or 30 mm	
Left Ventricular Strain -ST Depression and T wave Inversion	3
Discordant to the QRS Complex	
With Digitalis	1
LAE: More Than One Box in Depth (0.1mV) and duration (1mm)	3
Left Axis Deviation	2
QRS Duration > 90 ms	1
Intrinsicoid Deflection in V5 or V6 >50 ms	1
Maximum	13

LVH = 5 points or greater. Possible LVH = 4 points

Sokolow-Lyon LVH criteria
S in V1 + R in V5 or V6 ≥ 3.5 mV or 35 mm in Height
Or
R in Lead V5 or V6 > 2.6 mV or 26 mm

Cornell LVH criteria
Females: R in aVL + S in V3 > 2 mV or 20 mm
Males: R in aVL + S in V3 > 2.8 mV or 28 mm

CHAPTER 5. CARDIAC ENLARGEMENT

P, QRS, and ST-T Morphology Between RVH and LVH (Fig: 05.10)

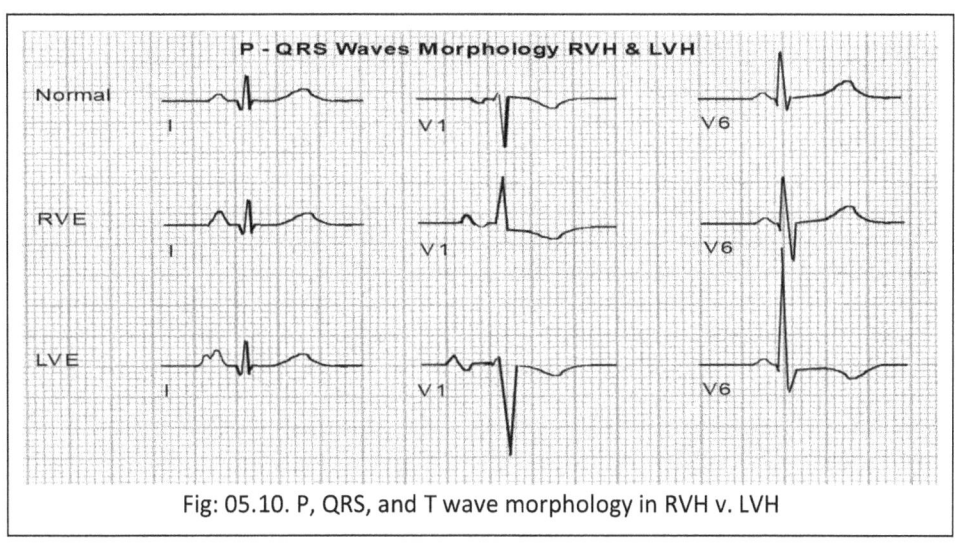

Fig: 05.10. P, QRS, and T wave morphology in RVH v. LVH

Causes: Left Ventricular hypertrophy or dilatation occurs in a variety of conditions, such as hypertension, aortic stenosis, congestive heart failure, hypertrophic cardiomyopathy, or infiltrative cardiomyopathies. When choosing drugs for treating hypertension, we should look at drugs that not only control the blood pressure but also reduce the left ventricular hypertrophy. Hence, ACE/ARBS are very important drugs in the management of hypertension. In a patient with dilated cardiomyopathy, the choices will be dictated by the left ventricular ejection fraction and other manifestations of congestive heart failure. In patients with hypertrophy cardiomyopathy, the focus should be on drugs that reduce left ventricular contractility and the intracavity gradients.

Biventricular Hypertrophy: It is seen in patients with advanced cardiomyopathy, where all the cardiac chambers are markedly dilated. In this situation, we may see findings of both atrial enlargements, and increased voltage on both the right and the left side of the chest.

CLINICAL EKG INTERPRETATION

Hypertrophic Cardiomyopathy (HCM): It can produce unique electrocardiographic changes related to the hypertrophic myocardium. There may be narrow and deep Q waves in leads II, III, and aVF. The leads I and aVL may show T wave inversion. Anterior chest leads may show increased voltage due to septal hypertrophy. They may also have T wave inversion in leads V1 and V2. You may also see left atrial enlargement due to a non-compliant left ventricle. The Q waves noted in the inferior leads in patients with HCM are called "pseudo-Infarct" Q waves.

These patients are prone to sustained atrial and ventricular tachyarrhythmias. They are at an increased risk of sudden death. All the family members should be scanned to make sure they don't have hypertrophic cardiomyopathy. They also should have a complete cardiovascular evaluation, echocardiography, and electrophysiological studies if needed. Please note the absence of typical Electrocardiographic changes doesn't exclude HCM.

LV Apical Hypertrophy (Fig: 05.11)

- Seen in Young people
- Prone to serious ventricular arrhythmias and sudden death.
- Many need Intra cardiac defibrillator (ICD) placement

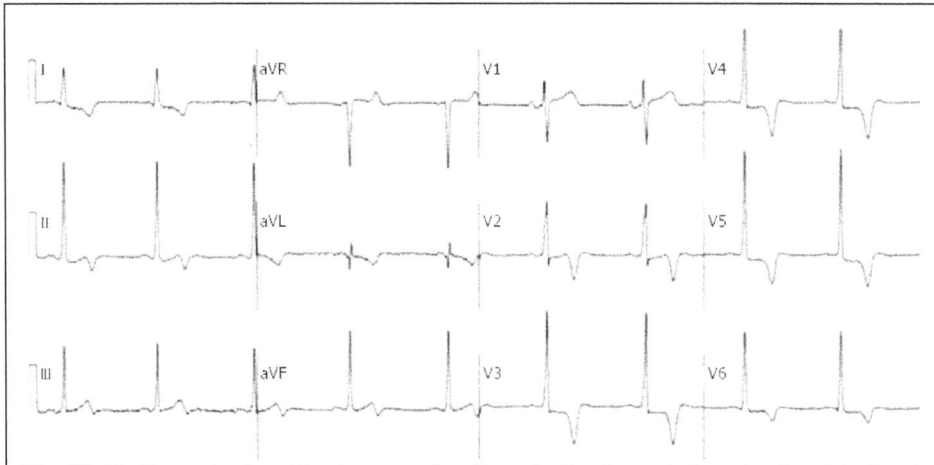

Fig: 05.11. Sinus rhythm. The increased voltage in the lateral chest leads with deeply inverted T waves.

CHAPTER 5. CARDIAC ENLARGEMENT

EKG QUIZ

EKG 5.1

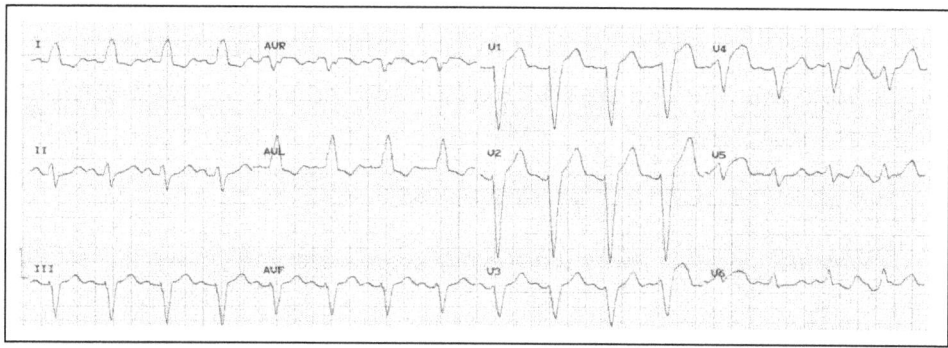

EKG 5.2

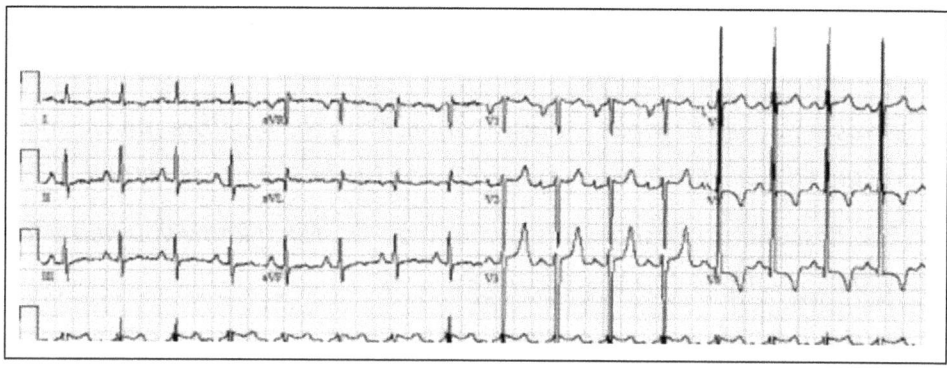

EKG 5.3

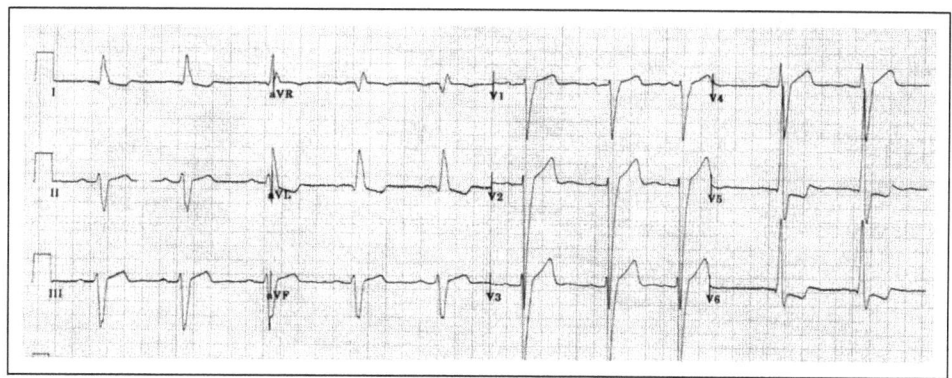

CLINICAL EKG INTERPRETATION

COMIC HOUR

Speech

Some time ago, I was getting ready to give a speech in Toastmasters Club. I went to freshen up a little before the speech. Mrs. Wanda, the club president, pulled me to the side and asked, "Hey! Dr. Nik, do you always get nervous, before you give a speech?'

"Not really," I said, "But, why do you ask?"

"I was just curious. I was wondering what were you doing in the ladies' room."

I didn't like her then, but now I like her because she always reminds me that getting nervous is counterproductive. It's not good for health.

Not now

I was supposed to make a presentation. The fellow before me was going on and on. I guess I must have dozed off, and the host was concerned.

The host shook my shoulders and asked, "Dr. Nik, I know you had a long trip. Would you like a cup of coffee?"

"No, not during his speech," I said, "I'm fine!" As I tried very hard to stay awake.

ACLS QUIZ:

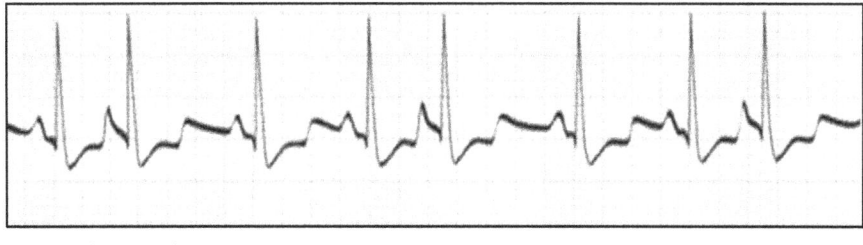

Extra beats? _____

Chapter 6 Sinus Node Dysfunction

- Sinus Pauses
- Sinus Exit Block
- Sinoatrial Block
- Sinus Arrhythmia
- Sick Sinus Syndrome
- Hyperdynamic Circulation

The sinus node is the main pacemaker of the heart maintaining varying heart rates to match all challenging situations in life. The autonomic nervous system controls the sinus node function. Sinus node also undergoes degenerative and fibrotic changes with age. Common sinus node dysfunctions include the following

- Sinus pauses
- Sinoatrial Block
- Sick Sinus Syndrome (SSS)
- Sinus Arrhythmia

Sinus node dysfunction (SND) includes disordered automaticity or impaired conduction of the impulse from the sinus node to the surrounding atrial tissue.

1. Extrinsic SND - Drugs, ANS influences that suppress automaticity and/or compromise conduction

2. Intrinsic SND - Degenerative SA node, fibrous replacement of the SA node or its connection to the atrium

SINUS PAUSE

There is a transient cessation of sinus node activity. This may appear as an absence of P waves on an electrocardiogram. This triggers the activity in the conduction system below resulting in a junctional or a ventricular escape rhythm. Sinus pause is not a multiple of PP interval (fig: 06.01).

Carotid artery pressure can slow the sinus node and create a temporary pause. Even, drugs used in the acute treatment of SVTs can cause a temporary sinus pause, before the rhythm resumes. A vasovagal attack is associated with a temporary sinus pause, lasting several seconds.

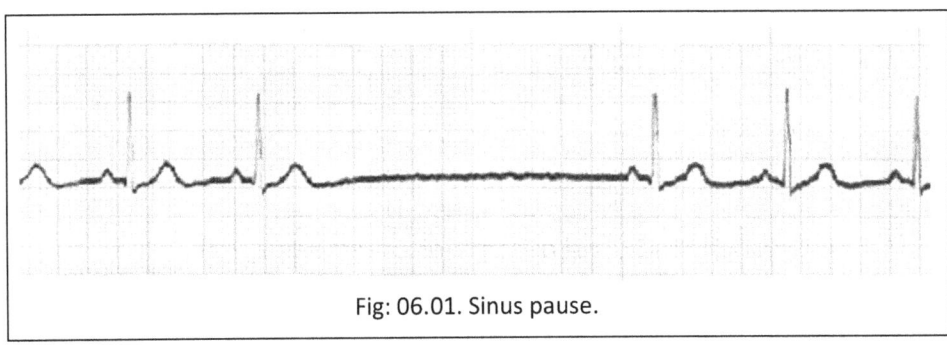

Fig: 06.01. Sinus pause.

Rate	**Varies**
P-P Regularity	Variable
R-R Regularity	Variable
P wave	Present, except during pause
P - QRS Ratio	1:1, 2:1, 3:1, 4:1, variable
PR Interval	Normal
QRS Width	Normal

CHAPTER 6. SINUS NODE DYSFUNCTION

SINUS EXIT BLOCK

Here the sinus node depolarizes, but the impulse is not able to reach the atrium.

In the 1st degree SA block, the SA node impulse slows and the electrocardiogram may appear normal.

SINOATRIAL (SA) BLOCK

SA block 2nd Degree - Type I (SA Wenckebach): Here the sinus impulse conduction slows until one is blocked. On the electrocardiogram, there is a progressive decrease in the P-P interval, before a P wave drops, creating grouped beats (Fig: 06.02).

- PP cycle becomes progressively shorter
- No P waves & QRS complexes
- Pause is less than twice the preceding PP cycle
- Gradual lengthening of conduction time from the SA node to the atria

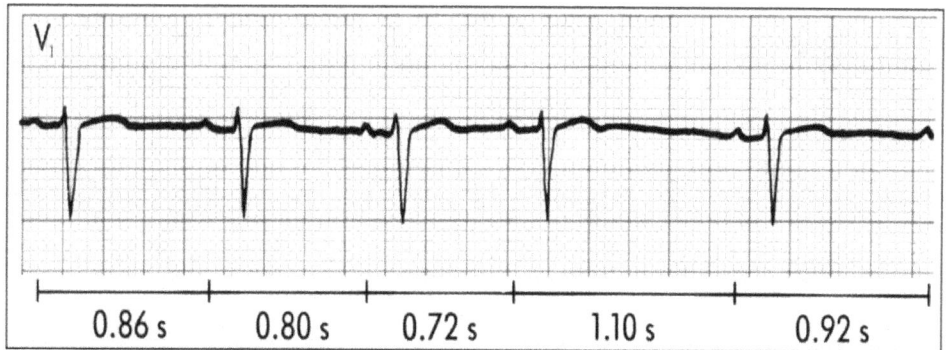

Fig: 06.02 Sinus rhythm Wenckebach Type I SA block. Note the progressive shortening of the PP interval as you would see a progressive shortening of the RR interval in AV node Wenckebach I block.

SA block 2nd Degree - Type II: Here the conduction of sinus impulses is blocked without slowing beforehand. It produces a pause that is a multiple (usually twice) of the P-P interval. You will also notice grouping of the beats (Fig:06.03).

CLINICAL EKG INTERPRETATION

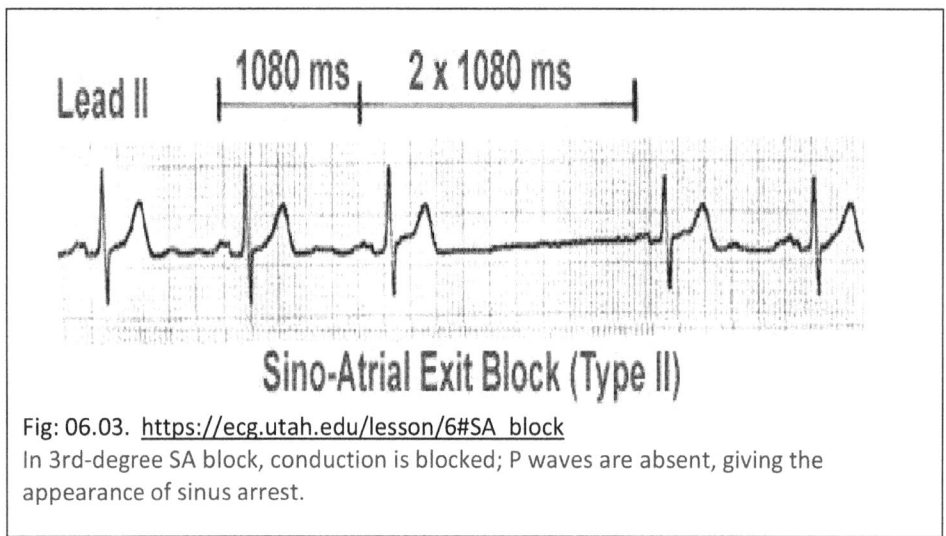

Fig: 06.03. https://ecg.utah.edu/lesson/6#SA_block
In 3rd-degree SA block, conduction is blocked; P waves are absent, giving the appearance of sinus arrest.

SA block 2nd Degree - Type II (Fig: 06.04):
- PP Cycles Are Constant
- No P Waves & QRS Complexes
- Pause is Twice the Preceding PP Cycle

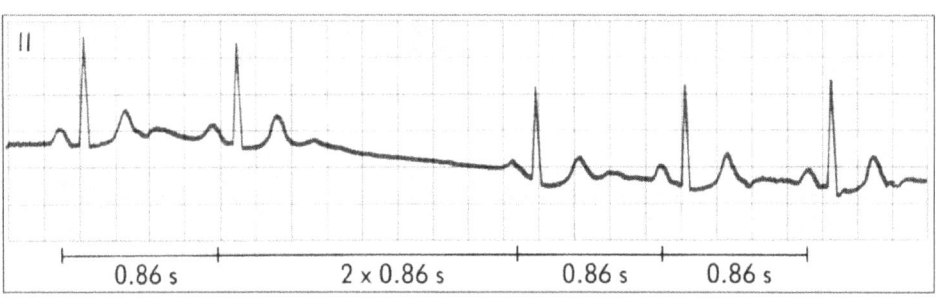

Fig: 06.04. Sinus rhythm with sinus block.

CHAPTER 6. SINUS NODE DYSFUNCTION

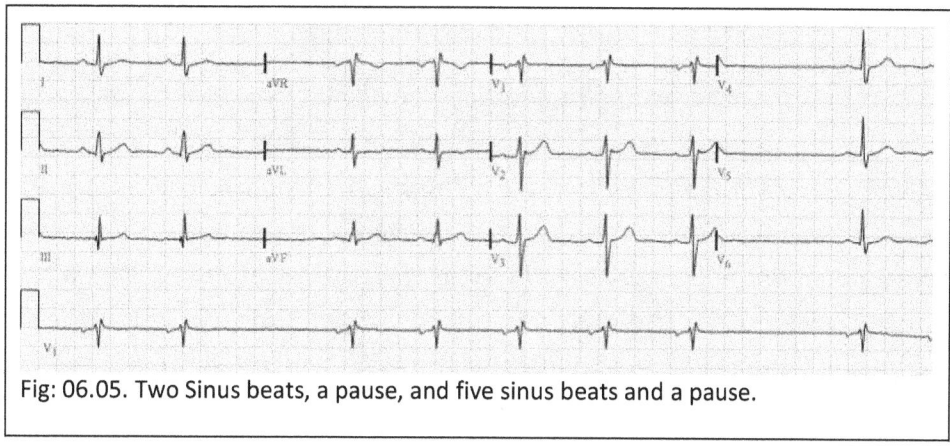

Fig: 06.05. Two Sinus beats, a pause, and five sinus beats and a pause.

Causes of sinus node dysfunction include idiopathic fibrosis, excessive vagal tone, ischemic, inflammatory, or infiltrative disorders.

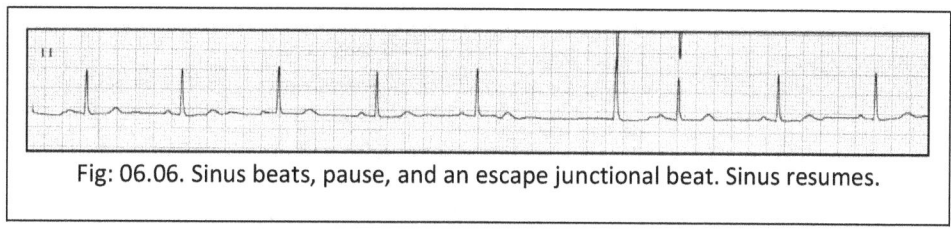

Fig: 06.06. Sinus beats, pause, and an escape junctional beat. Sinus resumes.

Treatment for sinus node dysfunction is a pacemaker. It is preferable if they have a dual chamber pacemaker to avoid atrial fibrillation.

Drugs like theophylline and hydralazine may be given orally can increase heart rate in young individuals with bradycardia without syncope.

Third Degree SA Block: This is similar to sinus pause, where none of the sinus impulses are reaching the atria. It is like a sinus arrest. There may be an action potential in the SA node, but it is not activating the atria or the ventricles.

SICK SINUS SYNDROME

Sick Sinus Syndrome (SSS) is characterized by tachyarrhythmia along with a dysfunctional sinus node causing bradyarrhythmia (Fig: 06.07). These patients have runs SVT with rapid ventricular responses with long sinus pauses where the sinus node fails to take over. Some of these patients may have palpitations and dizziness, and some may be asymptomatic. When these patients undergo Holter monitoring or event monitoring, we can appreciate tachyarrhythmia mixed long pauses. If the sinus pauses are longer than 2.5 seconds, it is an indication for a permanent pacemaker. The most common scenario is paroxysmal runs of atrial fibrillation with sinus pauses.

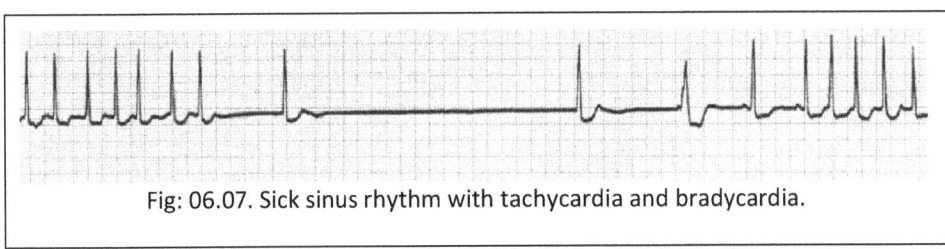

Fig: 06.07. Sick sinus rhythm with tachycardia and bradycardia.

Iatrogenic sick sinus syndrome can be related to beta-blockers and calcium channel blockers. Hence, these drugs should be used with extreme caution as they may worsen the bradyarrhythmia. If we do need to use them, we need to use the least amount needed and for the shortest duration of time. Better yet, insert a permanent pacemaker which can address the slow heart rates; and you can use the antiarrhythmic drugs to slow the rapid rates.

CHAPTER 6. SINUS NODE DYSFUNCTION

Multifactorial causes and mechanism of Sick Sinus Syndrome.

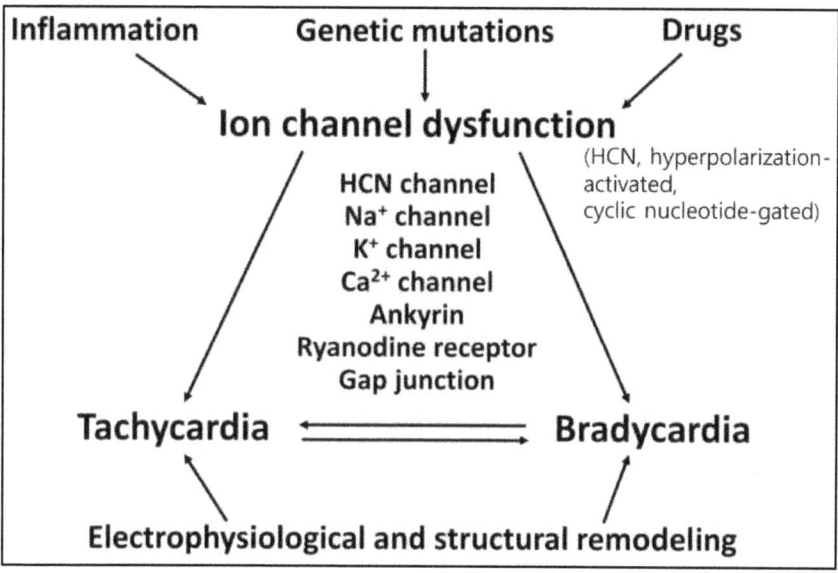

Patients with sleep apnea also may manifest with long sinus pauses, in the absence of significant sinus node dysfunction. So, if a patient has long pauses with a history of sleep apnea, proper treatment of sleep apnea with appropriate CPAP adjustments, may eliminate the sinus pauses.

SINUS ARRHYTHMIA:

It is commonly seen on the electrocardiogram, where the sinus rate may not be regular. The RR intervals may vary from beat to beat. The rate may also speed and slow down gradually, without the patient's awareness. It doesn't signify any organic heart disease. Respiratory sinus arrhythmia is seen more often in young healthy individuals. It's a pattern of gradual acceleration and deceleration of the heart rate (Fig: 06.08).

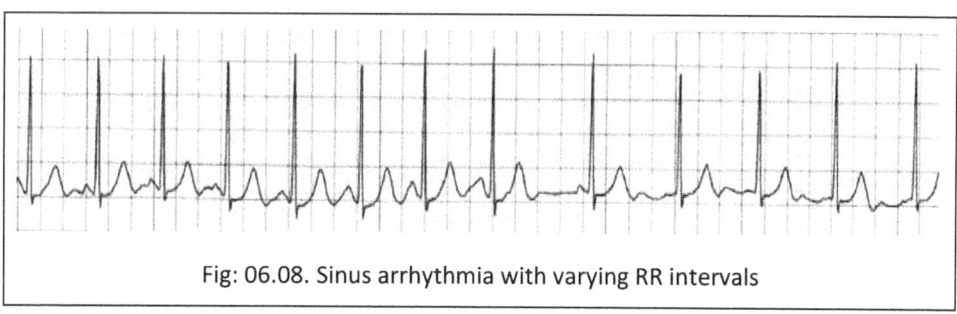

Fig: 06.08. Sinus arrhythmia with varying RR intervals

CLINICAL EKG INTERPRETATION

Hyperdynamic Circulation: This is a condition where some young people have a hyperdynamic circulatory state. They have rapid heart rates with a normal cardiovascular examination. They may have resting heart rates in the 100s. These young people have a normal cardiovascular examination and laboratory studies. Their echocardiogram may be entirely normal with normal ejection fraction.

We should always consider other conditions that cause rapid heart rates, such as hyperthyroidism, dehydration, anemia, and others.

COMIC CORNER

Grammar school

When I was attending a grammar school, I had to show my report card to my parents every month.

My mother looked at my report card and said, "With these grades, this kid doesn't know anything."

My father said, "With these grades, he doesn't even suspect anything!"

My mother said, "Then maybe, he will make a good doctor!"

How do you spell doctor?" I asked.

****

Jogging

The other day I was jogging around in the neighborhood with my younger daughter. A good-looking college girl passed by. I was looking. I admit, I look old and bald, but I was still looking.

My daughter said, "Daddy, you are looking at that lady like you have never seen a woman in 20 years!"

"That's exactly what I was thinking!" I said to myself.

Chapter 7 Bradycardia

- Sinus Bradycardia
- Slow Junctional Rhythm
- Ventricular Rhythm
- Idioventricular Rhythm
- Agonal Rhythm
- Asystole
- Lead Displacement

BRADYCARDIA

It is a condition where the heart rate is below 60 bpm. Even though this is an arbitrary number, a human body has an amazing capacity to function well with heart rates ranging from 40 bpm to 160 bpm without many symptoms (Fig: 07.01). However, there are certain times when the slow heart rate can be symptomatic. The main function of the heart is to pump a certain amount of oxygenated blood (5L/min) each minute to meet the metabolic demands of the heart during rest and stressful situations.

The bradycardia can be related to impulse generation or due to impulse conduction.

Conditions related to impulse generation could cause sinus bradycardia, chronotropic incompetence, and tachy-brady syndrome.

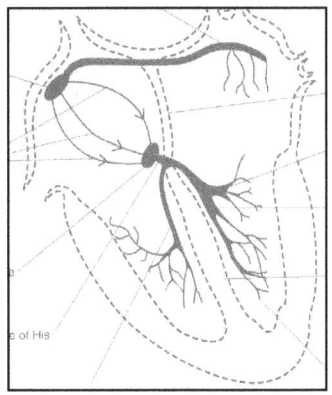

There is a multitude of factors that can slow the heart rate from physical training to advanced degeneration of the electrical grid of the heart. Many therapeutic drugs we use in our daily cardiology practice may also have a profound positive or negative effect on heart rates. Hence, it is of paramount importance not only to recognize the presence of bradycardia but also to look for conditions that are causing the bradycardia. The treatment of bradycardia depends on the etiology.

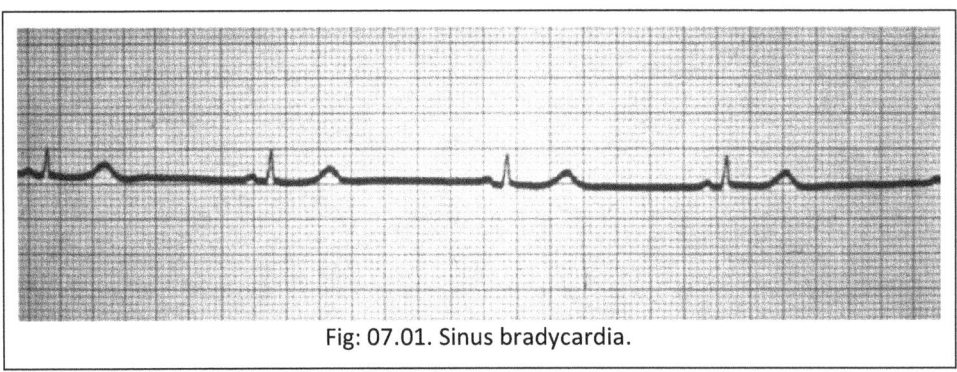

Fig: 07.01. Sinus bradycardia.

Symptoms related to bradycardia include dizziness or lightheadedness, fainting (syncope) or near-fainting, tiredness (fatigue), shortness of breath, palpitations, chest pain (angina), increased difficulty exercising, confusion or difficulty concentrating. Some patients may have no symptoms.

The slow heart rates can be physiological from training, they may be asymptomatic or symptomatic.

Athletes Heart: Well-trained athletes have a heart rate between 40 and 55 bpm. This comes from vigorous training over the years and they perform very well with those heart rates. To compensate for the increased demands during extreme physical activities, their hearts enlarge to accommodate more volume. So, it is common to see they have increased left ventricular voltage and left atrial enlargement. Once, they retire from active sports, their hearts may not revert to normal size and may in some cases lead to heart failure.

Causes of **acute** and **long**-term **bradycardias**: Some conditions that cause acute bradycardia include vagal vasodepressor syncope and drugs such as beta-blockers and calcium channel blockers.

Symptomatic Bradycardia: Symptomatic bradycardia or relative bradycardia is a term applied when the heart is inadequate to supply the metabolic needs of a patient, even if the heart rate is 60 to 80 bpm (Fig:07.02). If the person is running a fever or has anemia, then the normal heart rate may not keep up with the needs. Sometimes, a patient who has a pacemaker may not do well when their heart rates are set at 60 bpm. Increasing the heart rate to 70 or even 80 bpm may improve their weakness and fatigue.

Symptomatic Bradycardia
- ➤ **The Heart Rate is Slow**
- ➤ **The Patient Has Symptoms**
- ➤ **The Symptoms Are Related to the Bradycardia**

Vasovagal Attack: During extreme periods of stress the body responses with a "fight-or-flight," response. The flight activates the parasympathetic system, stimulates the Vagus nerve through the release of acetylcholine, which slows the heart rate, conduction through the AV node and sometimes causes sinus pauses lasting a few seconds. There is also profound vasodilatation in the limbs, which leads to hypotension. This is a classic example of acute symptomatic bradycardia.

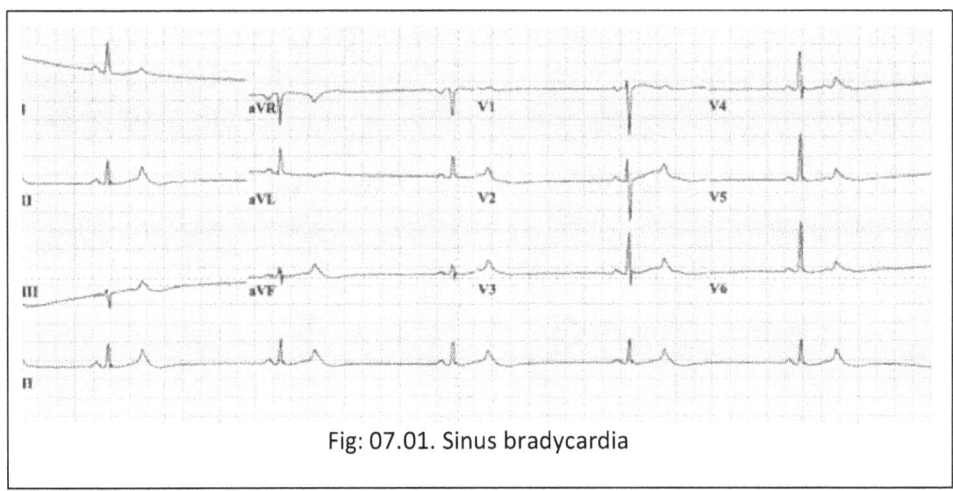

Fig: 07.01. Sinus bradycardia

This is a self-limiting condition, which improves as the effect of acetylcholine wears off. However, some symptoms can be minimized by placing the patient in a supine position, elevating the legs to improve venous return. In a hospital situation, administrating atropine to reverse the acetylcholine effects.

The best time to treat this is before it happens. Hence, you see anesthesiologists use atropine-like drugs pre-op to prevent a vagal attack and reduce secretions in the peri-operative periods.

Sinus Node conditions include sinus arrest, Sinoatrial block, Sick sinus syndrome, and atrial standstill (Fig: 07.03).

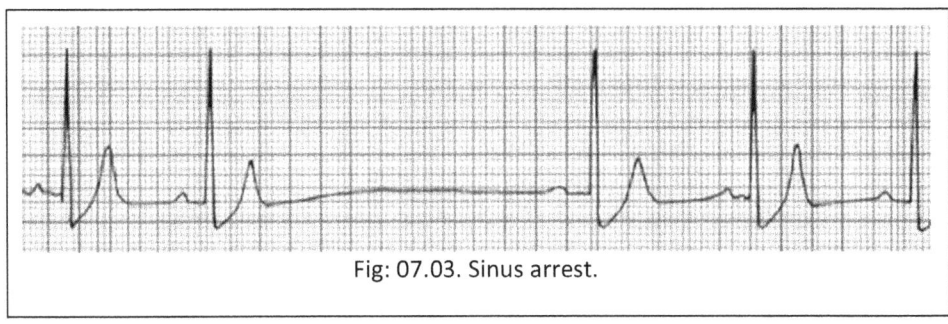

Fig: 07.03. Sinus arrest.

Drug-induced bradycardia can be from beta-blockers, calcium channel blockers, digoxin, clonidine, or reserpine. Metabolic conditions like hypothyroidism also can cause bradycardia. Cerebrovascular accidents are

CHAPTER 7. BRADYCARDIAS

volume. So, it is common to see they have increased left ventricular voltage and left atrial enlargement. Once, they retire from active sports, their hearts may not revert to normal size and may in some cases lead to heart failure.

Causes of **acute** and **long**-term **bradycardias**: Some conditions that cause acute bradycardia include vagal vasodepressor syncope and drugs such as beta-blockers and calcium channel blockers.

Symptomatic Bradycardia: Symptomatic bradycardia or relative bradycardia is a term applied when the heart is inadequate to supply the metabolic needs of a patient, even if the heart rate is 60 to 80 bpm (Fig:07.02). If the person is running a fever or has anemia, then the normal heart rate may not keep up with the needs. Sometimes, a patient who has a pacemaker may not do well when their heart rates are set at 60 bpm. Increasing the heart rate to 70 or even 80 bpm may improve their weakness and fatigue.

Symptomatic Bradycardia
- ➤ **The Heart Rate is Slow**
- ➤ **The Patient Has Symptoms**
- ➤ **The Symptoms Are Related to the Bradycardia**

Vasovagal Attack: During extreme periods of stress the body responds with a "fight-or-flight," response. The flight activates the parasympathetic system, stimulates the Vagus nerve through the release of acetylcholine, which slows the heart rate, conduction through the AV node and sometimes causes sinus pauses lasting a few seconds. There is also profound vasodilatation in the limbs, which leads to hypotension. This is a classic example of acute symptomatic bradycardia.

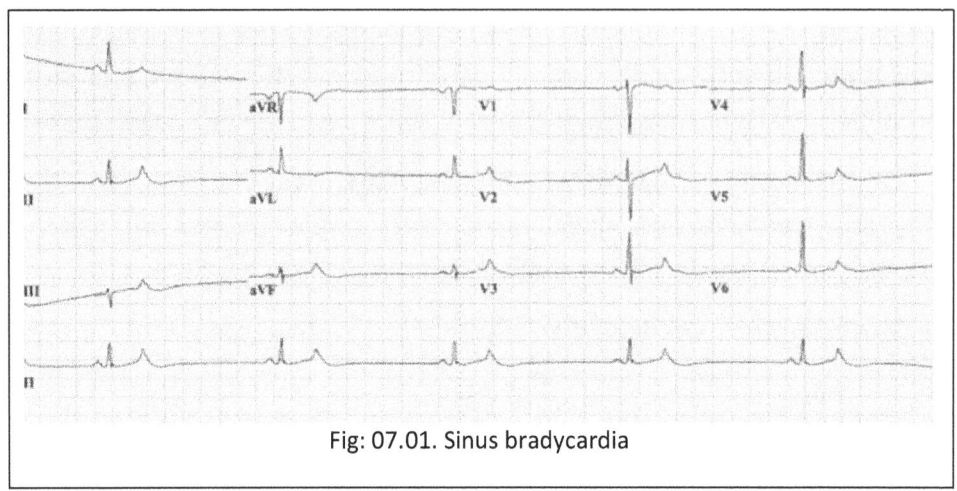

Fig: 07.01. Sinus bradycardia

This is a self-limiting condition, which improves as the effect of acetylcholine wears off. However, some symptoms can be minimized by placing the patient in a supine position, elevating the legs to improve venous return. In a hospital situation, administrating atropine to reverse the acetylcholine effects.

The best time to treat this is before it happens. Hence, you see anesthesiologists use atropine-like drugs pre-op to prevent a vagal attack and reduce secretions in the peri-operative periods.

Sinus Node conditions include sinus arrest, Sinoatrial block, Sick sinus syndrome, and atrial standstill (Fig: 07.03).

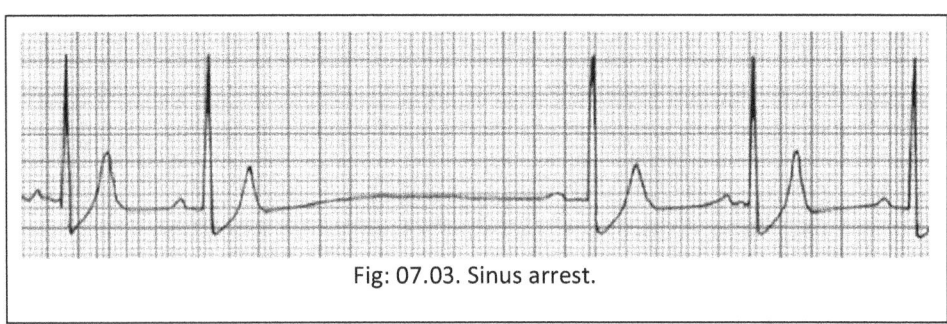

Fig: 07.03. Sinus arrest.

Drug-induced bradycardia can be from beta-blockers, calcium channel blockers, digoxin, clonidine, or reserpine. Metabolic conditions like hypothyroidism also can cause bradycardia. Cerebrovascular accidents are

CHAPTER 7. BRADYCARDIAS

frequently associated with bradycardias due to increased intracranial pressure.

Sleep Apnea: Sinus pauses of more than 3 seconds can be seen during sleep apnea. In fact, there may be several incidences where the sinus beats could be missing (Fig: 07.04). The treatment in these patients is not drugs or pacemaker. Treatment of sleep apnea with CPAP automatically corrects most of these rhythm changes.

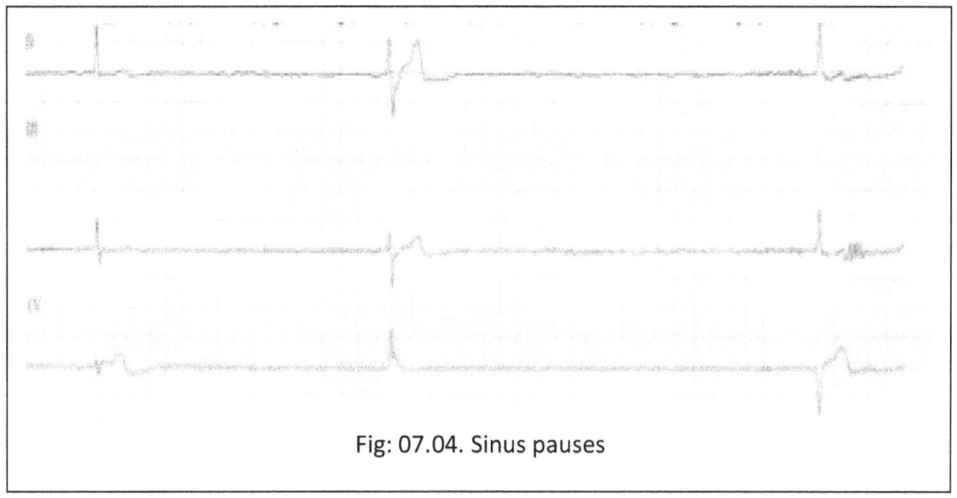

Fig: 07.04. Sinus pauses

AV blocks: AV blocks leading to bradycardia include second-degree heart block, high-grade AV block, and complete heart block.

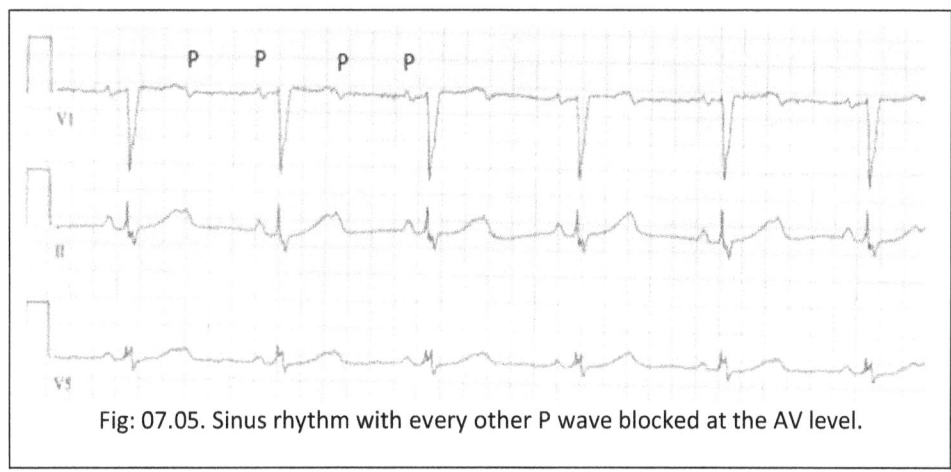

Fig: 07.05. Sinus rhythm with every other P wave blocked at the AV level.

CLINICAL EKG INTERPRETATION

Here is an example of complete heart block (Fig: 07.06). The P waves are marching independently. The is a narrow QRS rhythm which is most likely a junctional rhythm. There is AV dissociation and no sign of any atrial conducted beats.

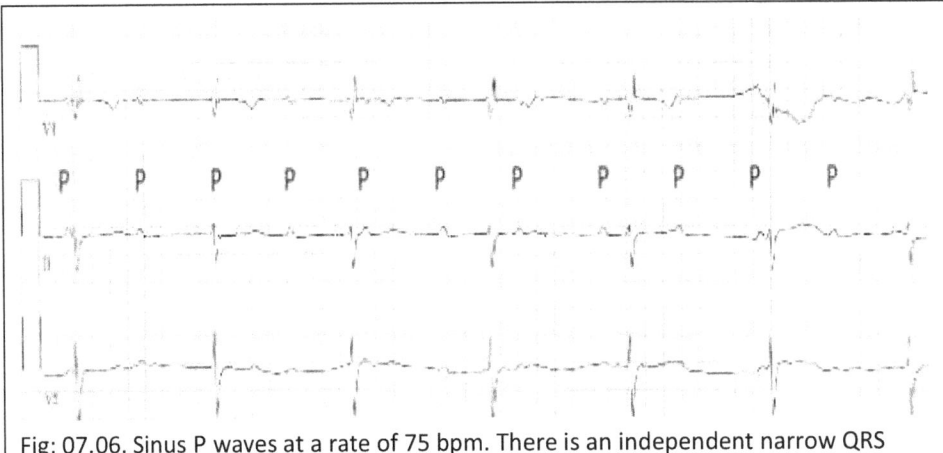

Fig: 07.06. Sinus P waves at a rate of 75 bpm. There is an independent narrow QRS rhythm with a rate less than 30 bpm. Nonspecific ST-T changes are also noted.

Both atrial and ventricular ectopic beats can lead to ineffective cardiac output, causing bradycardia as the heart may not be able to meet the body's oxygen and metabolic demand. Here are some common causes of ectopic beats:

- Acute myocardial infraction IMI.
- Degeneration of the electrical system of the heart, sinus node arrest, sinus bradycardia, AV nodal disease,
- Electrolyte abnormalities such as hyperkalemia, hypercarbia, and hypothyroidism

When dealing with patients with frequent PACs or PVCs we should be aware that they can develop into atrial fibrillation or ventricular tachycardia. All these patients should have:

- CBC, O2 Saturation, blood gases
- Electrolytes, Magnesium, & Serum Phosphate Level
- Ionized Calcium and Albumin level
- Thyroid Studies

CHAPTER 7. BRADYCARDIAS

- Blood Sugar Level
- Renal Function
- Acidosis or Alkalosis
- V/S: P, BP, R, and Urine Output

JUNCTIONAL RHYTHM

Junctional rhythm is characterized by a slow rate of 40 to 60 bpm. There P waves can be before the QRS or right after the QRS complexes. The QRS duration is <120 ms. The PR interval is variable. Junctional rhythm is usually an escape rhythm seen when there is a sinus node arrest or a long pause (Fig: 07.07).

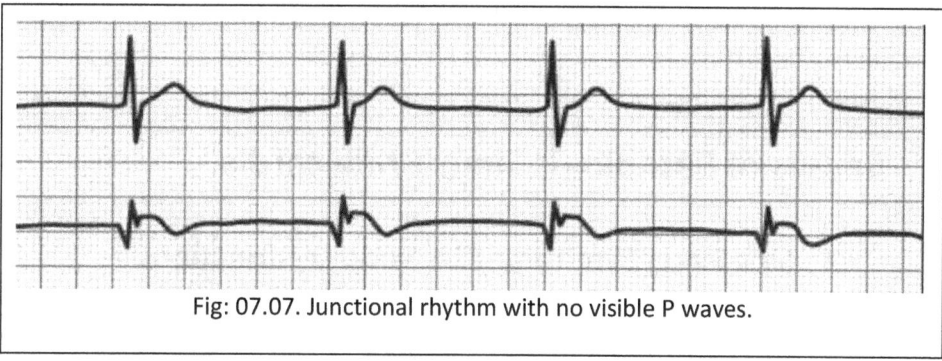

Fig: 07.07. Junctional rhythm with no visible P waves.

	Junction rhythm Points
Rate	40 - 60 bpm
P-P Regularity	None, or Regular if Antegrade or Retrograde
R-R Regularity	Regular
P wave	Variable (None, Antegrade, or Retrograde)
P - QRS Ratio	None, or 1:1 if Antegrade or Retrograde
PR Interval	None, Short, or Retrograde
QRS Width	Normal

Here is an example of atrial fibrillation with a pretty regular narrow QRS rhythm (Fig: 07.08). Whenever you see a regular ventricular rate in the presence of atrial fibrillation, you should always think of high-grade AV block with a junctional or a ventricular rhythm.

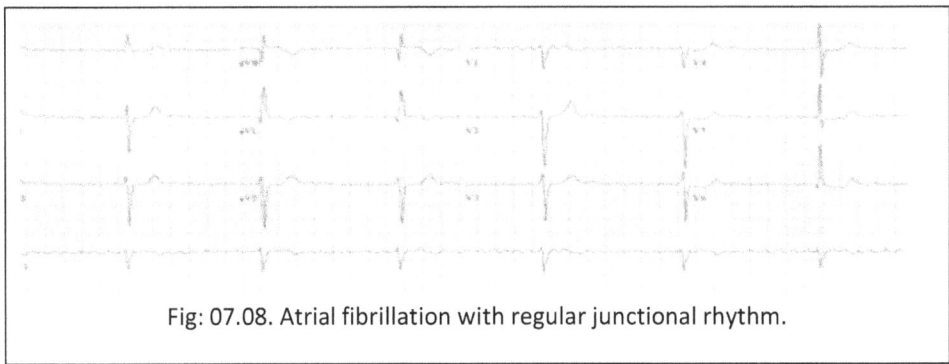

Fig: 07.08. Atrial fibrillation with regular junctional rhythm.

Causes of Pathologic Sinus Bradycardia

- **Sick Sinus Syndrome/SA Node Dysfunction**
- **Infarction or Cardiac Surgery**
- **Infiltrative Processes (Amyloidosis, Sarcoidosis)**
- **Increased Vagal Tone (Valsalva, Vomiting)**
- **Medications (i.e. BB, CCB)**
- **Genetic Diseases**

CHAPTER 7. BRADYCARDIAS

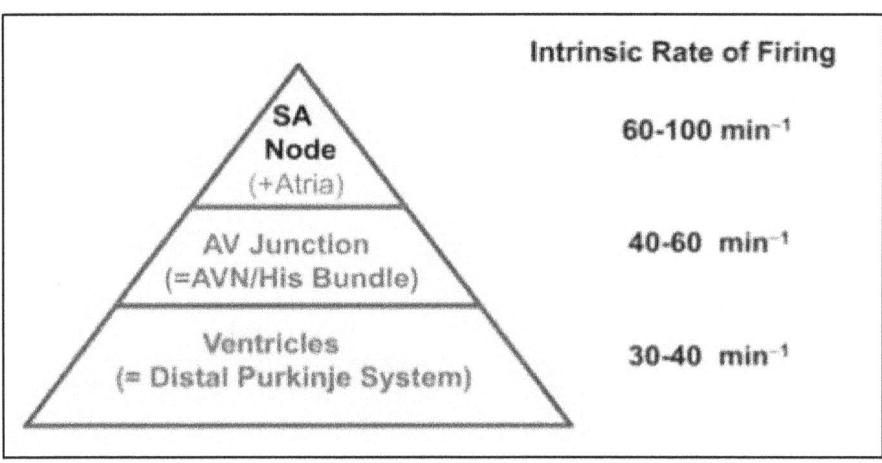

Treatment Algorithm for Symptomatic Bradycardia:

- **Prepare for transcutaneous pacing.**

- **Atropine 0.5 mg IV bolus, repeat up to a maximum of 3 mg**

- **Epinephrine 2 to 10 µg/min infusion.**

- **Dopamine 2 to 20 µg/kg/min infusion**

Atropine should be used with caution in patients with acute myocardial ischemia or infarction, as it accelerates the heart rate that can increase myocardial oxygen demand. It may also precipitate ventricular ectopic activity.

Atropine also may not be useful in second- or third-degree AV block, since the impulses from the sinus node or the atria cannot reach the ventricles.

NIK'S COMEDY RELIEF

Gall bladder attack

A young surgeon walks into a patient room and tells her, "Mrs. Garcia, we have some good news for you."

"What is it, I hope it's not cancer?"

"You are right! It's not cancer. All you had was a simple gall bladder attack with some big gallstones."

"So what? I had a gall bladder all my life. You call that good news?"

"The good news is that we can take out your gall bladder, and you won't be having the abdominal pain, bloating, and indigestion."

"I don't have any of those symptoms. Can you do something for my constipation?"

"Mrs. Garcia, we can schedule your surgery for tomorrow. It will only be a 45-minute procedure!"

"I don't know at my age, whether I need that surgery? For now, can you order something for my constipation?"

"You will be feeling much, much better after the surgery."

"Doc, do you think I will make it through the surgery? This will be my first surgery in years!"

"You better make it through the surgery, and we will make sure that you will make it through the surgery, because you are my first surgery patient, too!" Said the young doctor.

Chapter 8 Supraventricular Arrhythmias

- PACs
- Atrial Bigeminy
- Blocked Atrial Beats
- Sinus Tachycardia
- Paroxysmal Supraventricular Tachycardia (PSVT)
- Junctional Rhythm
- Junctional Tachycardia
- Atrial Fibrillation
- Atrial Flutter
- Multifocal Atrial Tachycardia

PREMATURE ATRIAL COMPLEXES (PACS)

These are very commonly seen in a patient, on a monitor, and after surgical procedures. These may be related to the stretching of the atria following volume overload. Fervently the PACs may progress to short runs of atrial beats and eventually into atrial fibrillation. Hence, when you see frequent PACs following surgery, look for correctable causes such as electrolyte abnormalities, ischemic, and volume overload (Fig: 08.01).

The beats arrive before the next P wave or they may be hidden in the T wave of the beat. The QRS complex if similar to that of the normal beat. There is generally a pause following the PAC.

CLINICAL EKG INTERPRETATION

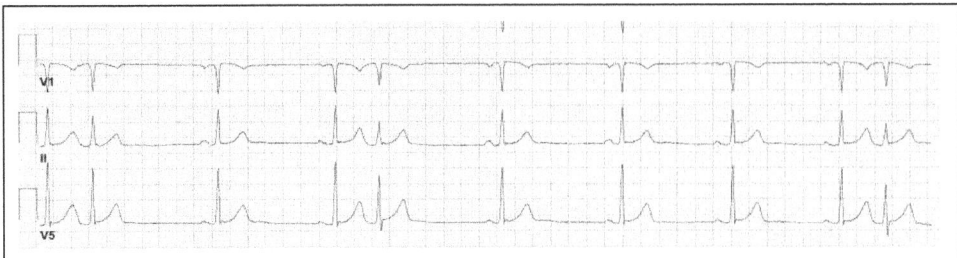

Fig: 08.01. Sinus rhythm with premature atrial complexes. Note the deformity of the preceding T waves and the pause following the PAC.

Blocked PAC

If you don't see a distinct P wave, look for deformities of the T wave. Compare the T wave to the other T waves without a pause (Fig: 08.02). If there is a minor change, most likely that represent the blocked P wave. This will also help us to differentiate it from 2:1 AV block. In 2:1 conduction, the blocked P wave should arrive on time at the next PP interval.

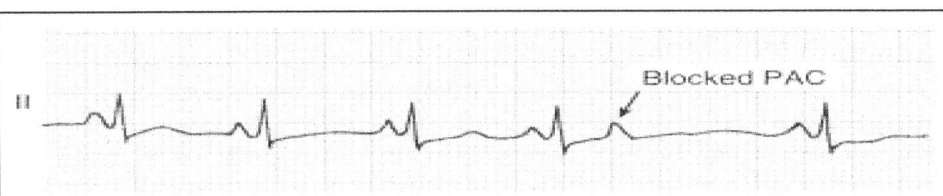

Fig: 08.02. Sinus rhythm with blocked premature atrial complexes. Note the deformity of the preceding T waves and the pause following the PAC.

Atrial bigeminy: Look for grouped beats with an alternative long-short cycle. Here it starts with a normal beat. Then, we have premature beat either atrial or ventricular, followed by a pause and the cycle repeats. A visual clue will be runs of two beats with short and long cycles (Fig: 08.03). The QRS complexes will be very similar.

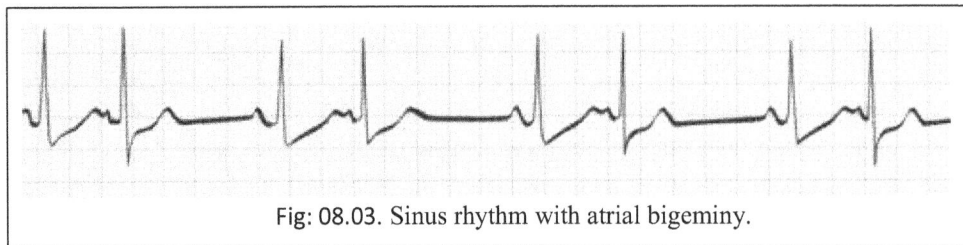

Fig: 08.03. Sinus rhythm with atrial bigeminy.

CHAPTER 8. SUPRAVENTICULAR ARRHYTHMIAS

The P wave of the short cycle will be closer to the preceding T wave, which is another clue that it is ectopic and premature. The P wave morphology may also be different.

Sinus rhythm with premature atrial complexes (PACs).

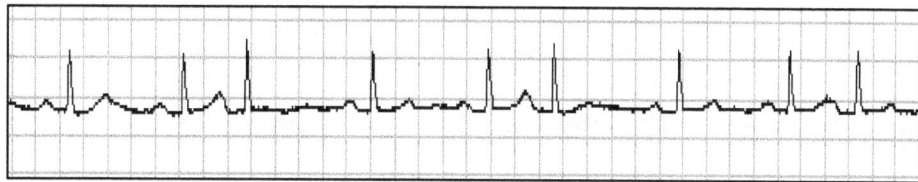

Atrial Bigeminy

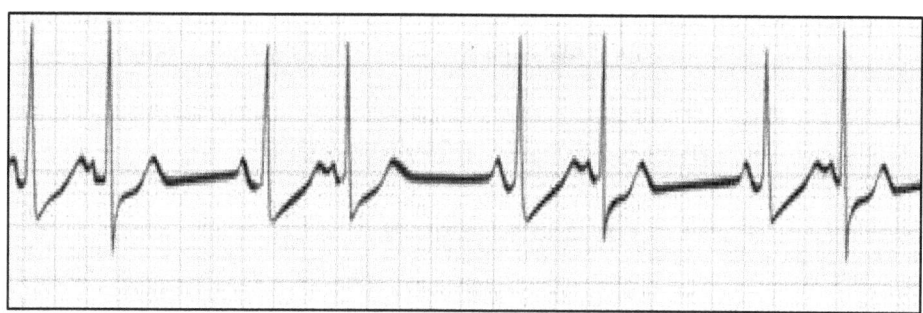

Atrial Trigeminy

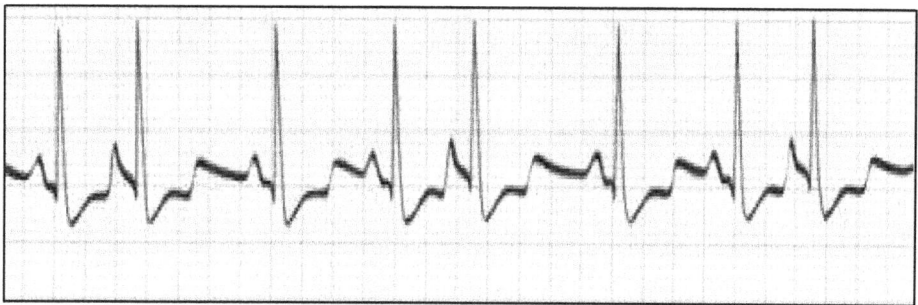

CLINICAL EKG INTERPRETATION

JUNCTIONAL PREMATURE COMPLEX (JPC)

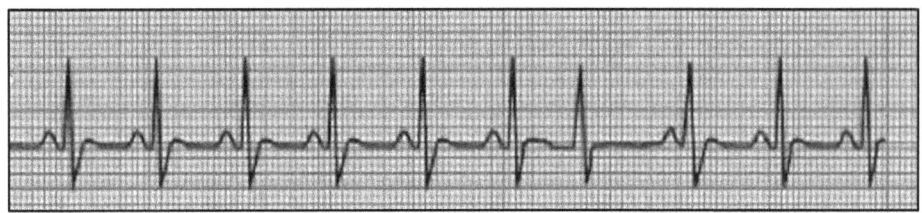

SUPRAVENTRICULAR TACHYCARDIA (SVT):

This refers to tachyarrhythmias arising above the ventricle. They can arise from the:

SUPRAVENTRICULAR TACHYCARDIA (SVT)

- **Sinus Node: Sinus Tachycardia**
- **Atrial**
  - **Atrial Tachycardias**
    - Paroxysmal Atrial Tachycardia or PSVT
    - Atrial Flutter
    - Atrial Fibrillation
    - Multifocal Atrial Tachycardia
- **Junctional Tachycardia.**
- **Wolff Parkinson White (WPW) Tachycardia.**

Mechanism of Tachyarrhythmias:
- Automaticity
- Reentry

CHAPTER 8. SUPRAVENTICULAR ARRHYTHMIAS

Mechanism of supraventricular Tachycardias: Mainly there are two mechanisms by which a supraventricular tachycardia originates and sustains the rapid rhythms.

Automaticity	Re-entrant
PSVT	Atrial Flutter
Sinus Tachycardia	Atrial Fibrillation
Junctional Tachycardia – JT	AVNRT - Nodal Re-entry
Multi-focal Atrial Tachycardia - MAT	AVRT–Atrioventricular Re-entry

The mechanism by which a supraventricular tachycardia makes a difference in terms of how it behaves and what is the most effective way to terminate a tachyarrhythmia.

Automaticity: As the name indicates, these arrhythmias are initiated by an automatic impulse from within the tissue, be it atrial muscle or the AV node. This irritable focus fires at a rapid rate and sustains the impulse. If the conduction system distal to the site can handle the rapid rate, there will be one-to-one conduction. However, if the rate is very rapid and the conduction system is unable to recover to conduct the next impulse, it may result in rate-dependent aberrant conduction or wide QRS tachycardia.

These tachyarrhythmias can initiate spontaneously and terminate spontaneously. Patients may experience palpitations and dizziness if the rates are very high. Some older patients may have chest pain and shortness of breath.

*****

ACLS QUIZ:

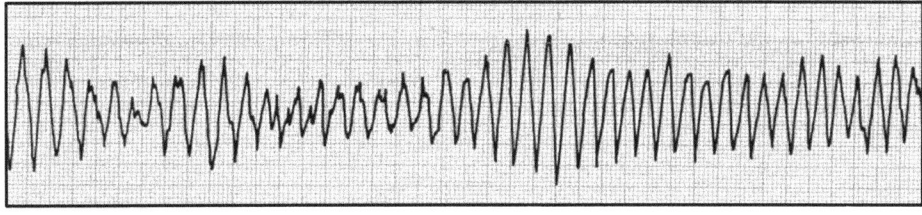

What is your diagnosis? _____

It can also be secondary to increased sympathetic or parasympathetic nervous system stimulation brought about by an electrolyte, metabolic, or hemodynamic changes in the body. Common examples of this include ectopic beats following myocardial infarction, low potassium, low calcium levels, or chronic lung disease (MAT).

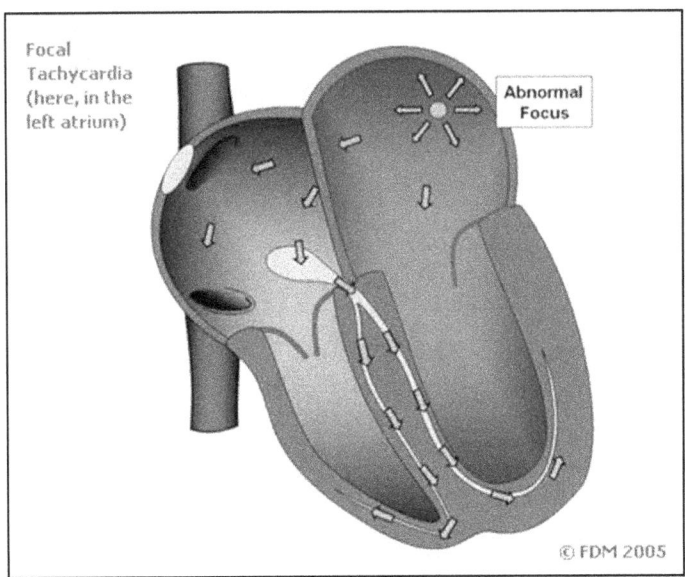

Re-entrant Tachycardia: Here, the ectopic impulse arises from a focus. This impulse may be transmitted back to the site by alterations in the tissue so they act like microcircuits to set up a circus movement of the electrical impulse. This circus movement can occur at the atrial tissue level (micro circuits), at the AV nodal level, where part of the AV node may be blocked in one direction, or at the ventricular level, where the impulses arrive from the site to the AV node, and through the ventricular myocardium reach an atrial site to a set of a macro circuit to sustain the tachyarrhythmia.

- The re-entrant circuit within the atrial tissue
- The re-entrant circuit at the AV node AVNRT
- Re-entrant circuit

CHAPTER 8. SUPRAVENTICULAR ARRHYTHMIAS

For unknown reasons, the conduction system such as the AV node (AV nodal reentry) develops two pathways, one conducting the impulse from the atrium at a slower pace and the other one at a faster pace.

When an impulse arrives from the atrium the slow conduction pathway, which has a shorter refractory period conducts the impulse (Path A).

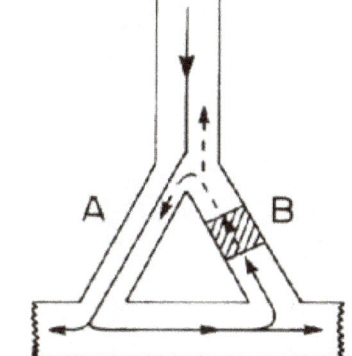

The impulse travels a short distance within the AV nodal tissue and finds the fast pathway now able to transmit the impulse in the opposite direction (Path B).

The impulse from the fast pathway reaches the top of the AV node and finds the slow pathway ready to conduct again.

As a result, the impulse goes through this circular movement while at the same time activating the ventricles, setting up a reentry tachycardia.

Most supraventricular tachycardias have narrow QRS complexes unless there is an underlying bundle branch block (BBB) or there is a tendency for rate-dependent BBB. Unlike patients with ventricular tachycardia, most people with SVT, tolerate the rhythm fairly well, unless the rates are so high, they may feel dizzy or even pass out.

Carotid Sinus Pressure: Carotid sinus pressure is applied in patients with supraventricular tachycardias in order to get a better understanding of the atrial rhythm or mechanism.

Carotid sinus pressure triggers the Baroreceptor reflex and activates the Vagus nerve and vagal discharge. This slows the conduction through the AV node. As a result, the ventricular rate slows. That might be enough to unravel the hidden P waves in atrial flutter or PSVT.

CLINICAL EKG INTERPRETATION

Before applying any carotid sinus pressure, listen to both carotid arteries for any loud bruits, which may signal carotid artery stenosis. Place the index and middle fingers on top of the carotid artery just below the jaw and locate the strongest carotid pulse. The fingers should be over the carotid body near the bifurcation where the Baroceptor is located.

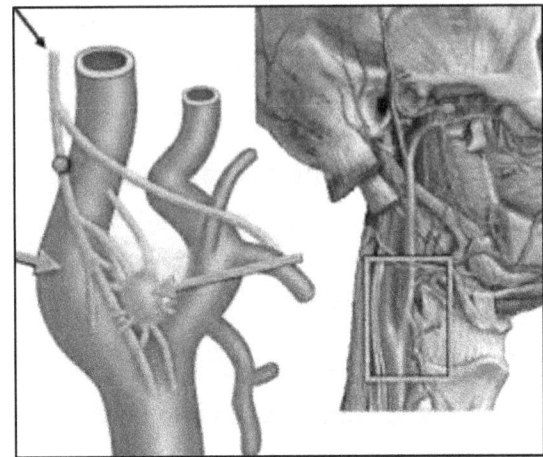

While the EKG paper is running and while you are watching the monitor, apply gentle pressure until you see a slowing of the ventricular rate unmasking the P waves or atrial activity. Make sure two over jealous trainees are not doing simultaneous carotid artery pressure on both sides of the neck at the same time.

In some cases of PSVT, it is possible to terminate the tachyarrhythmia with carotid artery pressure.

Valsalva Maneuver: If the carotid artery pressure doesn't work, we can try Valsalva maneuver, where a patient is asked to bear down as though having a bowel movement. It also slows the heart rate and occasionally may terminate the PSVT. Eyeball pressure should not be used to initiate a vagal response.

Beta-Blockers: If the above techniques fail to reveal the underlying atrial rhythm, we also can try a bolus of a beta-blocker such as 5 mg of Lopressor or Metoprolol IV, which can temporarily slow the heart rate and assist in identifying the rhythm. Before administering a beta-blocker, make sure the blood pressure is adequate or administer a fluid bolus to support borderline blood pressure if needed.

CHAPTER 8. SUPRAVENTICULAR ARRHYTHMIAS

SVT– DIAGNOSTIC APPROACH

SVT– Diagnostic Approach

- Underlying EKG, P Wave, and QRS Morphology

- What Are the Atrial and Ventricular Rates?

- What is the Relationship Between P and QRS Complexes?

- What is the Morphology of the P and QRS Complex: Narrow or Wide? Varying P Wave Morphology?

- Origination and Termination

- Symptomatology: Fine, OK, Dizzy, Weak, low BP, etc.

- Look for Hidden Waves: P Waves in the QRS or in the ST Segments.

- ST-T Changes Which May Suggest Ischemic Underlying Cause.

ACLS QUIZ:

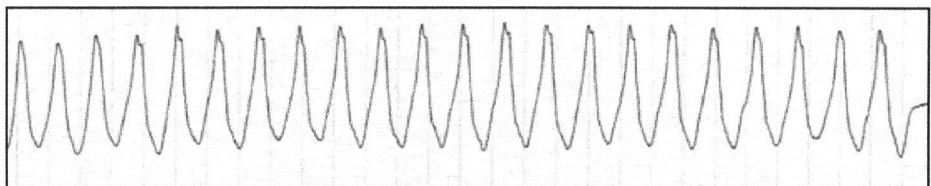

What is your diagnosis? _____

CLINICAL EKG INTERPRETATION

Here is a table covering the salient features of various SVTs

SVT	Atrial Rate bpm	Conduction	RR INT	P waves	QRS
Sinus	100-160	1:1	Regular	Upright	Narrow
PSVT	160-225	1:1, 2:1	Regular	Variable	Narrow
At. Flutter	225-320	1:1, 2:1, 4:1,	Variable	Sawtooth	Narrow or wide
At. Fib	>320	Variable	Variable	Not clear	Narrow or wide
MAT	100-250	1:1	Variable	Multiform	Narrow
Junctional	100-180	1:1 2:1	Regular	Inverted	Narrow
WPW	100-300	1:1, 2:1	Variable	Upright	Delta wave

SINUS TACHYCARDIA

This is one of the most common tachyarrhythmias we encounter in medical practice. It can result from physiological demands such as exercise, stress, and others. Often in a hospital situation, the sinus tachycardia is an indirect marker for much more significant underlying pathology that needs immediate attention. Such situations could include bleeding, pain, infection, hypotension, etc. (Fig: 08.04).

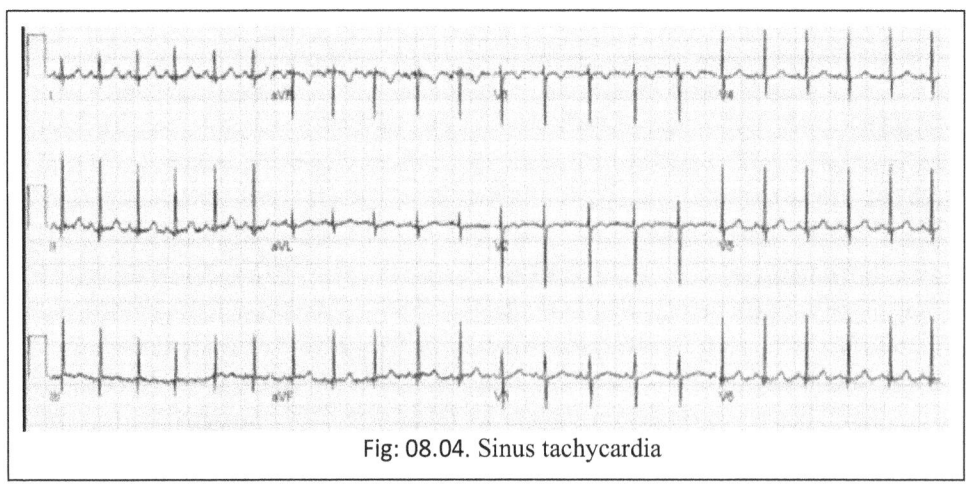

Fig: 08.04. Sinus tachycardia

CHAPTER 8. SUPRAVENTICULAR ARRHYTHMIAS

The sinus tachycardia rate varies from 100 to 160 bpm. The QRS complexes are narrow unless the patient has an underlying BBB. The P waves are upright in I, II, and lateral chest leads. The PR intervals are constant and the RR intervals are constant. It is not terminated by carotid artery pressure or Valsalva maneuver even though they may slow the heart rate transiently.

When the heart rate approaches 150-160 bpm, we must keep in mind other differential diagnoses such as PSVT, Junctional tachycardia, or atrial flutter with 2:1 conduction. In these circumstances, Valsalva maneuver can be tried to slow the rate to look for hidden clues.

The sinus tachycardia is an important signal and we must look for the causes and correct the causes as sinus tachycardia increases cardiovascular demand and compromise cardiac function in a critically ill patient in an in the intensive care unit.

Look for other pieces of evidence on the electrocardiogram that can shed some light on the underlying conditions such as an old MI, recent ischemic changes, or a new onset BBB.

PAROXYSMAL ATRIAL TACHYCARDIA (PSVT)

This rhythm is characterized by an impulse arising from the atria with a heart rate ranging from 160 to 225 bpm. As the name implies, the tachyarrhythmia is paroxysmal in nature and can terminate spontaneously. It is generally seen in younger individuals. The term paroxysmal refers to the periodic sudden onset of a tachyarrhythmia.

PSVT is related to increased excitability at an atrial site. Certain situations like stress, excess caffeine, drugs, may increase this excitability and precipitate an episode of tachyarrhythmia. Even a premature beat from the atria or the ventricle can provoke the irritable foci and set off a PSVT.

PSVT Rate: When the ventricular rate is more than 200, it becomes challenging to determine the rate. You can use the following chart to determine the ventricular rate. If the RR intervals cover 5 small boxes, the rate is 300 bpm. If the RR intervals cover 10 boxes the rate is 150 bpm.

CLINICAL EKG INTERPRETATION

Small Boxes	Rate
5	300 bpm
6	250 bpm
7	214 bpm
8	187 bpm
9	166 bpm
10	150 bpm

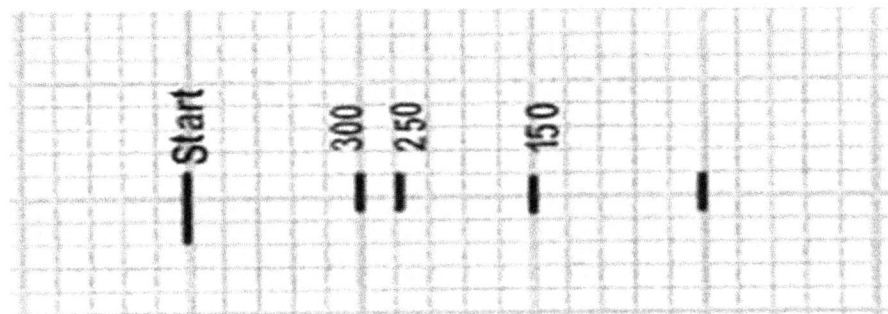

As the name implies, the tachyarrhythmia is paroxysmal in nature and can terminate spontaneously. At rates below 200 bpm, we may be able to see distinct P waves with uniform morphology throughout the tachycardia (Fig: 08.05). The QRS complexes are narrow unless there is a preexisting bundle branch block or WPW.

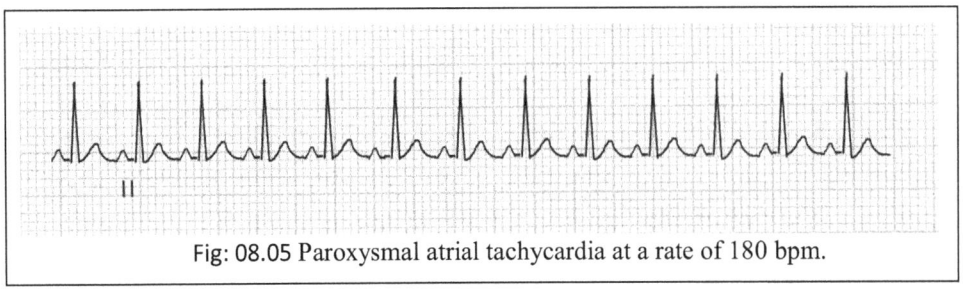

Fig: 08.05 Paroxysmal atrial tachycardia at a rate of 180 bpm.

CHAPTER 8. SUPRAVENTICULAR ARRHYTHMIAS

It may be confused with a sinus tachycardia at lower heart rates, but generally, there is a history of paroxysmal episodes of palpitations that may terminate spontaneously or by vagal maneuvers. On the other hand, the sinus tachycardia is gradual in onset and typically related to an underlying treatable cause such as fever, anemia, hypotension, or an acute myocardial infarction. Sinus tachycardia responds to measures taken to treat the underlying causes.

At faster rates, it may be confused with atrial flutter, which has a different mechanism of action, and a different mode of onset and termination. Vagal maneuvers can slow the ventricular rate and uncover the flutter waves (Fig: 08.06).

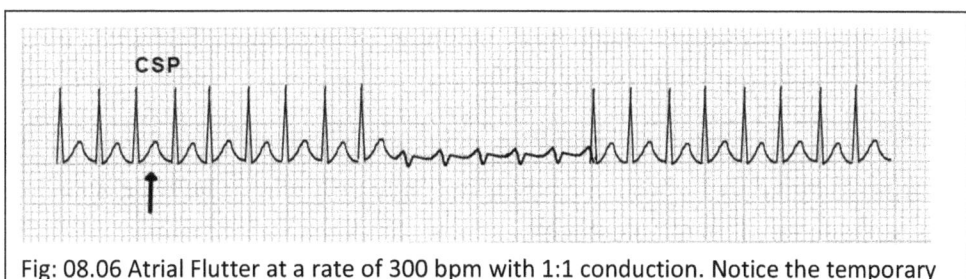

Fig: 08.06 Atrial Flutter at a rate of 300 bpm with 1:1 conduction. Notice the temporary absence of R waves following carotid sinus pressure and uncovering of the flutter waves.

Occasionally, we may come across a PSVT with 2:1 conduction. Whenever we see PSVT or PAT with 2:1 block we should always consider digitalis toxicity if the patient is on digoxin (Fig: 08.07).

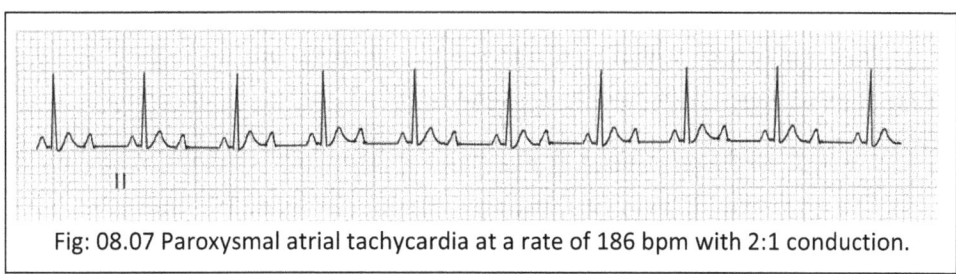

Fig: 08.07 Paroxysmal atrial tachycardia at a rate of 186 bpm with 2:1 conduction.

A PSVT usually terminates with a vagal maneuver such as straining. However, if the ventricular rates are fast and the episodes are prolonged, patients may experience palpitations or pounding in the chest along with chest pain, shortness of breath, or dizziness.

Electrocardiographically it is a narrow QRS tachycardia with a preceding P wave for each QRS complex. The PR and the RR intervals are constant. Occasionally the P waves may be buried in the preceding T waves, especially at rates above 200 bpm.

If the heart rates are more than 180 bpm and the arrhythmia is sustained, these patients may end up in the emergency rooms.

Management: Management of PSVT depends on the symptoms, ventricular rate, blood pressure, and any ischemic changes on the electrocardiogram.

A vagal maneuver such as straining sometimes terminates the arrhythmia. Make sure the patient is in a supine position.

Similarly, carotid sinus pressure may terminate a PSVT. Listen to the carotids to make sure there are no bruits. Only one side to be tried at a time and no more than for 5-10 seconds.

Ice cold towel could be applied to the face in an attempt to terminate the PSVT.

If there is no response to the above physiological measures, the patient may be treated with 6 mg of adenosine given rapidly intravenously (in 1-2 sec). It should be followed by a bolus of saline fluid to make sure the drug reaches the heart. Adenosine often terminates the tachyarrhythmia.

If the first dose doesn't terminate the arrhythmia, a second dose of adenosine (12 mg) can be given intravenously.

If the second dose, doesn't convert the rhythm, a third dose of adenosine 12 mg can be given intravenously, up to a maximum dose of 18 mg IV.

It has a short half-life and the most common symptom is flushing. It has a success rate ranging from 78% to 96%.

Intravenous Beta blockers, verapamil, or Cardizem can be tried in patients with no evidence of WPW syndrome.

CHAPTER 8. SUPRAVENTICULAR ARRHYTHMIAS

If all measures fail and if the patient's blood pressure in unstable, you can attempt electrical cardioversion using 25 to 50 watts power. Make sure the patient is adequately sedated. Rarely, do we need to use the electrical cardioversion for PSVT?

Oral beta-blockers, verapamil, or diltiazem may be useful for control of SVT on an outpatient basis.

Acute treatment SVT Flow Diagram:

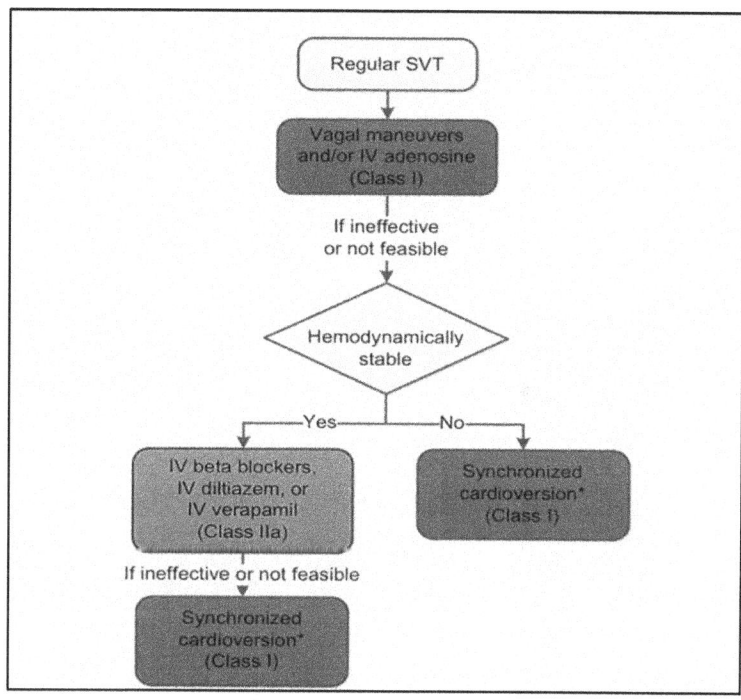

Ref: https://www.heartrhythmjournal.com/article/S1547-5271(15)01189-3/pdf

ACLS QUIZ:

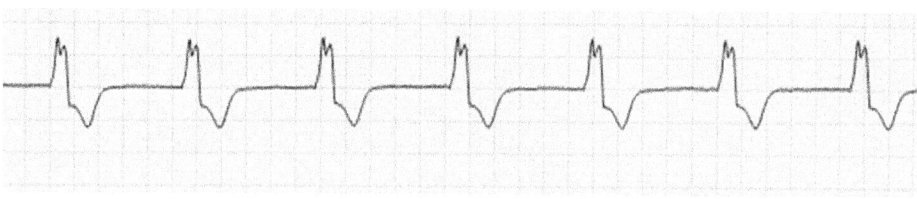

What is your diagnosis? _____

CLINICAL EKG INTERPRETATION

Long Term Management of SVT of Unknown Mechanism

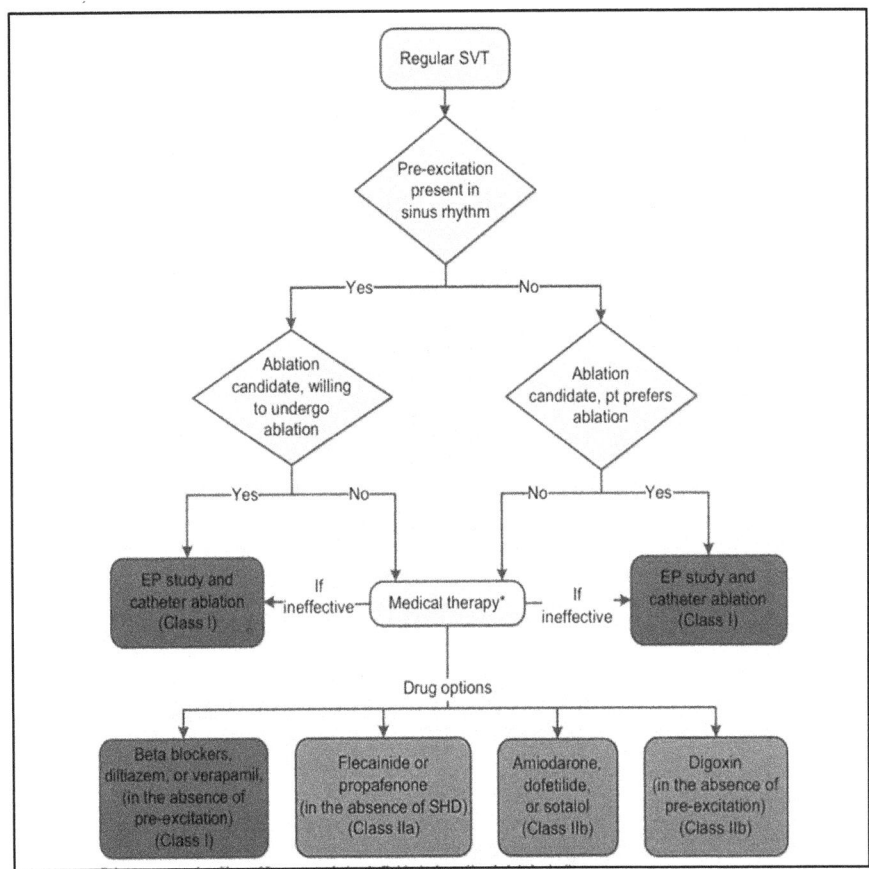

Ref: https://www.heartrhythmjournal.com/article/S1547-5271(15)01189-3/pdf

ACLS QUIZ:

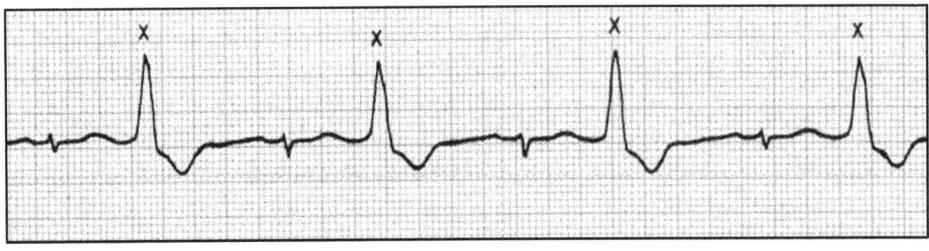

What is your diagnosis? _____

CHAPTER 8. SUPRAVENTICULAR ARRHYTHMIAS

ATRIAL FLUTTER:

It is a re-entrant tachyarrhythmia which is commonly seen in medical practice. It arises from an atrial ectopic focus and sets of a circuit through accessory pathways within the atrial myocardium. It produces the characteristic Flutter waves that look like undulating waves with the peaks pointing up or down depending on the direction of the impulse propagation in the accessory pathway.

While it activates the atria, it also activates the ventricle and it is not uncommon to see a 1:1 conduction. More often, there may be 2:1 conduction, where it may be mistaken for other supraventricular tachycardias such as atrial tachycardia, sinus tachycardia, or even junctional tachycardia, especially when the flutter waves are not clearly seen or hidden in the T waves. When the conduction is 3:1 or 4:1 the flutter waves can be easily seen. In an emergency situation, when the ventricular rates are rapid and the flutter waves are hidden in the QRS and T waves, vagal maneuvers such as carotid sinus pressure or straining may temporarily slow the ventricular rate and uncover the flutter waves.

The atrial flutter can be paroxysmal or chronic. There is a tendency for a blood clot formation if the atrial flutter lasts for more than 48 hours.

There are two types of atrial flutter based on the direction of the impulse propagation and the morphology of the flutter waves (atrial activity).

A Typical Atrial Flutter the electrical impulse travels in a counter-clockwise fashion along the septal wall of the right atrium.

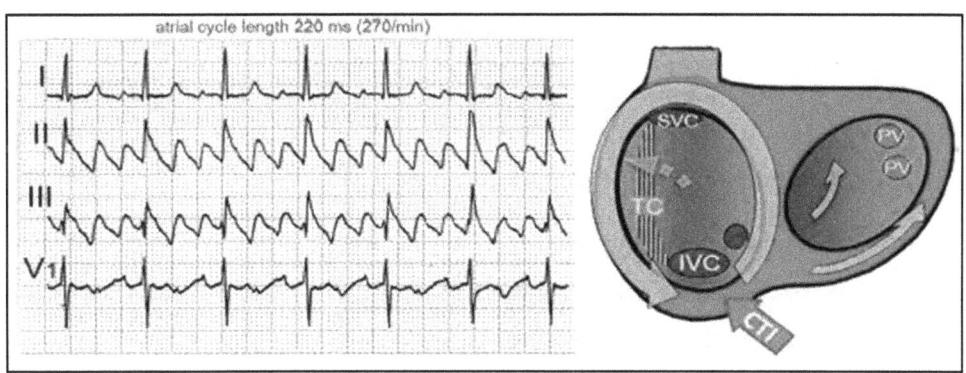

https://www.aerjournal.com/articles/atrial-flutter-typical-and-atypical-review

CLINICAL EKG INTERPRETATION

Typical (counterclockwise) flutter is associated with a regular typical 'sawtooth pattern' of continuous undulation characterized by negative deflections in leads II, III and aVF

Atrial flutter waves in V1 can be positive, biphasic or negative. The flutter rates vary from 240 to 350 bpm.

Reverse Typical Atrial Flutter: It shows rounded or bimodal positive deflections in inferior leads II, III and aVF. The flutter waves in V1 also can show a very bimodal negative wave-like 'W' wave in V1.

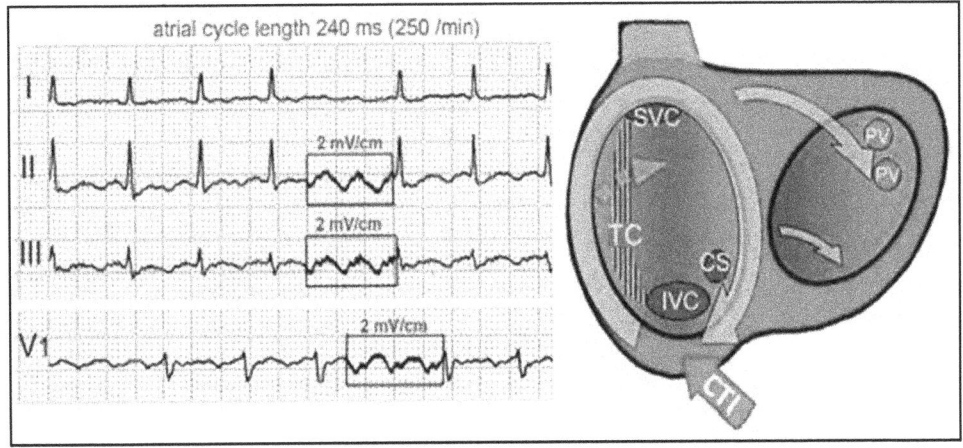

https://www.aerjournal.com/articles/atrial-flutter-typical-and-atypical-review

Patients can have varied presentations with atrial flutter. Some patients may have an atrial flutter on a routine electrocardiogram in an office setting, with no symptoms, while others may present to the emergency departments with palpitations, chest pain and shortness of breath.

When we are faced with a patient with atrial flutter we need to focus on some important historical data and clinical findings in order to best serve the patient. Remember to treat the patient, not just the flutter.

- Is this a new onset atrial flutter or did the patient have this before?
- How long did the patient have this rhythm?
- Is the patient on any treatment?
- Precipitating factors?

CHAPTER 8. SUPRAVENTICULAR ARRHYTHMIAS

- Underlying cardiac findings such as CAD, HTN, CHF, others.
- Is the patient on blood thinners?

Next, we need to focus on the ventricular rate. If the rate is too fast and the patient is hypotensive, quick cardioversion using 25 to 50 watts might be in order.

If we are in doubt about the diagnosis, a carotid pressure may slow the ventricular response and reveal the real flutter waves to confirm the diagnosis.

Often, we may come across atrial flutter with 2:1 conduction (Fig: 08.08)

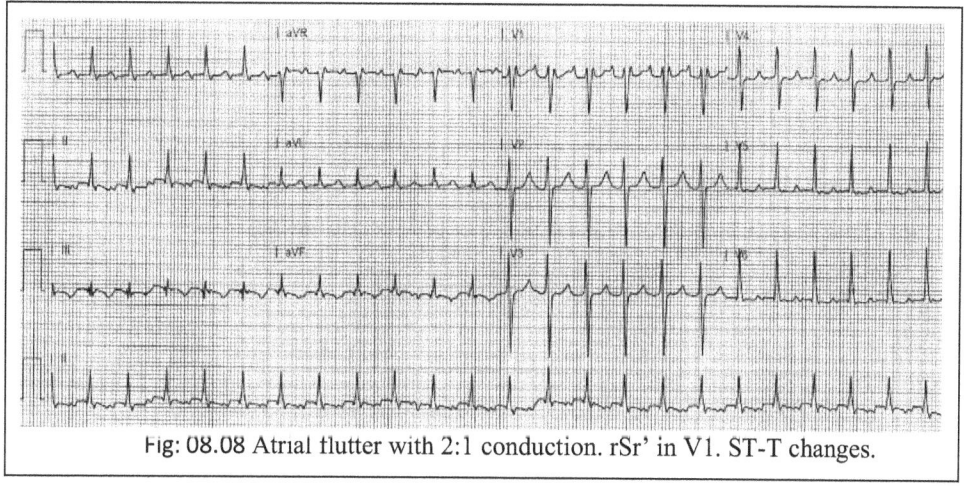
Fig: 08.08 Atrial flutter with 2:1 conduction. rSr' in V1. ST-T changes.

If the patient had an atrial flutter for several days, there is a tendency for development of a blood clot in the left atrial appendage. If we do attempt to restore the rhythm to sinus with drugs or cardioversion, we risk the development of a stroke. Hence, it is very important to reduce the ventricular rate, stabilize the patient, and perform a TEE to exclude any blood clots in the left atrial appendage, before attempting cardioversion to restore normal sinus rhythm.

If the patient does have blood clots in the left atrial appendage, it is reasonable to keep the patients on anticoagulants for 4-6 weeks before attempting cardioversion to sinus rhythm.

Atrial flutter is one arrhythmia, which has a very high success rate with ablation. Hence, all patients with atrial flutter should be evaluated for ablation treatment.

Atrial flutter has a single site of origin, so the flutter waves look very similar in tracing as opposed to AF or MAT where the P wave morphology can be varying from beat to beat.

Acute Treatment of Atrial Flutter: Patients with atrial flutter can present with very rapid ventricular rates and older patients may have several c-morbid conditions which may complicate the management. The immediate goal is to convert the rhythm to sinus if possible if the flutter had been there for less than 48 hours.

If the patient is suitable for cardioversion, we can attempt pharmacological cardioversion. The drug of choice for cardioversion in atrial flutter is oral or intravenous ibutilide. Please refer to the ACC/AHA/HAS 2015 guidelines at the end of this chapter for proper dosages.

If the atrial flutter onset time is uncertain, it complicates the matters, as those patients who had flutter for more than 48 hours are at increased risk of left atrial thrombus and any cardioversion could potentially dislodge the thrombus and cause a serious cerebrovascular occlusive event in the form of a major stroke or a peripheral arterial blockage. Hence, if we do need to attempt, cardioversion, those patients may undergo TEE to exclude left atrial thrombus. If there is no left atrial thrombus, we could proceed with either pharmacological or electrical cardioversion. However, if there is a definite thrombus, then these patients need to be on anticoagulants for 4-6 weeks before attempting any type of cardioversion.

If immediate cardioversion is not a choice, then we need to focus on controlling the ventricular rates in the presence of persistent atrial flutter. We could consider Intravenous or oral beta-blockers, diltiazem, or verapamil. Please refer to the table at the end of this chapter for drug dosages.

We also have an option to place a pacemaker catheter in the right atrium and attempt rapid atrial pacing at a rate of 400-800 bpm for a few seconds under cardiac monitoring in the intensive care unit or in the Cath lab. This

CHAPTER 8. SUPRAVENTICULAR ARRHYTHMIAS

technique only has a 50% success rate. It may also be possible in patients who have a pacemaker with an atrial electrode in place.

In any case, if these patients have not been on anticoagulants in the past, they should be started on anticoagulants as soon as the condition permits.

Of course, the most definitive treatment for atrial flutter is catheter ablation with a success rate in excess of 90%.

Drugs such as Amiodarone, Dofetilide, and Sotalol may be useful on a long-term basis to maintain sinus rhythm.

Acute IV Drug Therapy for Flutter
2015 ACC/AHA/HRS Guidelines

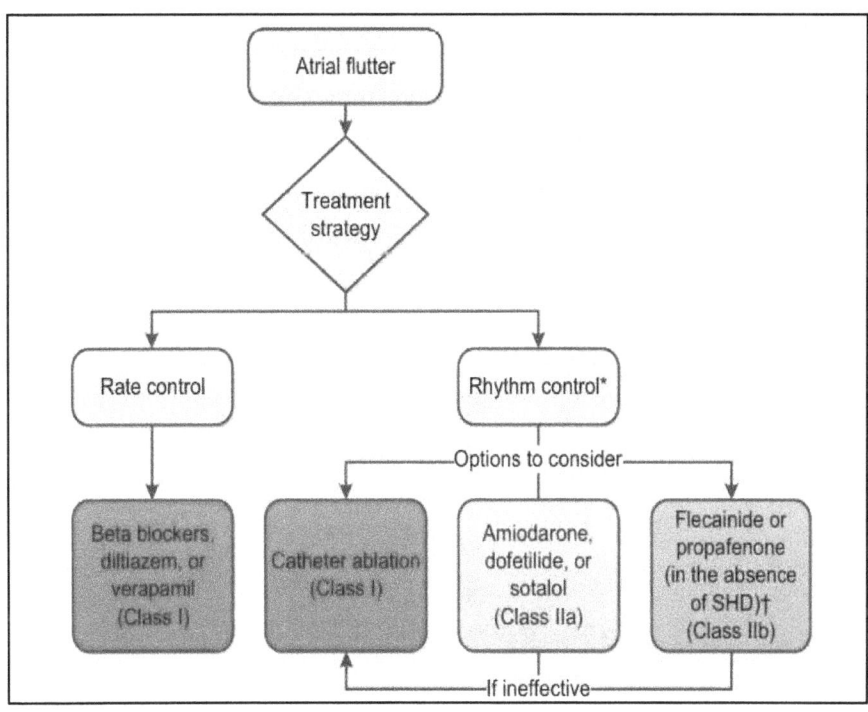

Ref:https://www.heartrhythmjournal.com/article/S1547-5271(15)01189-3/pdf

ATRIAL FIBRILLATION

Atrial fibrillation is the most common arrhythmia, we encounter in cardiology practice. The incidence of atrial fibrillation or At. Fib goes up significantly after age 60 years.

Atrial fibrillation is characterized by an atrial rate between 340-600 bpm along with variable ventricular rates. As demonstrated in the image the atria may be activated from multiple sites, with impulses traveling in many directions. Hence, Atrial fibrillation is the most common irregularly irregular rhythm we will encounter in our medical practice.

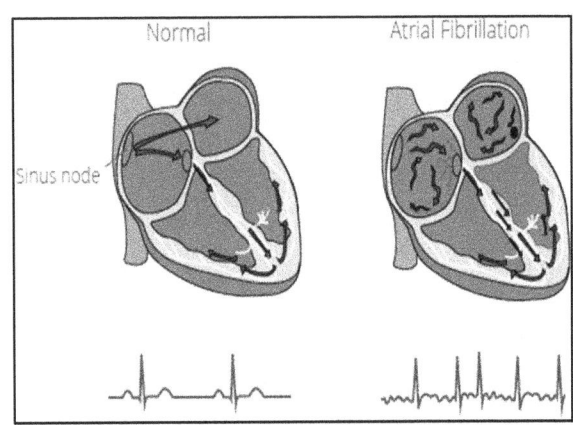

Instead of well-defined P waves, we may see fine undulating waves in place of P waves. The RR intervals vary from beat to beat (Fig: 08.09). During periods of hemodynamic stress, the ventricular rates can be very high in the range of 150-250 bpm. Occasionally, the ventricular rates can be as high as 300 bpm. It is not uncommon to see almost flat lines at the site of supposed P waves.

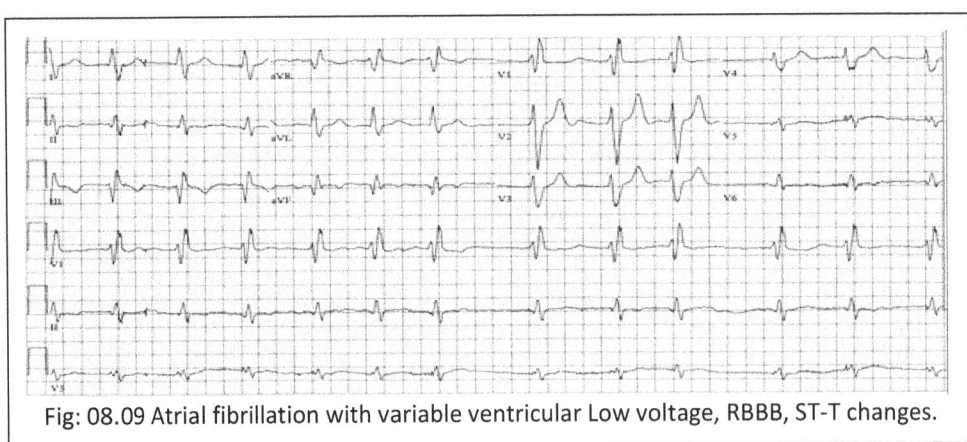

Fig: 08.09 Atrial fibrillation with variable ventricular Low voltage, RBBB, ST-T changes.

CHAPTER 8. SUPRAVENTICULAR ARRHYTHMIAS

When the atrial rates are around 300 bpm, we can see some fib waves with some amplitude which can mimic MAT or flutter. However, the flutter waves are more consistent throughout the tracing at a constant rate. So, pay attention to the PP intervals, and if they are consistent, then you may be dealing with atrial flutter.

Atrial fibrillation can occur in the presence of many other electrocardiographic abnormalities such as BBB, hypertrophy, or acute myocardial infarction. Hence, we need to focus on the electrocardiogram, beyond the atrial fibrillation and see what other changes are visible, which can be a clue to the rapid ventricular rate.

Whenever there is a fairly regular ventricular rate in the presence of atrial fibrillation, always consider a complete heart block with junctional escape rhythm or an idioventricular rhythm if the QRS is wide. It may also suggest possible pacemaker failure if you do see some pacemaker spikes (fig: 08.10).

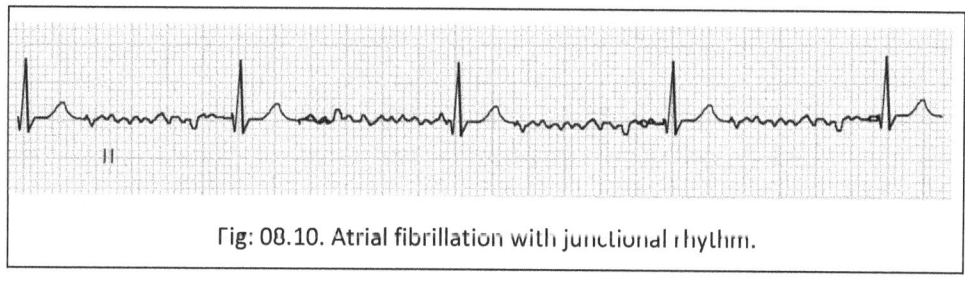

Fig: 08.10. Atrial fibrillation with junctional rhythm.

The Atrial fibrillation can be chronic or paroxysmal. It is often associated with left atrial enlargement. In fact, in the presence of increased left precordial voltage, the accompanying atrial fibrillation is considered an indirect marker for left atrial enlargement and carry the same points as a left atrial enlargement.

Occasionally, the QRS complexes can be wider if the underlying rhythm has BBB. Sometimes, the rate dependent BBB can result in a wide QRS tachycardia with rapid ventricular rates.

Atrial fibrillation is always pathological and its presence should alert you to the next question, "What is causing it?" An echocardiogram could be very useful in looking at structures such as chambers, walls, and valves to establish an etiology for the atrial fibrillation (Fig: 08. 11).

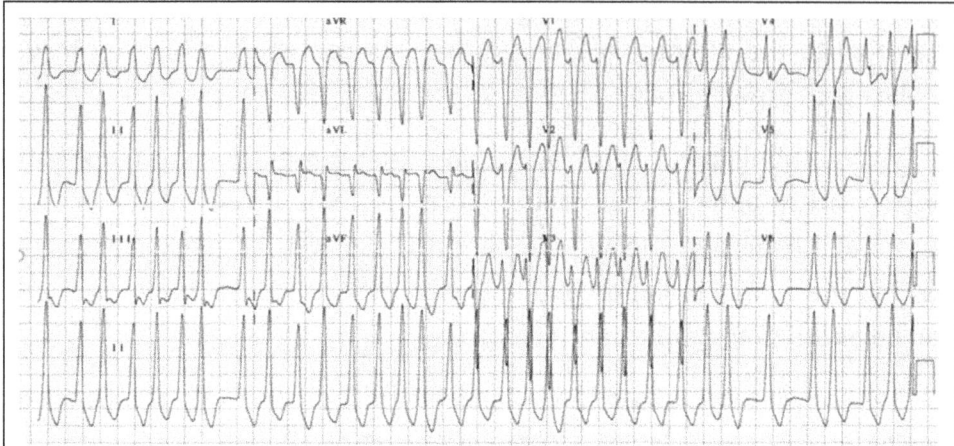

Fig: 08.11 Atrial fibrillation with very rapid ventricular rate, LVH with strain, along with ST depression in the inferior leads.

Atrial fibrillation should draw our attention to many things. We should not only be concerned about the mere presence of atrial fibrillation, but also the effect of a rapid ventricular rate on hemodynamics in each situation.

- The ventricular rate control is of utmost importance in an acute situation to reduce myocardial oxygen demand.
- Next, we focus on common conditions triggering the rapid ventricular response, such as infection, hemorrhage, acute myocardial infarction, volume depletion, congestive heart failure, valvular heart disease, thyrotoxicosis, cardiac surgery, chronic lung disease, among others.
- In the long run, conversion to sinus rhythm by using drugs or ablation should be considered as atrial contribution can significantly improve symptoms, especially in patients with myocardial infarction or heart failure. Pharmacological cardioversion of atrial fibrillation has very low yields. However, there are drugs which can maintain sinus rhythm in patients with paroxysmal atrial fibrillation.

CHAPTER 8. SUPRAVENTICULAR ARRHYTHMIAS

- In case of a medical emergency, when the ventricular rate compromises the hemodynamics in a patient with marginal cardiac function, or if there is hypotension, a direct electrical synchronized cardioversion using 50 to 100 watts, may restore the sinus rhythm and help us to stabilize the patient.
- Patients with atrial fibrillation are at increased risk for stroke or peripheral emboli and need to be on anticoagulants.

If you notice a regular ventricular response in the presence of atrial fibrillation, consider the following conditions:

- Complete Heart Block (CHB)
- Paced Rhythm
- Digitalis Toxicity

In complete heart block, the ventricular rhythm could be from the AV nodal site, in which case the QRS complex can be narrow. However, if the QRS is wide, it could be coming from the ventricular site where the rate can be below 45 bpm and suggest more advanced conduction problems, requiring a permanent pacemaker.

If you see a paced ventricular rhythm, look for the pacer spike in all leads. Sometimes, the spikes may be difficult to detect. A sharp deflection prior to the QRS complex could be your only clue on the electrocardiogram.

As the digitalis use is on the decline, it is uncommon to see digitalis toxicity. However, if a patient is on digoxin, it is recommended to check the digoxin level along with electrolytes and renal function.

Occasionally, atrial flutter and fibrillation can occur in the same patient and sometimes on the same EKG tracing. It is important to identify which is the dominant underlying rhythm as atrial flutter has a very high success rate with radiofrequency ablation.

> **Differential Diagnoses of Atrial Fibrillation Include:**
>
> - WPW With Rapid Ventricular Rate, SVT
>
> - VT When There is Underlying BBB
>
> - Paced Rhythms with no Visible P Waves
>
> - Sinus Rhythm with Frequent PACs
>
> - Multifocal Atrial Tachycardia (MAT)

- Consider elective cardioversion:
    - If the duration Atrial fib is <48hrs, you can proceed with DCCV
    - If duration >48hrs or unknown: anticoagulate for 3+ weeks prior to DCCV, or anticoagulate then TEE to rule out intracardiac thrombus prior to DCCV
    - Anticoagulation must continue after cardioversion for 4 weeks

Long-term Anticoagulation for Atrial Fibrillation:

- All patients with rheumatic heart disease should be anticoagulated
- If <65 yrs. and has h/o DM, HTN, CHF, CVA, prosthetic valves, thyrotoxicosis, LV dysfunction or LA enlargement, then give coumadin
- If no risk factors, do nothing. This is very unusual in patients over 60 years.

65-75 yrs. With any of the above risk factors, give coumadin; if no additional risk factors, give coumadin or aspirin

CHAPTER 8. SUPRAVENTICULAR ARRHYTHMIAS

- \>75 yrs. Give coumadin but keep INR 2-2.5 due to increased risk of bleeding

CHA2DS2-VASc Score for Anticoagulation

RIKS FACTOR	SCORE
CHF with EF ≤ 40%	1
Hypertension	1
Age >≥ 75 Yr.	2
Diabetes mellitus	1
Stroke/TIA/thromboembolism	2
Vascular disease	1
Age 65-74 Yr.	1
Sex (female)	1

If a person has a score of ≥ 2, that person needs to be on anticoagulants long-term.

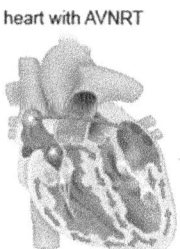
heart with AVNRT

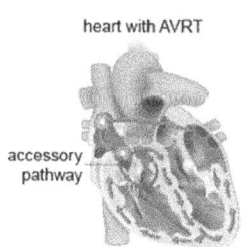
heart with AVRT
accessory pathway

Multifocal Atrial Tachycardia (MAT)

Multifocal Tachycardia (MAT) is commonly seen in patients with chronic lung disease (Fig: 08.12). The hallmark of multifocal atrial tachycardia is the varying morphology of well-defined P waves. In many ways, it resembles atrial fibrillation.

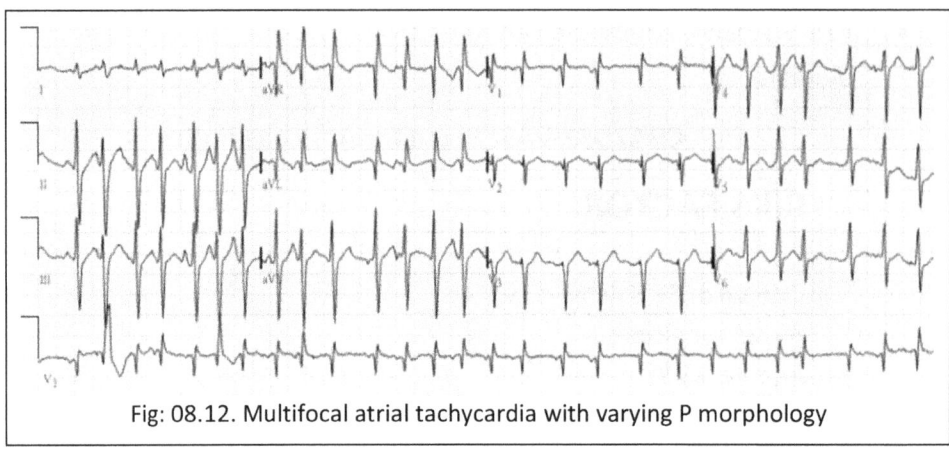
Fig: 08.12. Multifocal atrial tachycardia with varying P morphology

The atrial impulses arise from different foci. It is also called as the wandering pacemaker. The P-P, P-R, and R-R intervals vary from beat to beat. Again, they are associated with rapid ventricular response and other findings such as right axis deviation, right ventricular hypertrophy, and strain.

Multifocal atrial tachycardia can occur in the setting of acute myocardial infarction, congestive heart failure, pulmonary embolus, infection, Hypokalemia, or sepsis.

We need to differentiate it from atrial flutter or atrial fibrillation as the management may be different in these conditions.

The treatment needs to be focused on improving the oxygenation and controlling infection, among others, which will automatically bring the ventricular rate down. Multifocal atrial tachycardia may not respond to usual drugs used in atrial fibrillation to reduce the ventricular response. Beta-blockers may be contraindicated due to underlying chronic lung disease. Once the pulmonary condition improves, the rhythm may revert to sinus.

CHAPTER 8. SUPRAVENTICULAR ARRHYTHMIAS

JUNCTIONAL TACHYCARDIA

The main purpose of the AV node is to delay the sinus impulse from reaching the ventricles and allow adequate time for the ventricles to completely fill before the ventricular depolarization beings.

The Junctional tachycardia is characterized by a narrow QRS complex and perhaps a retrograde P wave which may appear at the end of the QRS complex (fig: 08.13). Since the Atrial impulse is traveling upward and to the right, it appears negative in most leads. Sometimes, the P waves may appear just before the QRS complex with a very short PR interval or it may be completely hidden in the QRS complex.

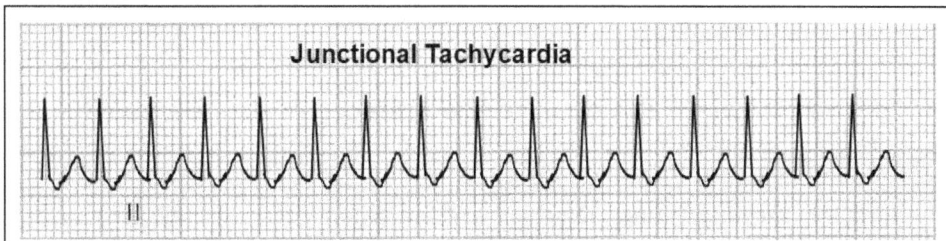

Fig: 08.13. Junctional tachycardia with a ventricular rate of 214 bpm and retrograde P wave coming after the narrow QRS complexes.

The QRS complex is usually narrow (<120 ms) unless there is a disease in the bundle branches.

The AV junction intrinsic rate varies between 40 and 59 bpm. The rate in accelerated Junctional rhythm varies from 60 to 100 bpm. The junctional tachycardia rate varies between 120 and 220 bpm.

The very proximal part of the AV node has no spontaneous automaticity. It is the middle and the distal third of the AV node that can generate an impulse.

Junctional tachycardia also can have a preceding P wave with a short PR interval (Fig: 08.14).

CLINICAL EKG INTERPRETATION

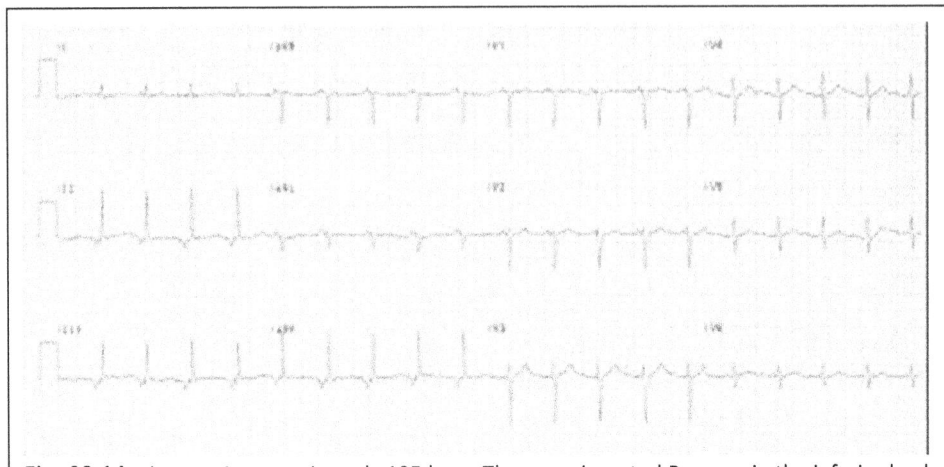

Fig: 08.14. The rate is approximately 125 bpm. There are inverted P waves in the inferior leads just before the narrow QRS complexes. Ref: https://emedicine.medscape.com/article/155146-overview

Junctional rhythm can occur in the presence of digitalis toxicity, sinus node disease.

Accelerated Junctional rhythm is seen most often in the presence of acute inferior wall myocardial infarction, digitalis toxicity, myocarditis, valvular heart disease, and cardiac surgery. The morphology of accelerated junctional rhythm is very similar to the junctional tachycardia.

It is often confused with paroxysmal supraventricular tachycardia when the P waves are not clear. Carotid sinus pressure or Valsalva maneuver may slow that rate and reveal the nature of the P waves.

At this rate, it needs to be differentiated from atrial flutter with block, sinus tachycardia, atrial tachycardia, or atrioventricular reentrant tachycardia (AVRT) involving retrograde condition.

The presence of P waves can help us to identify the origin of the tachycardia. It is not unusual to see a tiny P wave following the QRS complexes. Always, look for deformities of the terminal QRS and you might detect a P wave.

In atrioventricular reentry tachycardia, the RP interval is fixed am a little more prolonged compared to that of AVRT

CHAPTER 8. SUPRAVENTICULAR ARRHYTHMIAS

In atrial flutter, we will often see 2 flutter waves for each QRS complex. If you detect flutter waves in any of the leads that would exclude the AVRT.

It may be challenging to differentiate between atrial tachycardia and AVNRT unless we have a tracing with the origin and termination of the tachyarrhythmias (Fig: 08.15). In AVNRT, due to simultaneous activation of the atria and the ventricles, there is absence of P waves, the presence of a "Pseudo S" in II, II< aVF, or "pseudo r prime," in V1.

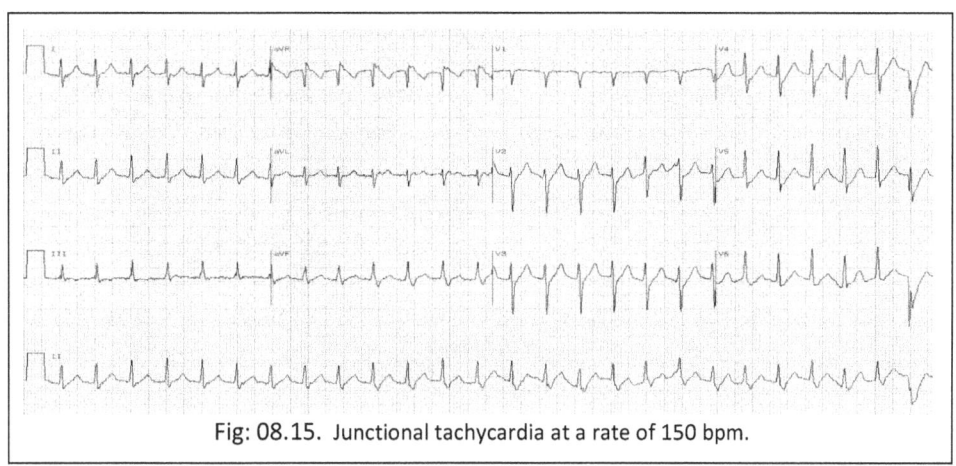

Fig: 08.15. Junctional tachycardia at a rate of 150 bpm.

Adenosine test: When adenosine is administered it may abruptly terminate the AVNRT or AVRT by changing the refractory period of the electrical circuit. Whereas in case of atrial tachycardia (from an excitable focus) or atrial flutter may slow the ventricular response and reveal the atrial activity. Carotid sinus may also produce a similar result.

Differential Diagnosis of Narrow QRS Tachycardia

- **Sinus Tachycardia**
- **AVNRT**
- **AVRT**
- **Atrial Tachycardia**
- **Atrial Flutter**
- **MAT**

Drug Therapy for Junctional Tachycardia
2015 ACC/AHA/HRS Guidelines

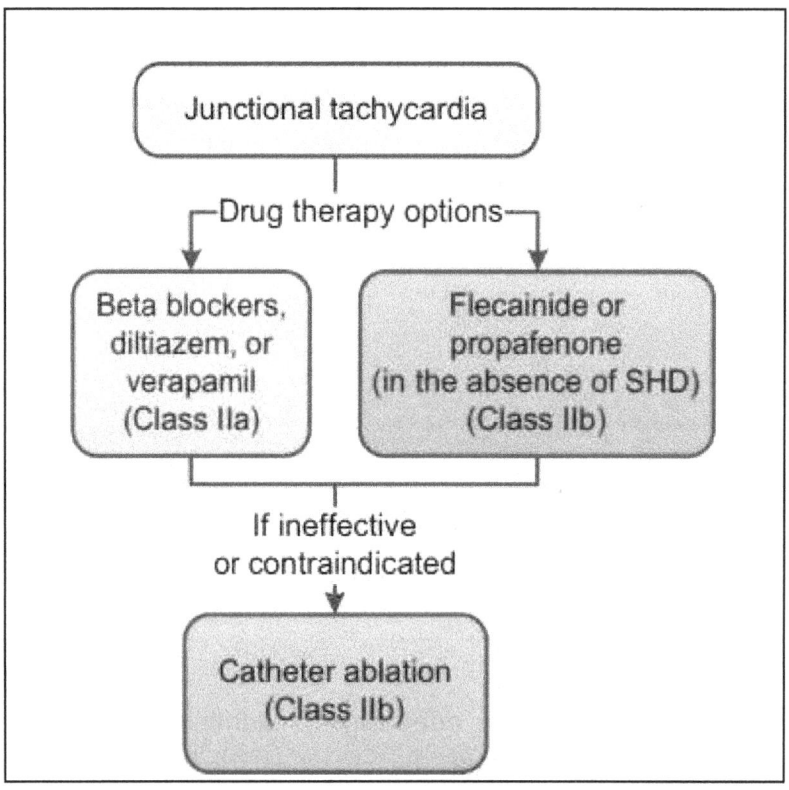

Ref:https://www.heartrhythmjournal.com/article/S1547-5271(15)01189-3/pdf

WPW TACHYCARDIA

Orthodromic Tachycardia: Here, the initial impulse travels through the AV node, and normal conducting pathway. Then, it activates the atrial free wall accessory pathway and sets off a re-entry tachycardia. The QRS complexes are narrow and the rates can vary between 200 and 300 bpm. It may have reciprocal ST-T changes (Fig: 08.16).

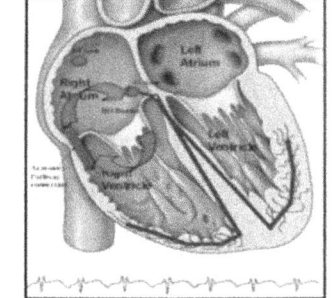

Asymptomatic patients with WPW: These patients may benefit from event monitoring over a period of a few weeks to

CHAPTER 8. SUPRAVENTICULAR ARRHYTHMIAS

determine the frequency and the nature of tachyarrhythmia if any. Based on the type and duration of arrhythmias, a treatment plan can be formulated. We also need to ascertain whether the tachycardia is conducting through the normal pathway or through the accessory pathway.

Electrophysiological Evaluation: These patients can benefit from EP studies to determine if they are suitable candidates for ablation as it can eliminate or drastically reduce the frequency of serious supraventricular arrhythmias. If a correctable pathway is easily identified, isolated and treated with ablation, we should be able to abolish the tachyarrhythmias related to that accessory pathway.

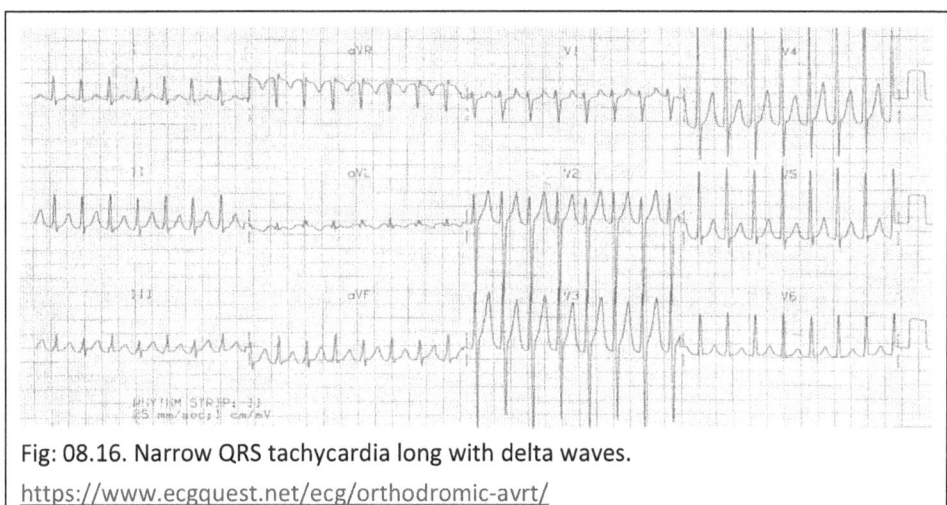

Fig: 08.16. Narrow QRS tachycardia long with delta waves.
https://www.ecgquest.net/ecg/orthodromic-avrt/

COMPLETE COMIC BLOCK (CCB)

"As we get older, we lose three things in a sequence. Of course, the first one is the memory. And I can't remember the other two."

Acute IV Drug Therapy for Orthodromic AVRT
2015 ACC/AHA/HRS Guidelines

Ref:https://www.heartrhythmjournal.com/article/S1547-5271(15)01189-3/pdf

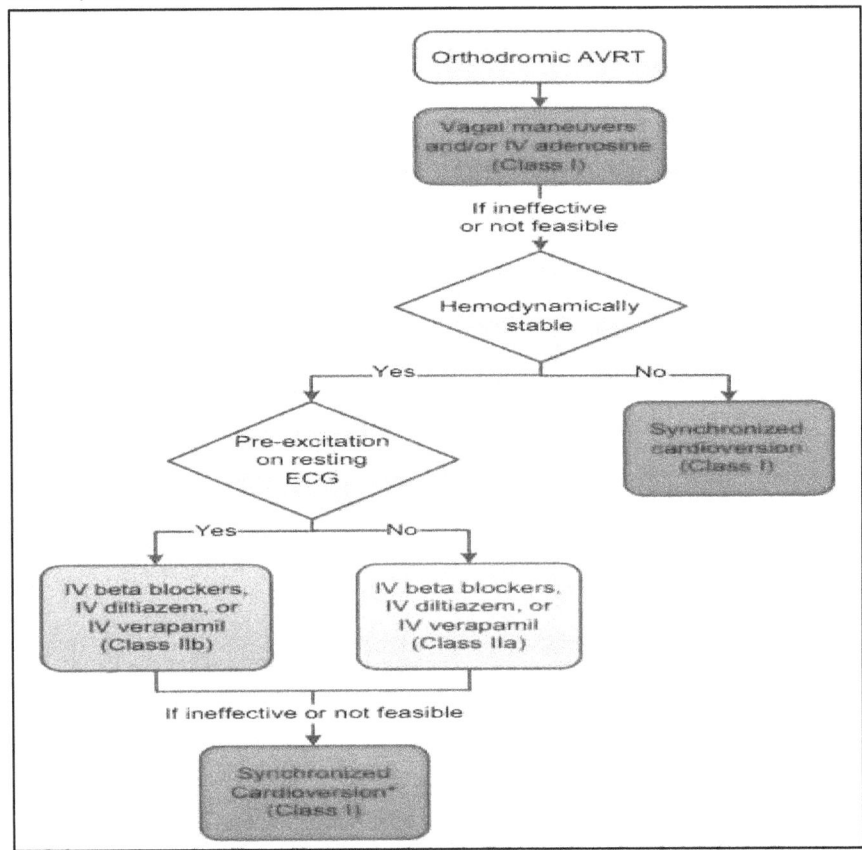

ACLS QUIZ:

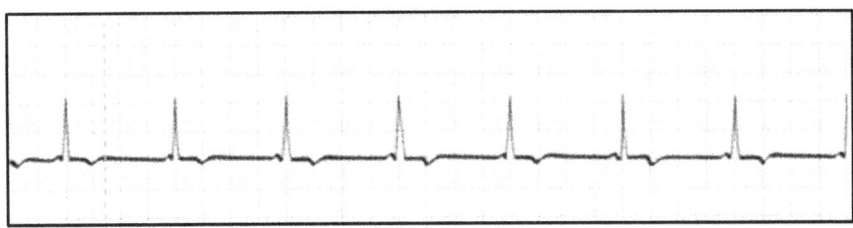

What is your diagnosis? _____

CHAPTER 8. SUPRAVENTICULAR ARRHYTHMIAS

Antidromic Tachycardia: Here, the initial impulse travels through the accessory pathway, activates the ventricles through the Purkinje system producing a wide QRS tachycardia, then travels in a retrograde fashion through the AV nodes and sets of a re-entry circuit (Fig: 08.17).

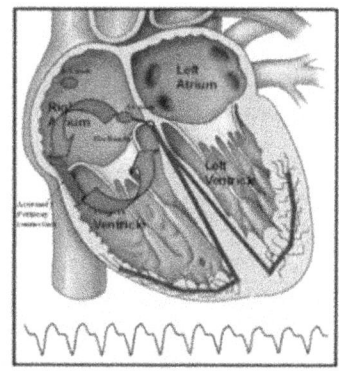

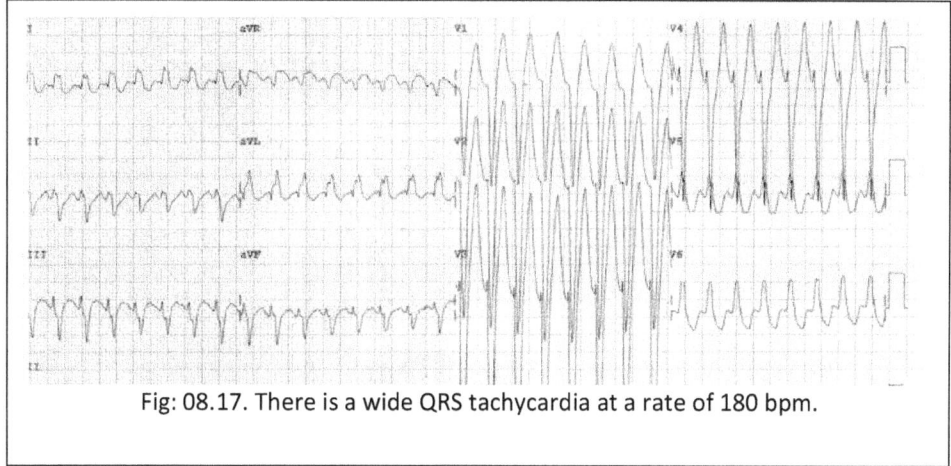

Fig: 08.17. There is a wide QRS tachycardia at a rate of 180 bpm.

When a patient with WPW develops atrial fibrillation, they are prone to very rapid ventricular rates with wide QRS complexes due to the rapid and erratic conduction through the accessory pathway

CLINICAL EKG INTERPRETATION

Ongoing management of orthodromic AVRT
2015 ACC/AHA/HRS Guidelines

Ref:https://www.heartrhythmjournal.com/article/S1547-5271(15)01189-3/pdf

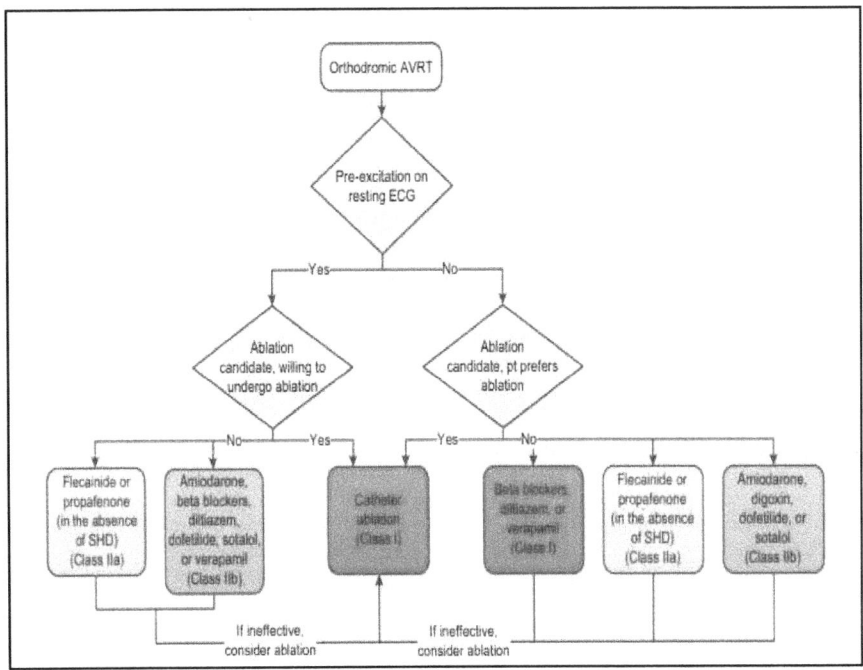

For individual drug dosages, please look at the charts at the end of this chapter.

QUIZ:

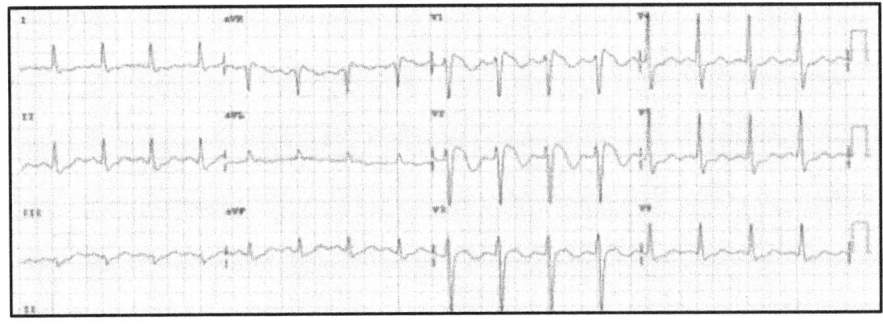

What is your diagnosis? _____

CHAPTER 8. SUPRAVENTICULAR ARRHYTHMIAS

Acute IV Drug Therapy for SVT
2015 ACC/AHA/HRS Guidelines

Ref:https://www.heartrhythmjournal.com/article/S1547-5271(15)01189-3/pdf

Drug	Initial	Subsequent
Adenosine	6 mg IV over 1-2 sec. Rapid saline flush	12 mg IV bolus in 1-2 min. 12 mg IV bolus Max 18
Esmolol	500 mcg/Kg IV over 1 min	Infusion 50-300 mcg/Kg/min
Metoprolol	2.5-5.0 mg IV bolus over 2 min	2.5-5.0 mg IV bolus in 10 min up to 3 doses
Diltiazem	0.25 mg/Kg IV bolus over 2 min	5-10 mg/h. Max 15 mg/h
Verapamil	5-10 IV boluses over 2 min	10 mg IV 30 min after the first dose. Infusion 0.0 mg/kg/min
Digoxin	0.25 to 0.5 mg IV bolus	Can repeat 0.25 mg IV up to a max of 1.0 mg over 24 given every 6 h.
Amiodarone	150 mg IV over 10 min	Infusion 1 mg/min for 6 h. 0.5 mg/min over 18 h.
Ibutilide	1 mg over 10 min. If <60 Kg, then 0.01 mg/kg. Can repeat 1 mg after 10 min.	Contraindicated if QTC > 440 ms.

CLINICAL EKG INTERPRETATION

Ongoing Oral Drug Therapy for SVT
2015 ACC/AHA/HRS Guidelines

Ref:https://www.heartrhythmjournal.com/article/S1547-5271(15)01189-3/pdf

Drug	Initial	Max Doses
Atenolol	25-50 mg QD	Max: 100 mg QD
Metoprolol Tartrate	25 mg BID	Max: 200 mg QD
Nadolol	40 mg QD	Max: 320 mg QD
Propranolol	30-60 mg daily	40-160 mg daily long-acting
Diltiazem	120 mg daily in divided doses or a single dose	Max: 360 mg daily
Verapamil	120 mg daily in AN extended release form	Max: 480 mg daily
Digoxin	0.25 to 0.5 mg PO Loading dose	Can repeat 0.25 mg PO up to a max of 1.0 mg over 24 given every 6 h. Maintenance: 0.125 to 0.25 mg daily PO
Amiodarone	150 mg IV over 10 min	Infusion 1 mg/min for 6 h. 0.5 mg/ min over 18 h.
Flecainide	50 mg Q 12 h	150 mg Q 12 h Atrial flutter
Propafenone	150 mg Q 8 h.	Max: 300 mg Q 8 h Atrial Flutter

CHAPTER 8. SUPRAVENTICULAR ARRHYTHMIAS

Ongoing Oral Drug Therapy for SVT
2015 ACC/AHA/HRS Guidelines

Ref:https://www.heartrhythmjournal.com/article/S1547-5271(15)01189-3/pdf

Drug	Initial	Max Doses	
Amiodarone	400-600 mg QD in divided doses	Max: 1200 mg QD	
Dofetilide	500 mcg Q 12 h	If CrCl > 60 mL/min	
	250 mcg Q 12 h	If CrCl 40-60 mL/min	
	125 mcg Q 12 h	If CrCl <40 mL/min	
Sotalol	40-80 mg Q 12 h	Max: 160 mg Q12 h Avoid if QTC >450 ms	
Ivabradine	5 mg BID	7.5 mg BID	

LOWN-GANONG-LEVINE (LGL) SYNDROME

- PR interval < 0.12 sec (Fig: 08.18)
- Normal QRS width
- No delta waves

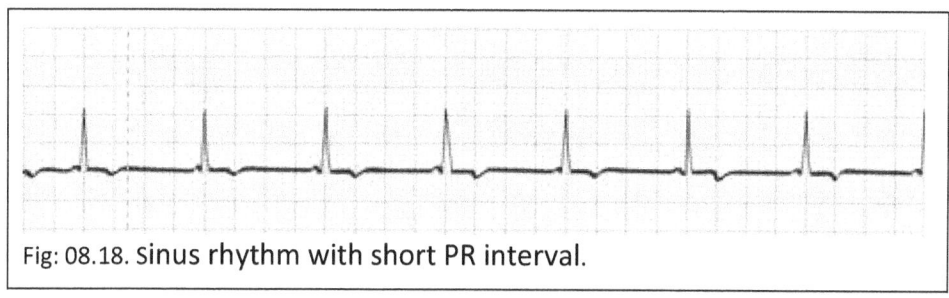

Fig: 08.18. Sinus rhythm with short PR interval.

CLINICAL EKG INTERPRETATION

COMIC RELIEF: IT IS THE PEN!

People always ask me, "Do you doctors get special training for your handwriting in the medical schools?"

I always tell my patients, "No, as a matter of fact, I had excellent handwriting before I started my medical school. But later on, they told me that I could keep either my handwriting or my medical diploma. It was a hard decision. I had to let go of my print-like handwriting. I still worry about that."

The other day, I was waiting near an elevator at the hospital. A young nurse came running down the hall. She asked, "Dr. Nikam, could you please verify this order?"

I looked at the order but I couldn't make any sense out of it. I said, "Ma'am, I have no idea what is on this order sheet. Why are you asking me?"

She said, "You are the one who wrote it!"

Come to think of it, I quite like my medical degree.

******

ACLS QUIZ:

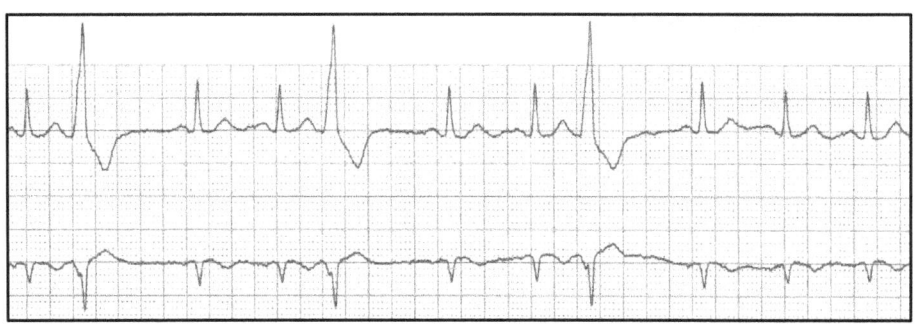

What is your diagnosis? _____

Chapter 9 Ventricular Arrhythmias

- PVCs
- Ventricular Bigeminy
- Idioventricular Rhythm
- Ventricular Tachycardia
- Ventricular Fibrillation
- Ventricular Flutter
- Agonal Rhythm

Ventricular arrhythmias are very common in everyday cardiology practice. Ventricular arrhythmias arising from the ventricle could be due to automaticity, excitation, or reentry.

Premature ventricular complexes are frequently found patients with the Cardiovascular problems the premature ventricular complexes could arise from the right or the left ventricle. Depending on the relationship between the sinus beats and the ventricular premature complexes, we can have:

- Isolated ventricular complexes
- Ventricular bigeminy
- Ventricular trigeminy
- Short bursts of ventricular tachycardia (VT)

CLINICAL EKG INTERPRETATION

PREMATURE VENTRICULAR COMPLEXES (PVC)

They are wide, with a QRS duration of >120 ms. The ST segment is sloping in the opposite direction with T wave inversions. There is a compensatory pause following the PVC before the next sinus impulse appears (Fig: 09.01).

PVCs arising from the left ventricle will have RBBB pattern, PVCs arising from the right ventricle will have an LBBB, while those arising from the septum will have a hybrid morphology.

PVCs arising from the top of the ventricle traveling toward the apex will have positive deflection in the inferior leads, which are also called the "outflow tract" PVCs. Outflow tract PVCs arising from the right ventricular outflow tract (ROVT) or the left ventricular outflow tract (LVOT) are of benign in nature.

The coupling interval refers to the interval between the PVC and the preceding QRS complex.

Multiform PVCs have varying morphology in the same lead. Generally, they are multifocal in origin and usually, represent organic heart disease.

R on T phenomenon: when the PVCS fall on the T wave of the preceding sinus beat, it is called the R on T phenomenon. It may precipitate TV or VF.

If PVCs occur more than 6 bpm, they suggest more serious underlying problems and they need to be suppressed.

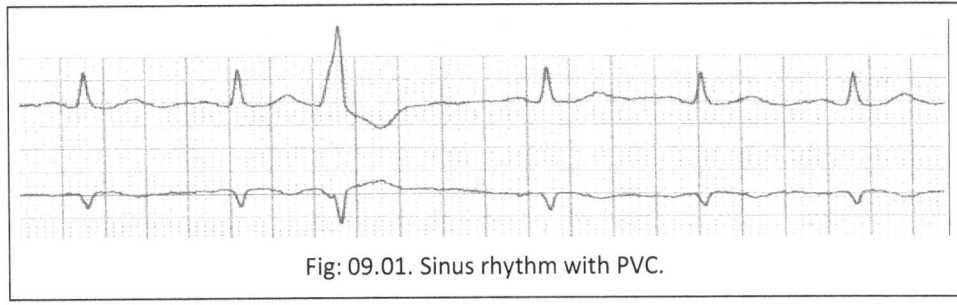

Fig: 09.01. Sinus rhythm with PVC.

CHAPTER 9. VENTICULAR ARRHYTHMIAS

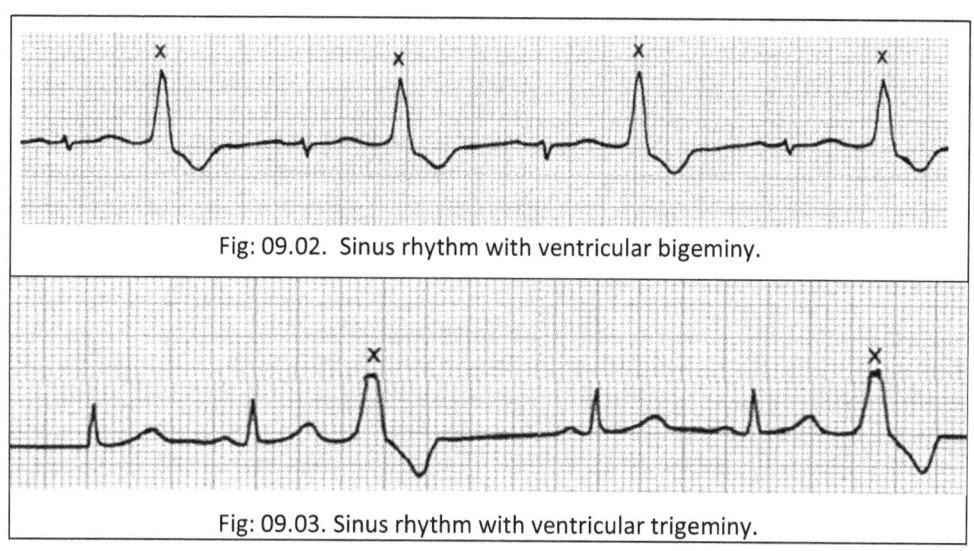

Fig: 09.02. Sinus rhythm with ventricular bigeminy.

Fig: 09.03. Sinus rhythm with ventricular trigeminy.

PVCs are very common in normal people and in people with structural heart disease. They represent increased myocardial automaticity due to stress, caffeine, drugs, and electrolyte changes such as hypokalemia or hypomagnesemia.

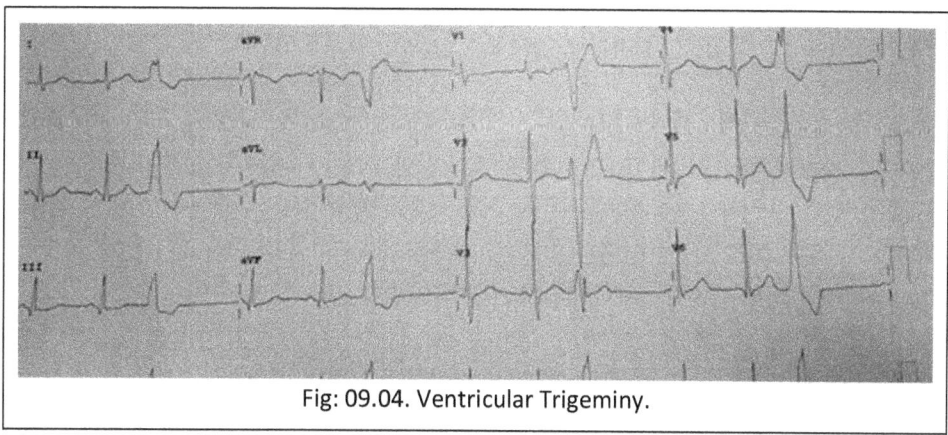

Fig: 09.04. Ventricular Trigeminy.

PVC Induced Cardiomyopathy: PVCs are ineffective beats that fail to generate significant stroke volume. Hence, very frequent PVCs (as much as 30% of total heart beats in a day) can lead to cardiomyopathy. Controlling PVCs can lead to improvement in heart failure symptoms and clinical picture.

CLINICAL EKG INTERPRETATION

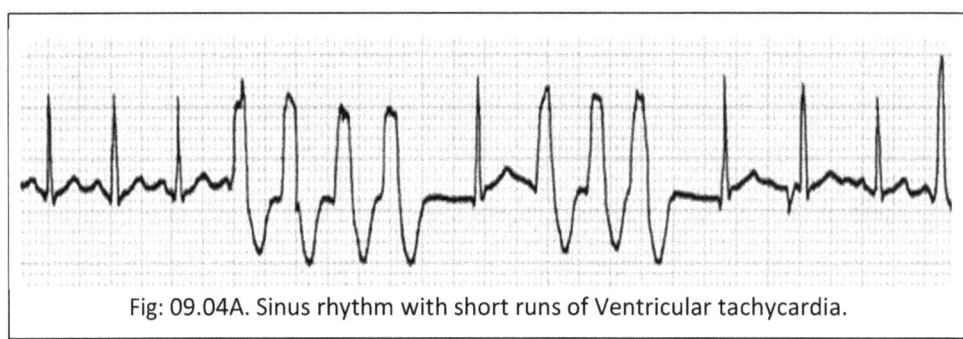

Fig: 09.04A. Sinus rhythm with short runs of Ventricular tachycardia.

The PVCs can arise from the right ventricle, which will have a LBBB pattern and the PVCs arising from the left ventricle will have a RBBB pattern.

PVCs appear earlier than the anticipated next sinus beat. PVCs originating from different foci can have varying morphology and RR intervals. They are also called multifocal PVCs, which may suggest a widespread underlying cardiac disease.

With unifocal PVCs, the RR relation between the normal beat and the PVC remain constant in each situation.

IDIOVENTRICULAR RHYTHM

It is an escape rhythm when all other sources of impulse generators fail to produce a rhythm. The rate varies from 30 to 45 bpm. It has a wide QRS morphology. This is an ineffective rate to sustain normal cardiac function. Hence, it may signal the need for a temporary pacemaker to allow time to evaluate the rest of the electrical system of the heart.

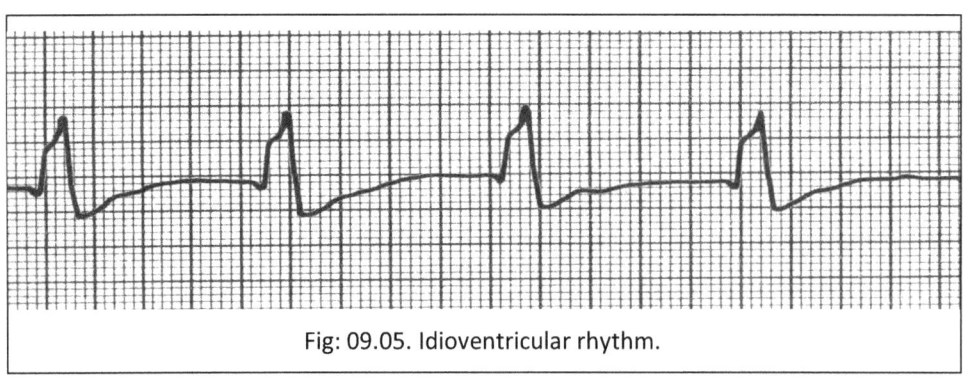

Fig: 09.05. Idioventricular rhythm.

CHAPTER 9. VENTICULAR ARRHYTHMIAS

Accelerated Idioventricular Rhythm: It is like the idioventricular rhythm, but the rate can be between 40 and 100 bpm.

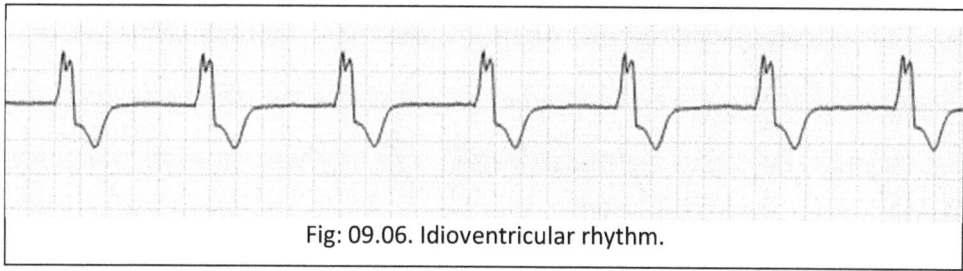

Fig: 09.06. Idioventricular rhythm.

VENTRICULAR TACHYCARDIA (VT)

It is a wide QRS rhythm. It can be paroxysmal or sustained (Fig: 09.05). If not treated promptly with DC shock, it may deteriorate into more serious ventricular fibrillation (V. Fib). They are commonly seen in acute myocardial infarction, cardiomyopathies, myocarditis, among many other conditions.

The site of origin can be guessed based on the direction of the QRS complex on a 12-lead electrocardiogram. The management of VT can be quite challenging and some patients may need the insertion of an intracardiac defibrillator (ICD) in addition to antiarrhythmics to present recurrent episodes. Most of the deaths in the early hours of myocardial infarction are due to serious ventricular arrhythmias such as VT or V. Fib.

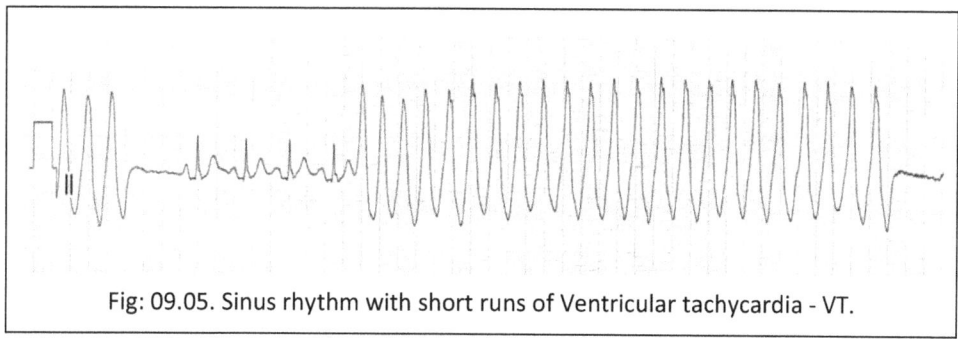

Fig: 09.05. Sinus rhythm with short runs of Ventricular tachycardia - VT.

VT is a wide QRS tachycardia varying from 150 to 200 bpm. There is P wave dissociation. We can occasionally see a captured beat where the supraventricular beat fusses with the ventricular beat and it will have a hybrid morphology. The presence of a fusion beat is another sign of VT as we don't see that in an SVT with BBB or aberration.

It is usually associated with dizziness, weakness, and sometimes syncope.

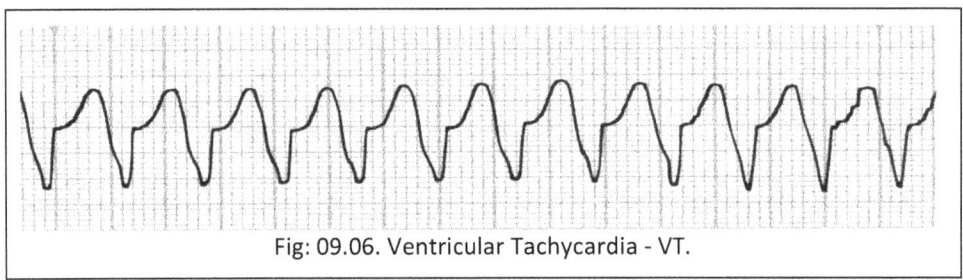

Fig: 09.06. Ventricular Tachycardia - VT.

It can lead to more serious ventricular fibrillation. Ventricular tachycardia occurs in the presence of an acute myocardial infarction and severe heart failure. It may also be seen in patients with hypertrophic cardiomyopathy and in a patient with a prolonged QT interval.

The LBBB pattern VT will have deep rS complexes in V1 with a slurred S descend and a qR pattern in V6.

The LBBB SVT will have a steep S descend in V1. There is no Q wave in V6. The R in V6 is notched.

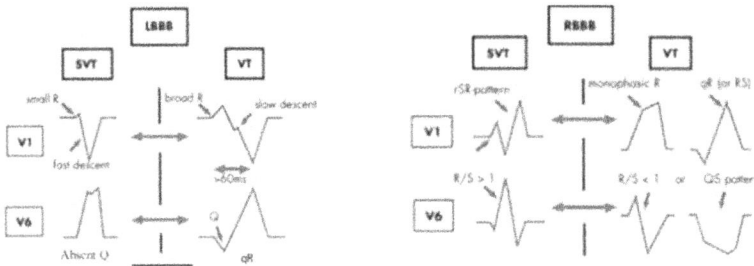

The RBBB pattern VT will have a monophasic or qR complex in V1 with a rS or qS descend in V6.

The RBBB pattern SVT may have an rSr' in V1. The V6 may show a qRs with a slurred S wave.

CHAPTER 9. VENTICULAR ARRHYTHMIAS

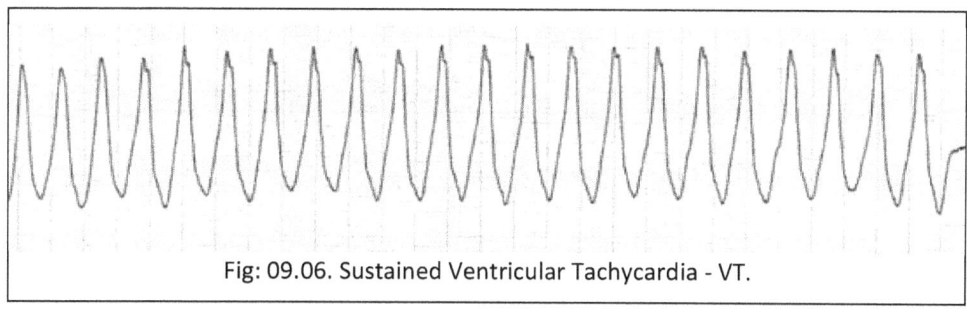

Fig: 09.06. Sustained Ventricular Tachycardia - VT.

Classification of VT

There are two types of VT: Monomorphic VT & Polymorphic VT.

Morphology
- Monomorphic
- Polymorphic
- Bidirectional

The Monomorphic VT can arise from a variety of sources:
- Scar VT
- DCM
- ARVC

Idiopathic
- Outflow tract VT
- Fascicular VT
- Other focal VTs
- Bundle branch reentry

Polymorphic VT
- Torsades de Pontes
- LQTS
- Drugs

Catecholaminergic PMVT
Ischemia

Mechanism
- Reentry
- Automaticity

CLINICAL EKG INTERPRETATION

- Triggered activity

- **Inherited arrhythmia syndromes**
    - Long QT syndrome -> Torsades
    - Short QT syndrome -> atrial fib, VT/VF, SCD
    - Brugada syndrome -> VF, SCD
    - Catecholaminergic polymorphic VT -> polymorphic or bidirectional VT during exercise/stress, SCD
    - ARVC -> epsilon waves, monomorphic VT

First, recognize the VT and differentiate it from SVT with aberration. Next, determine the site of origin of the VT. The mechanism of the VT can be determined in the EP lab, where we also can determine how the VT responds to certain maneuvers and treatment options.

Answers to these questions not only will help us to differentiate an SVT with wide QRS from real VT, but also pinpoint the underlying rhythm, initiate prompt and appropriate treatments, and stabilize the hemodynamic situation.

Recognition: It is fairly easy to spot a wide QRS tachycardia with a rapid rate. The VT is fairly regular with very minor variations. There is AV dissociation. We may see fusion bests when one of the sinus impulses manages to capture the ventricle causing a different type of QRS complex called the fusion beat.

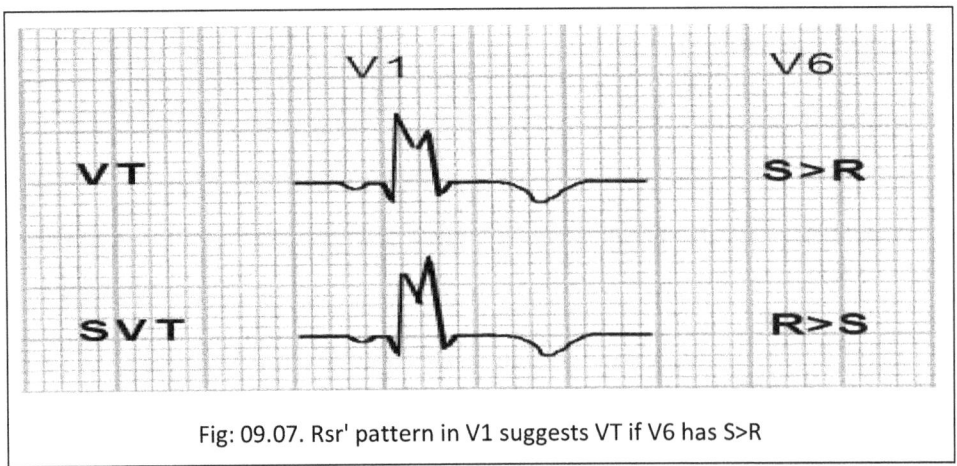

Fig: 09.07. Rsr' pattern in V1 suggests VT if V6 has S>R

CHAPTER 9. VENTICULAR ARRHYTHMIAS

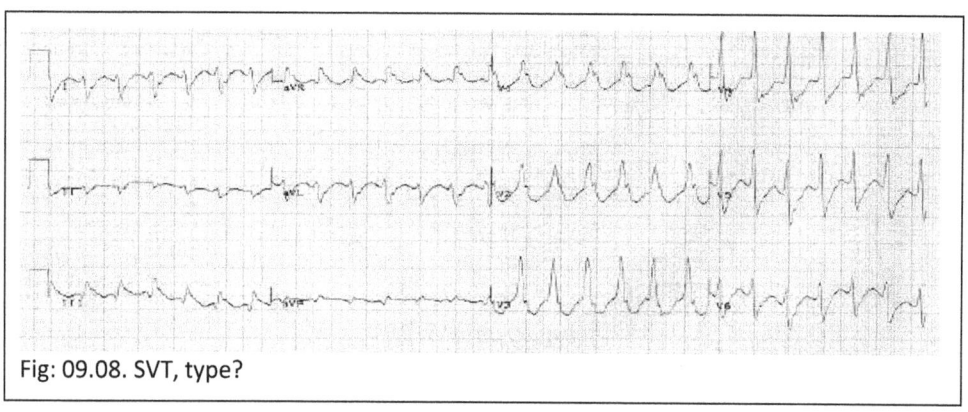

Fig: 09.08. SVT, type?

Morphology	Site of Origin
RBBB	LV Origin
LBBB	RV or Right Septal Origin
Frontal axis	
Inferior	Outflow Tract
Superior	Inferior Wall
North-West	Lateral Wall
Chest lead Transition	
QS in V6	Apical
V1 is +ve	Posterior Origin
Q V1	Septal Origin

Scar VT is a **reentrant arrhythmia**: The impulse enters the region close to the scar. Then it goes around the scar and the circuit.

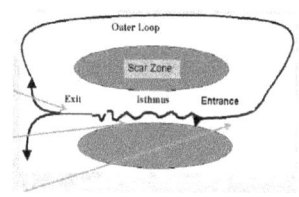

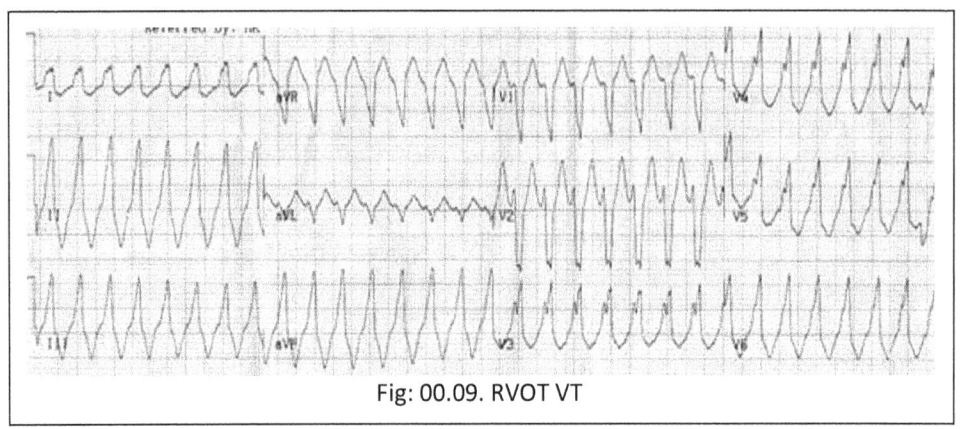
Fig: 00.09. RVOT VT

Since the SVT with aberration goes through the normally functioning bundle branch, it has a typical RBBB or LBBB pattern.

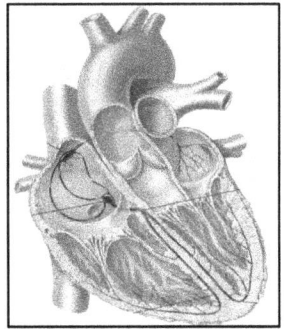

Bidirectional Ventricular Tachycardia: Occasionally, we can see a run of bidirectional ventricular tachycardia, mostly brought on by stress, exercise, or excess catecholamine (Fig.: 09.10). This VT is characterized by a 180-degree shift in the frontal plane QRS axis from one beat to the other. It may also be seen with digitalis toxicity which rare as the use of digoxin in on the decline. These patients may benefit from amiodarone.

CHAPTER 9. VENTICULAR ARRHYTHMIAS

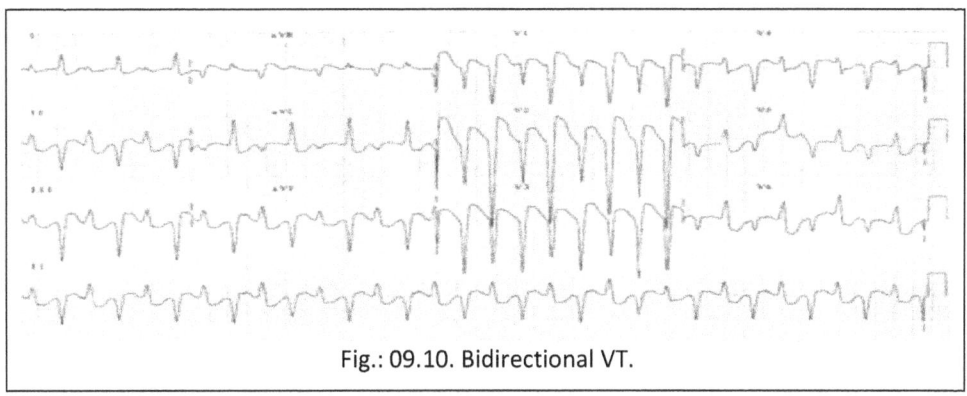

Fig.: 09.10. Bidirectional VT.

Arrhythmogenic Right Ventricular Cardiomyopathy (ARVC): This is a rare genetic disorder involving the right ventricular outflow tract, where the heart muscle is replaced by fibrofatty tissue. This leads to recurrent ventricular arrhythmias and increased sudden death risk.

The criteria for the diagnosis of ARVC include:

- Inverted T waves in V1, V2, and V3
- Epsilon wave in V1, V2, and V3
- Terminal QRS of > 55 ms from the S wave nadir to the end of QSR wave.
- Sustained or nonsustained VT with LBBB morphology and superior axis (negative QRSs in II, III, and aVF. Positive QRS in aVL).
- Sometimes sustained or nonsustained VT with RVOT configuration. LBBB pattern with positive QRS complexes in the inferior leads (Fig.:09.06).
- Frequent ventricular extrasystoles, greater than 500 in 24 hours.

CLINICAL EKG INTERPRETATION

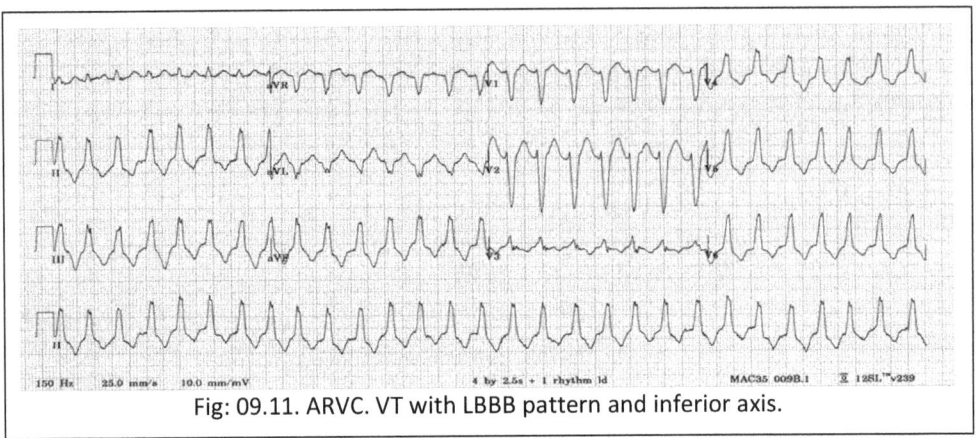
Fig: 09.11. ARVC. VT with LBBB pattern and inferior axis.

Ventricular Fibrillation: The ventricular rate is in excess of 300 bpm or more. The QRS complexes appear like a wiggly line with the fibrillatory waves varying in morphology. This rhythm is generating any blood flow. If not treated immediately with DC cardioversion, the prognosis is grim.

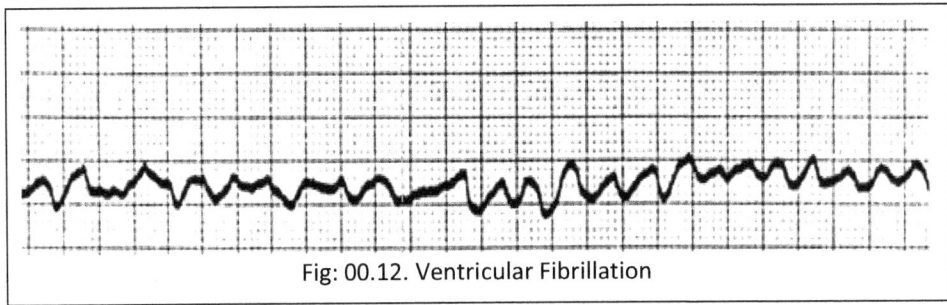
Fig: 00.12. Ventricular Fibrillation

Torsades de Pointe: This is a form of polymorphic tachycardia, which is seen in patients who are on certain antiarrhythmic drugs like quinine. It is also seen in association with hypokalemia, hypomagnesemia, and congenital long QT.

Here the QRS axis waxes and wanes. Magnesium can also be given as 1 g IV over 10 minutes.

It is also a serious rhythm problem and needs immediate DC cardioversion followed by Amiodarone IV or orally. Magnesium also can be given as 1 g IV over 10 minutes.

CHAPTER 9. VENTICULAR ARRHYTHMIAS

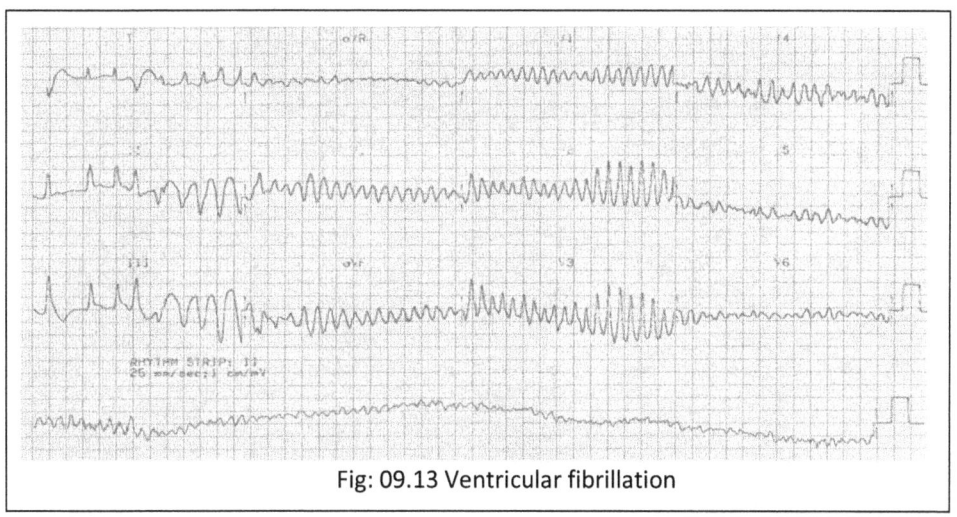

Fig: 09.13 Ventricular fibrillation

The treatment options for VT or V. Fib includes:

DC cardioversion if the patient is symptomatic – 200 to 360 watts

IV Lidocaine 50 mg bolus followed by 1-4 mg/min infusion.

Amiodarone infusion

Amiodarone 400 mg PO every 8 hours

In addition to DC shock and drugs to control VT, some patients may respond to VT ablation

Long term management includes ICD placement and in rare, focused radiation treatment.

Implantable Cardiac Defibrillators (ICD): These in patients with inducible VT and low left vernacular ejection fraction (<35%) have been shown to reduce one-year mortality by 50%. They are superior to drug treatment in preventing sudden death without the drug side effects.

Antiarrhythmic Drugs

CLINICAL EKG INTERPRETATION

Vaughan-Williams Classification	Mechanism of Action	Examples	Effect	Use
Class IA	Na-channel blockade, some K-channel blockade	Quinidine, procainamide, disopyramide	Slows conduction, prolongs repolarization	Preexcited afib, SVT, ventricular arrhythmias
Class IB	Na-channel blockade	Lidocaine, mexiletine, phenytoin	Slows conduction in diseased tissues, shortens repolarization	Ventricular arrhythmias
Class IC	Na-channel blockade	Flecainide, propafenone	Markedly slows conduction, slightly prolongs repol	Afib, aflutter, SVT, ventricular arrhythmias
Class II	Beta blockade	Metoprolol, propranolol,	Suppresses automaticity and slows AV nodal conduction	Rate control of arrhythmias, SVT, ventricular arrhythmias
Class III	Potassium channel blockade	Sotalol, amio, dofetilide, dronedarone	Prolongs action potential duration	Afib, aflutter, ventricular arrhythmias
Class IV	Calcium channel blockade	Verapamil, diltiazem	Slows SA node automaticity and AV nodal conduction	SVT, rate control of atrial arrhythmias, triggered arrhythmias
	A1 receptor agonist	Adenosine	Slows or blocks SA node automaticity and AV node condunction	Termination of SVT
	Increasing vagal activity	Digoxin	Slows AV nodal conduction	Rate control of arrhythmias

VENTRICULAR ASYSTOLE:

Here we see a straight line with an occasional ventricular complex (Fig: 09.14. The mediate action is to initiate a CPR.

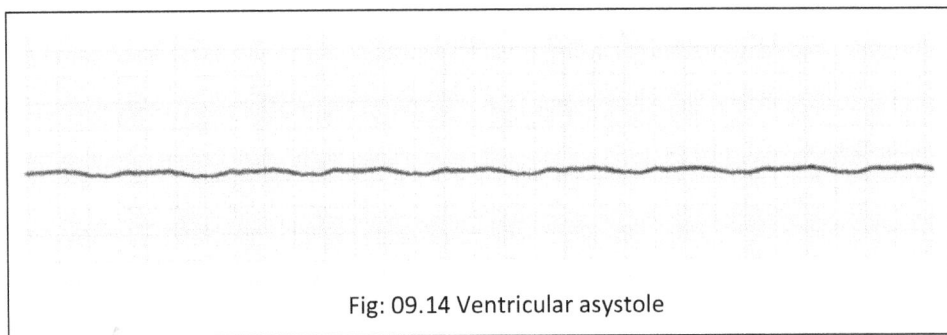

Fig: 09.14 Ventricular asystole

QUIZ:

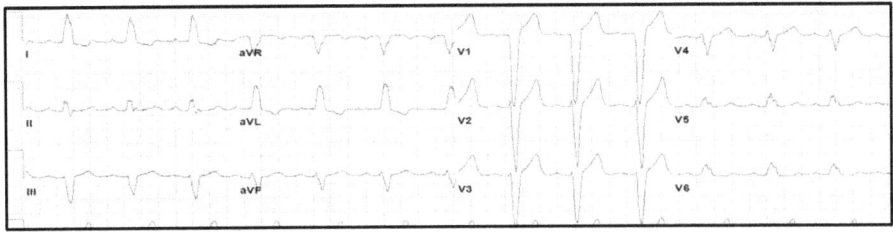

Can you list all the abnormal findings?

CHAPTER 9. VENTICULAR ARRHYTHMIAS

Asystole/PEA ACLS Protocol Summary

Asystole/PEA ACLS Protocol Summary

- ✓ CPR 2 min
- ✓ IV/IO access
- ✓ Epinephrine every 3-5 min.
- ✓ Consider advanced airway
- ✓ Capnography
- ✓ If rhythm shockable ->follow that rhythm protocol

- ✓ CPR 2 min
- ✓ Treat reversible causes
- ✓ If rhythm shockable ->follow that rhythm protocol
- ✓ If no signs of a return to a spontaneous circulation – CPR
- ✓ If ROSC – go to post-cardiac care unit.

ACLS QUIZ:

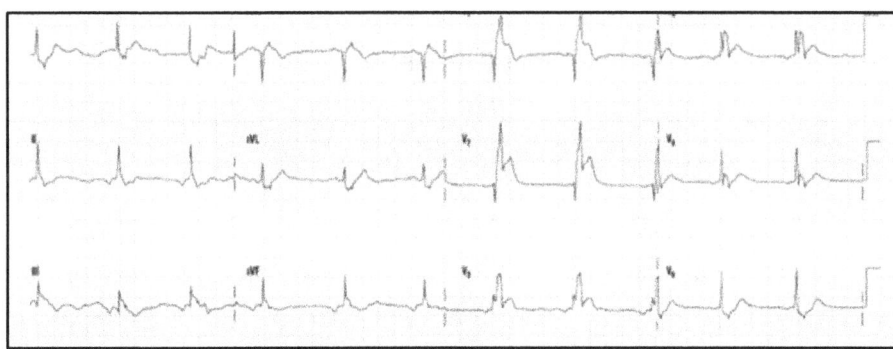

What's happening inside the heart? _____

CLINICAL EKG INTERPRETATION

DIFFERENTIAL DIAGNOSIS OF WIDE QRS TACHYCARDIA

Very often we come across a wide QRS tachycardia with a rate of 150 to 300 bpm and we are not sure if this represents ventricular tachycardia or supraventricular tachycardia with aberration or underlying bundle branch block. The treatment option for each could be different and could be deleterious to the others. Hence, it is essential to take a systematic approach to arrive at a correct diagnosis in short order.

	Supraventricular	Ventricular
Rate	160-300	160-250
Irregular	Atrial Fib Atrial Flutter MAT WPW	V. Tach
Regular	Junctional Atrial Tachycardia	V. Tach
Fusion Beats	No	YES
Carotid Pressure	May Reveal Atrial Activity	No Response

First, we need to ascertain whether the patient is stable or unstable. If the patient is unstable with hypotension, hypoxia, or symptoms, the right treatment is a DC shock to restore a stable rhythm. Then, we can work on the possible origin of the wide QRS tachycardia.

Once, the patient is deemed stable, the next thing we need to focus on the rate. The faster the ventricular rate, the more urgency in establishing the diagnosis.

Once, you determine the underlying site of origin of the tachyarrhythmia, the long-term treatment options, and preventive measure can be contemplated.

CHAPTER 9. VENTICULAR ARRHYTHMIAS

Differential Diagnosis of Wide QRS Tachycardias

Supraventricular tachycardia with ventricular aberration can present as VT on the first glance. Point to look for:

- Hunt down the little pal P waves.
- Where is the little Ps? Could they be missing in atrial fibrillation?
- Is the P wave up or down? Anterograde or retrograde condition
- What is the relationship between the wide QRS and the little Ps?
- Was there an underlying BBB, which could explain SVT wide QRS complexes?
- What are the patient's clinical presentation, vital signs, and perfusion?
- Is there a rate dependent ventricular aberration causing wide QRS tachycardia?
- Is there a Delta Wave (WPW)?
- VT more likely when the interval between R and S is >100ms
- The irregular RR interval is suggestive of SVT
- AV dissociation with RR<PP interval is a hallmark of VT
- Typical RBBB or LBBB QRS morphology more likely SVT

Atrial Fibrillation with Aberration: If the person has an underlying RBBB or LBBB, and develops a rapid ventricular rate, it will look like a V. tach. When you see an irregularly irregular ventricular response, it should be a clue to the underlying atrial fib mechanism. It is uncommon for V. Tach to show so much RR variability. Also, the QRS morphology may vary from beat to beat which is not the case with V. Tach. The presence of old BBB may be useful. However, sometimes a BBB may be rate dependent. Hence, slowing the ventricular response may help to determine if the BBB is rate dependent. It also helps to establish the Atrial Fib diagnosis.

If the patient is stable and cardioversion is needed, synchronized cardioversion can be attempted. Note, that sometimes, the atrial fib and atrial flutter may coexist on the same tracing. The key is to first, stabilize the patient, slow the ventricular response with drugs, and then work on restoring normal sinus rhythm if that was the baseline rhythm. While cardioverting if the rhythm deteriorates to V. flutter or fib, an immediate shock is warranted.

Atrial Flutter with Aberrant Conduction: We see this from time to time and it is important to know what the rhythm and QRS morphology were before the patient developed the atrial flutter with a rapid ventricular response.

If the patient is stable, vagal maneuvers can slow the ventricular rates and uncover the flutter waves. Once atrial flutter diagnosis is established, we can follow the atrial flutter protocol to reduce the ventricular rate, first. Then, look at the possibilities for reestablishing the sinus rhythm. If the atrial flutter is chronic, it may not be possible.

The ultimate treatment option for these patients will be RF ablation of the accessory pathway. As you recall, the RF ablation of atrial flutter has more than 95% success rate and must be the choice of treatment not only for the arrhythmia, but also in for preventing atrial fibrillation and worsening heart failure symptoms. Always look for the underlying rhythm before the patient developed before the current episode began. How has the patient's response has been in the past? What worked and what did not work. All this information can greatly enable prompt diagnosis.

Multifocal Atrial Tachycardia: This is commonly seen in patients with congestive heart failure or chronic obstructive pulmonary disease (COPD). Hence, history could be an important clue to the origin of wide QRS irregularly irregular tachycardia. Since the arrhythmia arises from multiple excitable foci, the P wave morphology will be highly variable. The QRS morphology may also be variable from beat to beat depending on the refractory period of the previous cycle. This highly irregular tachycardia makes it unlikely to be V. tach, which is fairly regular. Again, by slowing the rate, you may be able to unravel the mystery.

Atrial Tachycardia (AT): AT, with its regular rhythm and wide QRS morphology may be indistinguishable from VT. Once, you have addressed the acuteness of the condition, look for a history of tachyarrhythmia in the past. Look at past EKGs for any evidence for BBB. Scan the rhythm trips before and

CHAPTER 9. VENTICULAR ARRHYTHMIAS

after the termination of similar but short runs. If they are preceded by frequent PACs, it could be a clue to an ectopic atrial origin. On the other hand, if there we frequent PVCs, it could point more in favor of VT. Try vagal maneuvers to slow the ventricular rate and look for P waves. Look at the medication list and see if the patient has been on digoxin and if so, consider digitalis toxicity producing AT. If you do see definite P waves before each QRS complex, it would be safe to try intravenous drugs used to terminate the AT. If that is unsuccessful, electric cardioversion could be attempted.

WPW with Tachyarrhythmia: This will be similar to atrial fibrillation with a very rapid ventricular response and very irregular RR intervals. The main differentiating points will be irregular RR intervals, varying QRS morphology and history of WPW in the past, or on the EKG strips before the arrhythmias started. It is of paramount importance to differentiate the WPW tachyarrhythmias from any other SVT as the drugs used in the SVT may make the WPW rhythm worse. Remember that IV procainamide is the only drug that slows the conduction through the accessory pathway and slow the ventricular rate is WPW patients. Of course, in the long run, RF ablation is the most definitive way to abolishing these life-threatening arrhythmias. Sometimes, the ablation has to be done more than once to freeze all the accessory pathways.

Junctional Tachycardia: It could be a real challenge as there are no definite P waves preceding the QRS complexes. Since they can respond to drugs affecting the AV node, it is important to look for any sign of P wave even if they are retrograde or appear after each QRS complex.

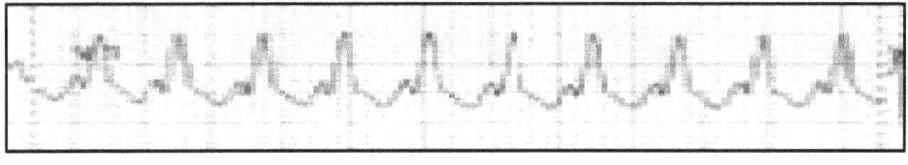

What is the rate and rhythm? _____

CLINICAL EKG INTERPRETATION

Ventricular Tachycardia (VT): Ventricular tachycardia (VT) is an ectopic rhythm that can develop anywhere along the right or the left ventricles or its conduction system.

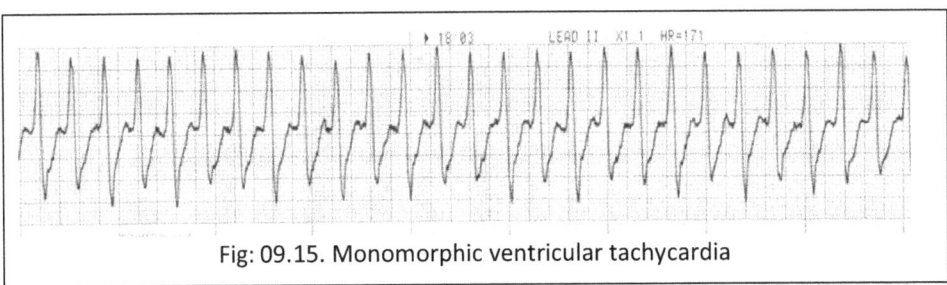

Fig: 09.15. Monomorphic ventricular tachycardia

Unlike the SVT, the VT is a life-threatening arrhythmia, especially, if it is sustained, as there is no effective cardiac output during VT. In addition, the arrhythmia has a tendency to suddenly deteriorate into Torsades de Pointe or ventricular flutter and fibrillation, leading to cardiac arrest. Hence, time is of the essence in establishing a diagnosis and initiating prompt treatment. If in doubt, perform DC shock and then sort out the points after establishing a stable rhythm. Whether the VT arises from the left ventricle or right ventricle is for a Monday morning debate. Establishing adequate circulation and perfusion by abolishing the VT should be the first order of business.

The second order of the business is to prevent it from happening again. That means we need to explore all the circumstances that lead to the VT, to begin with. Begin with a careful history, a complete physical examination, non-invasive studies such as EKG, event monitors, nuclear stress test, Echocardiogram, and complete lab studies. Correct all the metabolic and electrolyte disturbances. If there is evidence for stress-induced ischemia, cardiac catheterization and revascularization should be considered. If the arrhythmia is frequent, electrophysiological studies can be performed to look for inducible VT. If inducible VT found or if the ejection fraction is less than 35%, an ICD must be strongly considered.

CHAPTER 9. VENTICULAR ARRHYTHMIAS

NIK NIKAM AS AN AUCTIONEER

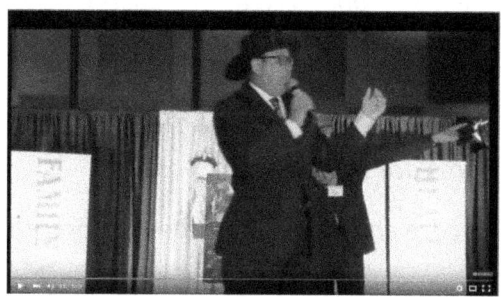

The auction is another passion of mine.

Ladies and gentlemen, let's start with 100

Do I hear a bid for 200, 200

Can you give me 200?

Who can give me 200?

The bid is on 200, 200,

Ok, now, we've 200.

200, now bidding 300, 300.

ACLS QUIZ:

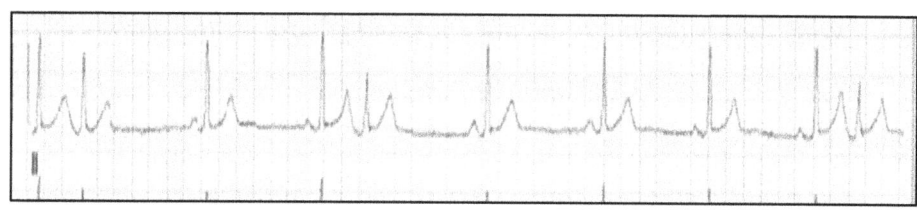

Concerned? _____

CLINICAL EKG INTERPRETATION

LAUGHTER THE BEST MEDICINE: CHEST PAIN?

A patient of mine was in the emergency room with chest pain. I examined him, looked at the EKG, and asked, "Hi Jason, what brought you to the hospital?"

He pointed the finger at his wife.

"What symptoms are you having?" I asked

"Chest pain, severe chest pain, shortness of breath, and sweating," as he grabbed his chest.

"Jason, do you know you are having a heart attack!"

"Are you asking me or are you telling me that I'm having a heart attack? You are the cardiologist! Don't you know how to read an EKG?

"Yes, I do, Jason, I'm telling you, you are having a heart attack, and this is the third one in less than a year. What's going on here?"

"She is the reason I am having the third heart attack!" As he pointed the finger at his wife, Sarah.

Sarah snapped back, "Yes, I'm the one sitting there smoking, eating greasy food, sipping Martinis, and skipping the medicines."

"No kidding, Sarah!" I joked.

Sarah said, "If I were not there when he had his first heart attack, he would have been dead, without my CPR."

"Now, what do you say to that?" I asked Jason.

"Well, that is the price you pay for saying, 'I do,' at the altar!"

"Are you sure? At this moment in your life, you need Sarah more than anyone else."

Jason said, "What I meant to say is, 'Yes, ma'am, I agree with you 100% if you just let me live my life!'"

"There you go again!" I said.

Chapter 10 Ischemia and Infarction

- Coronary Anatomy
- Acute Myocardial Infarction
    - ASMI
    - ALMI
    - IMI
    - Posterior MI
    - Right Ventricular MI

- Ventricular Ischemia
- Subendocardial Ischemia
- Giant Negative T Waves
- Nonspecific T Wave Changes
- Nonspecific ST-T Changes

As coronary artery disease accounts for more than 95% of the general cardiology practice, it is very important to master the EKG changes related to coronary artery disease, especially, myocardial ischemia and infarction.

CLINICAL EKG INTERPRETATION

CORONARY ANATOMY:

Knowledge of coronary anatomy is seminal to the understating of the electrocardiographic changes during an acute myocardial infarction, and at sites remote from the acute event. Acute myocardial infarction results from a total occlusion of a coronary artery or one of its branches. The location of the changes relates to the territory supplied by that branch. So, the electrocardiographic changes occur in a related group of leads that represent the area supplied by a coronary artery or one of its branches.

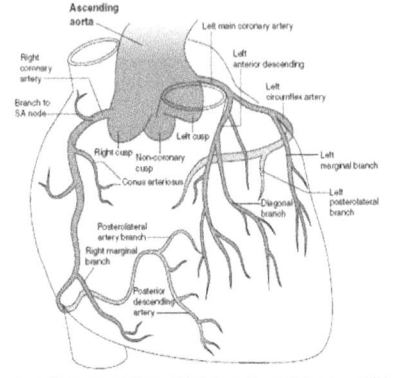

Left Main Coronary Artery: It arises from the left coronary cusp. It divides onto the Left Anterior Descending branch (LAD) and the Circumflex branches.

Left Anterior Descending Branch (LAD): It travels through the anterior interventricular groove toward the left ventricular apex. It wraps around the apex and supplies the tip of the left ventricle. It gives rise to the diagonal branches, which supply to the high anterior wall of the left ventricle. Hence, occlusion of a diagonal branch can reflect changes in I and aVL leads. The distal diagonal branches also supply the anterior and lateral walls of the left ventricle.

The LAD also gives rise to the septal branches which supply the interventricular septum. Occlusion of a proximal segment of a LAD can result in changes involving the lead I and aVL, along with changes in the anterior leads V1 to V6, depending on the area supplied by the LAD. If the LAD supplies the anterior wall, the septum, and the lateral wall, the changes related to its occlusion can be extensive. On the other hand, if mid LAD is occluded the changes may be more localized to the anteroseptal wall (V1 to V4). Similarly, if the distal LAD is blocked the changes may be localized to the lateral wall involving V5 and V6 (Fig: 10.01).

CHAPTER 10. ISCHEMIA AND INFARCTION

Also, as the proximal LAD supplies the interventricular septum, its occlusion leads to blockage of the left or the right bundle branches and such changes may suggest the location of the blockage and the prognosis, based on how proximal the blockage is.

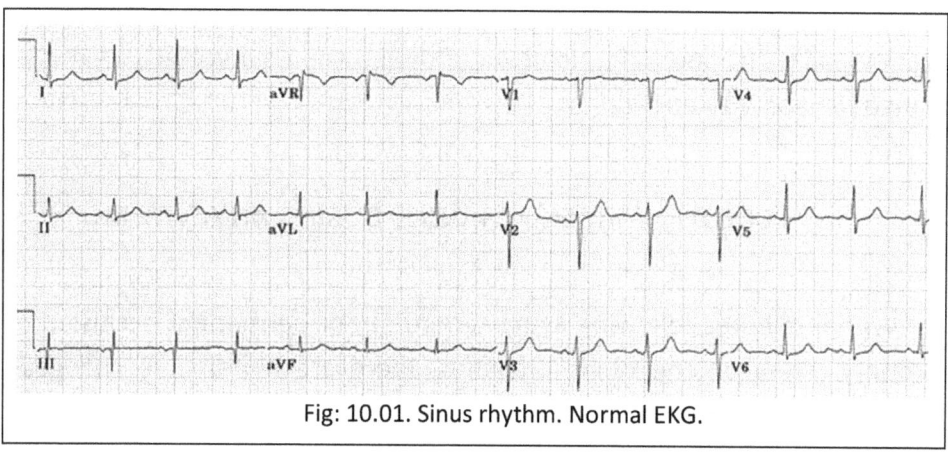

Fig: 10.01. Sinus rhythm. Normal EKG.

The Circumflex Branch: It arises from the Left Main and travels along the left atrioventricular groove and join the distal right coronary artery at the crux on the back of the heart. It gives rise to 2-3 marginal branches which supply the lateral wall of the left ventricle. Occlusion of the circumflex trunk or one of its branches can lead changes reflected in leads V4-V6.

In 15% of the cases, the circumflex trunk gives rise to the Posterior Descending Artery (PDA), which supplies the inferior wall of the left ventricle. When this artery is blocked, it can result in changes not only in the inferior leads (II, III, and aVF) but also in the lateral chest leads (V5 and V6). So, a combination of EKG changes can help us understand which coronary artery is the likely culprit and what more changes we could expect to see as the acute myocardial infarction evolves.

The Right Coronary Artery (RCA): The RCA arises from the right coronary cusp. It gives rise to the sinus node branch and the acute marginal branches. It travels through the right atrioventricular groove toward the crux of the heart where it joins the distal circumflex artery. RCA gives rise to the main branch, the Posterior Descending Artery (PDA), which supplies to the inferior wall of the left ventricle and sometimes the apex of the left ventricle.

CLINICAL EKG INTERPRETATION

As the RCA supplies the Sinus node, it is not uncommon to see bradyarrhythmia, when a proximal RCA is occluded. In addition, in 30% of the cases, the proximal RCA occlusion also can result in Right Ventricular wall infraction which can pose a different set of challenges in patient management. The changes related to occlusion of the RCA are localized to the interior wall (II, III, and aVF). However, if the LV apex is involved, we may see changes in lead V3V and V_4.

EVOLUTIONARY EKG CHANGES DURING AN ACUTE MI

Within minutes following acute temporary or permanent occlusion of a coronary artery or one of its branches, there are hyperacute changes of ischemia characterized by 'J' point elevation along with the ST segment.

The ST Segment: The ST segment elevation can vary from 2 to 10 mm from the baseline. If the ischemia is transient, these changes may revert to normal following the relief of acute ischemia. If the ST-segment elevation is due to total occlusion of a coronary artery, it may show progressive changes. The ST segment elevation also lifts the T waves from their baseline resulting in Hyperacute T waves, which are sometimes called, "Tombstone T waves".

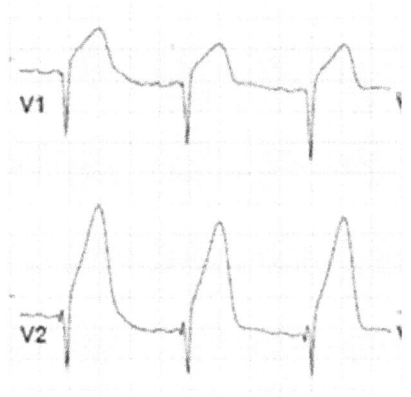

The ST segment may remain elevated for several hours depending on the extent of the MI. After 4-6 hours, the tall hyperacute T waves begin to invert. The ST segment may remain elevated for several days, even as the T waves become deeply and symmetrically inverted. The ST segment should return to baseline in 2-6 few weeks (Fig: 10.02).

CHAPTER 10. ISCHEMIA AND INFARCTION

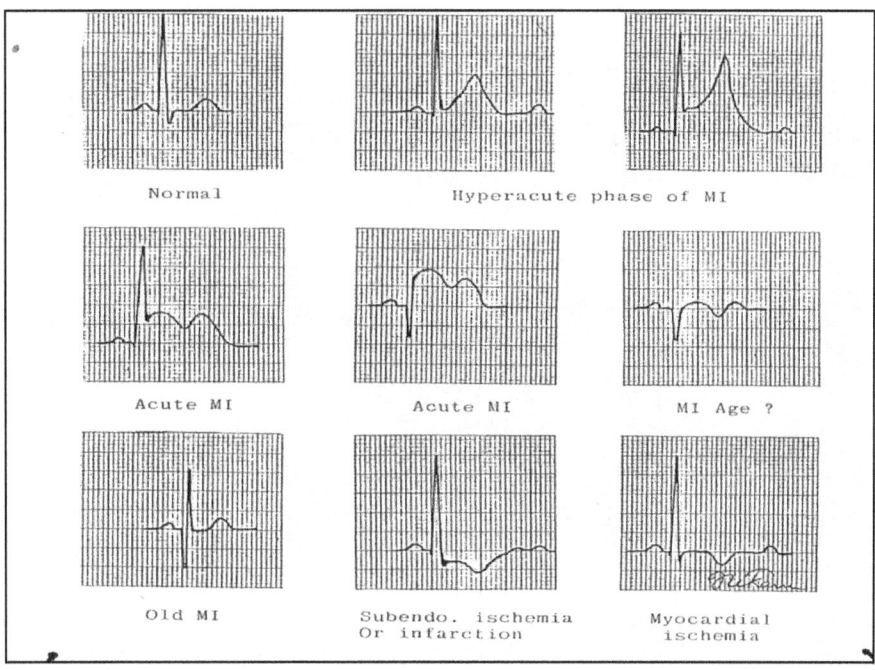

Fig: 10.02. Evolutionary changes of an Acute myocardial infarction and ischemia.

QRS Complexes: As the QRS complex reflects the electrical activity of the myocardium, the changes seen in the QRS complex are more permanent and it begins with the development of Q waves, a negative deflection in the opposite direction of the original QRS complex.

The Q waves appear approximately 6 hours after the onset of an acute MI. These Q waves are called pathological waves and are due to permanent necrosis of the myocardial tissue, which is eventually replaced by a scar tissue over a 6-week period. The Q waves develop in related lead groups like II, III, aVF, or V1 to V4, or V1 to V6, or I and aVL.

The Q waves become deeper as the R waves lose their amplitude. Eventually, the deep Q waves may completely replace the R waves, resulting in a QS complex. The Q waves resulting from myocardial necrosis are greater than 40 ms in duration and greater than 25% of the R waves as a contrast to the tiny Q waves related to the initial septal activation, which are less than 40 ms in duration.

In 15% of the cases, the R waves may reappear over a period of several months, even though their amplitudes may be much less compared to that of

CLINICAL EKG INTERPRETATION

the original R waves. So, the presence of R waves doesn't rule out an old myocardial infarction.

Based on the ESC and ACC guidelines:

Definition of a Pathologic Q Wave
- Any Q-wave in leads V2–V3 ≥ 20 ms or QS complex in leads V2 and V3

- Q-wave ≥ 30 ms and > 0.1 mV deep or QS complex in contiguous leads
    - I, II, & aVF
    - I, aVL, & V6
    - V4–V6

- R-wave ≥ 40ms in V1–V2 and R/S ≥ 1 with a concordant positive T-wave in the absence of a bundle branch block.

Notes

- An absence of pathologic Q waves does not exclude a myocardial infarction!
- Lead III often may have Q waves that are not pathologic as long as Q waves are absent in leads II and aVF (the contiguous leads)

Ischemic abnormalities in patients with no known history of myocardial infarction based on Novacode:

- High risk of ischemic injury/ Q wave MI:
    - Major Q waves: Q >= 50ms or Q >= 40 ms & Q greater than 25% or the R wave.
- Moderate risk of ischemic injury or possible Q wave MI:
    - Q >= 30 ms and ST deviation > 0.20 mV (minor Q waves with ST-T changes)

CHAPTER 10. ISCHEMIA AND INFARCTION

LV Aneurysm: It is characterized by persistent ST-segment elevation of more than 2 mm in the anterior or lateral lead, 6 weeks following an acute myocardial infarction. The ST segment may display convex or concave morphology. It is also associated with well-defined Q waves from the previous myocardial infarction. The T wave may have a smaller amplitude compared to the QRS complex.

LOCATION OF MYOCARDIAL INFARCTION

The myocardial infarction is usually localized to certain regions depending on the coronary artery or one of its branch's involvement.

LOCATION	ARTERY	LEADS
High Anterior MI	DIAG	I, aVL
Anteroseptal MI	LAD	V1-V4 (Fig: 10.03)
Lateral MI	LAD OR CIR	V5 to V6
Anterolateral MI	LAD	V1 to V6
Inferior MI	RCA OR CIR	II, III, and aVF. (Fig: 10.04)
Inferoapical MI	RCA	II, III, aVF, V3, and V4
Posterior MI	RCA OR CIR	V1- V3 R waves, ST ↑ and T ↑

Here is an example of a cross section of the left ventricle as seen on a 2D echocardiogram. From the orientation, it is easy to understand the location of the left ventricular segments.

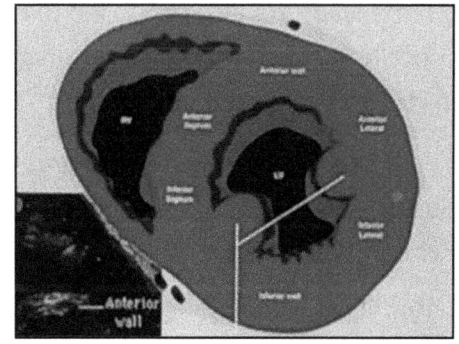

V1 and V2 represent the interventricular septum and also the right ventricle.

V3 and V4 represent the LV anterior wall &

V5 and V6 represent the LV lateral wall.

Of course, we don't see the high anterior wall which is higher up and is represented by I and aVL.

Anterior Wall MI: There is a lot of confusion regarding the terminology used by various authors in describing the location of an anterior infarction.

What someone calls a high anterior infarction may be called a high lateral infarction. In either case, they both are referring to occlusion of one of the proximal diagonal branches. They produce changes in lead I and aVL.

As to which leads represent the septum, the anterior wall, or the lateral wall, there is more confusion. First, if you see changes in the leads V1 to V6, it represents extensive anterior infarction and is likely related to occlusion of a proximal LAD.

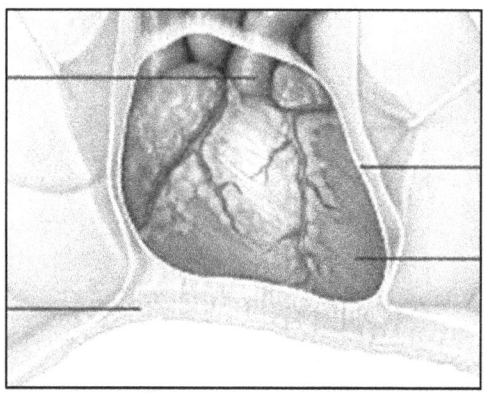

The actual orientation of the heart in the mediastinum is such that the right ventricle sits anterior to the left ventricle. The interventricular septum is behind the right ventricle and hence represented by lead leads V1 and V2. The anterior wall is located toward the left, which may be represented by leads V3 and V4. The same leads are also supposed to represent the left ventricular apex. Most LAD occlusion distal to the first diagonal branch results in anteroseptal MI with changes reflected in the leads V1 to V4.

The lateral MI produces changes in leads V5 and V6. This can result from occlusion of a large distal diagonal branch of a LAD or marginal branches of the circumflex artery.

Whenever we are dealing with an acute anterior MI, we need to anticipate certain future events that can challenge the patient's hemodynamics and lead to complications in due course. When the proximal LAD is occluded, it can lead to loss of LV systolic function by 30% to 40%. That can lead to cardiogenic shock and subsequent heart failure. The interventricular septum involvement can damage the conduction system,

CHAPTER 10. ISCHEMIA AND INFARCTION

leading to either the right or the left bundle branch block. The new onset left bundle branch block in the presence of an acute anterior MI carries a poor prognosis. In some cases, these bundle branch blocks could advance to complete heart block necessitating a need for a temporary or even a permanent pacemaker.

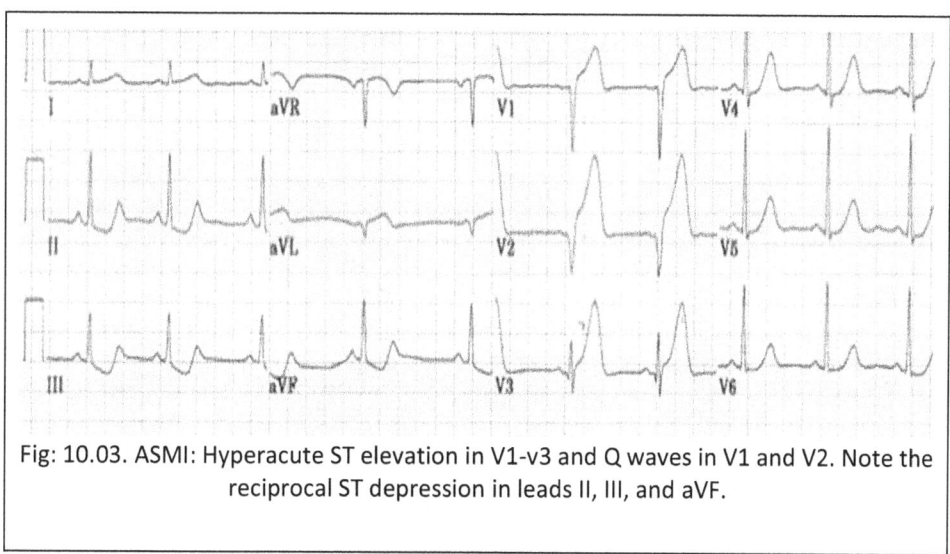

Fig: 10.03. ASMI: Hyperacute ST elevation in V1-v3 and Q waves in V1 and V2. Note the reciprocal ST depression in leads II, III, and aVF.

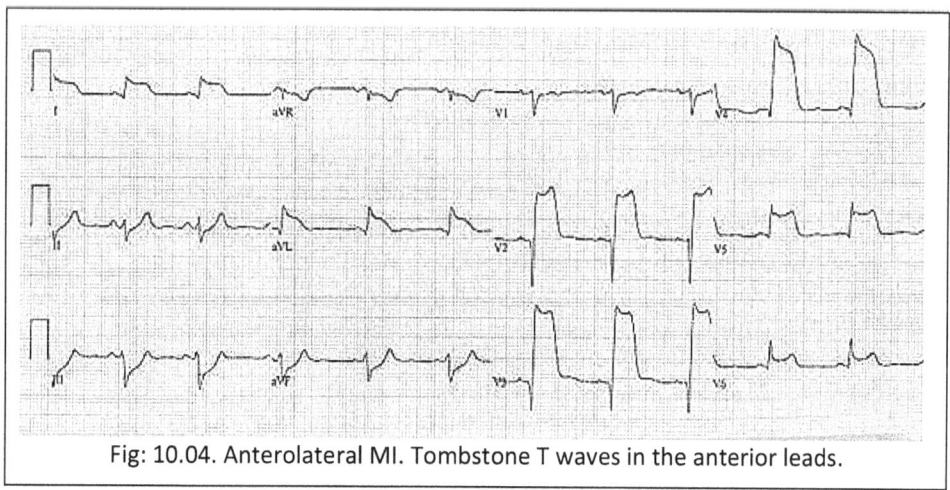

Fig: 10.04. Anterolateral MI. Tombstone T waves in the anterior leads.

CLINICAL EKG INTERPRETATION

Anterolateral MI: It Involves leads I, aVL, V2-V6. These hyperacute ST-T changes are referred to as Tombstone T waves, as they signify grave prognosis due to the extensive nature of the area involved (Fig: 10.05).

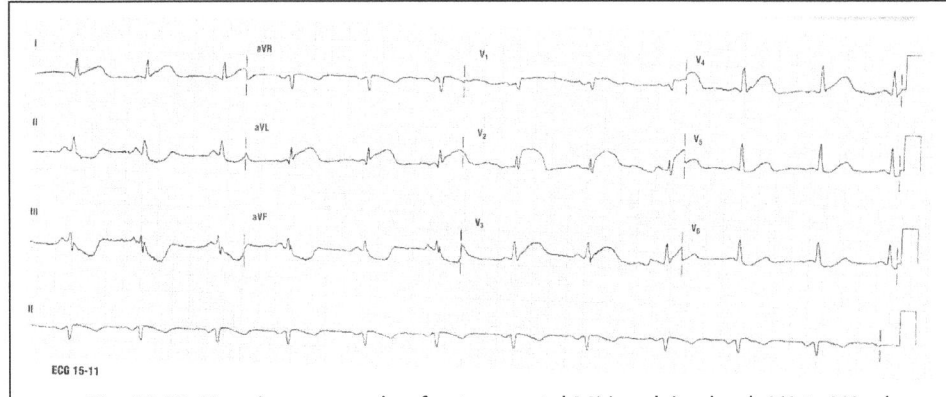

Fig: 10.05. Here is an example of anteroseptal MI involving leads V1 to V4, along with high anterior or lateral wall as we see changes in I and aVL. Note the reciprocal changes in leads II, III, and aVF.

The acute changes seen in V2-V6 in acute anterolateral MI are actually huge ST elevations. This ST pattern is technically a monophasic current of injury. When a needle used for pericardiocentesis, touches the epicardium, you will see a similar ST-T pattern. These changes may be mistaken for a bundle branch block. However, as the hyperacute ST elevation evolves, you will begin to appreciate the true nature of the QRS complex.

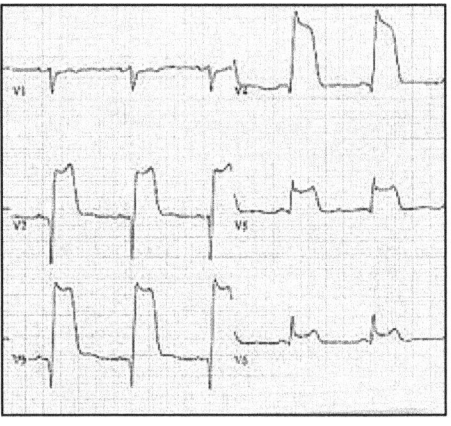

Inferior Wall MI: The Inferior wall MI poses its own challenges. We need to be cognizant of complications such as bradycardia, junctional rhythm,

CHAPTER 10. ISCHEMIA AND INFARCTION

hypotension, or involvement of the right ventricular wall. Anticipate and recognize them when they appear, and treat them appropriately.

Since the right coronary artery supplies the sinus node, you can anticipate bradyarrhythmia or even, accelerated junctional rhythm. In fact, the accelerated junctional rhythm which could last for several days may not have any significant long-term implications.

In addition, an absence of an atrial contribution can lead to reduced cardiac output that may require vasopressors for blood pressure support.

Right Ventricular Infarction: The proximal RCA occlusion may lead to right ventricular infarction. The ST-T changes can be appreciated by recording the right chest leads V1R to V6R, like that of the left chest leads. Look for ST elevation of >1 mm in the right leads (Fig: 10.06). As many as 30% of the patients with inferior myocardial infarction may have some degree of right ventricular infarction.

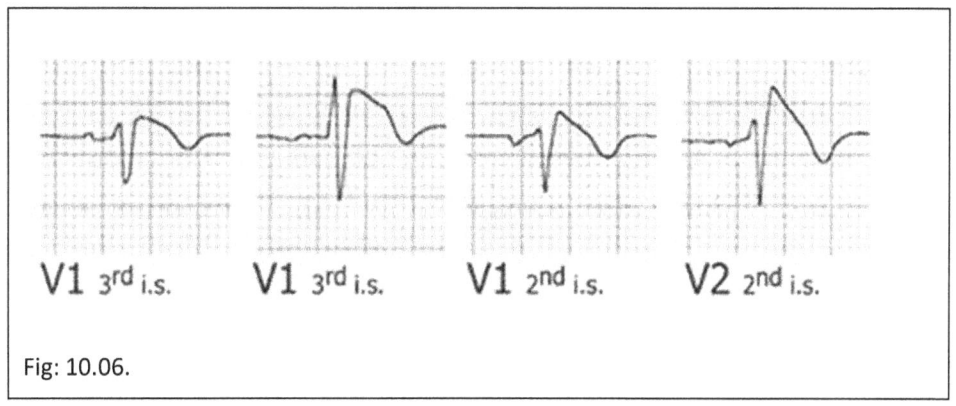

Fig: 10.06.

The hallmark of right ventricular infarction is persistent hypotension in the absence of pulmonary congestion. Confirming the presence of right ventricular infarction by an EKG and an Echocardiogram can aid us in appropriately treating these patients with volume expansion and vasopressors for several days, until the heart recovers.

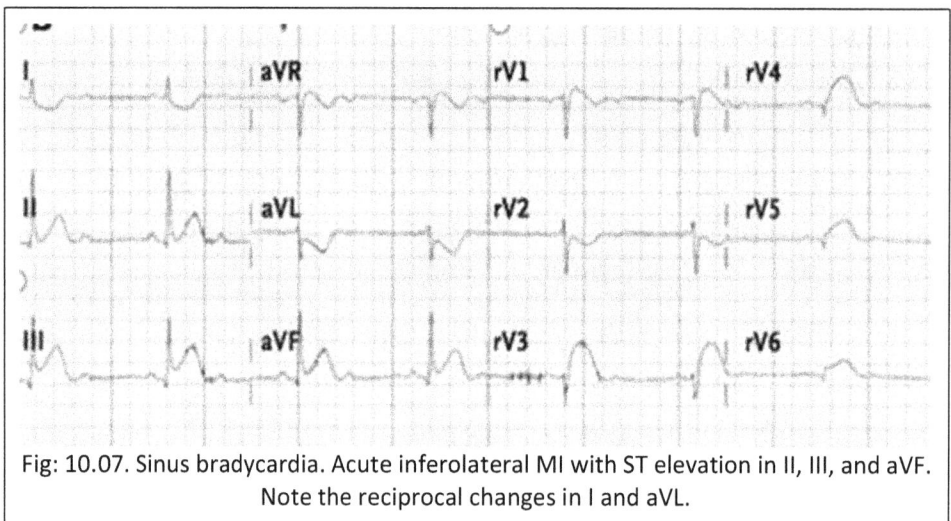

Fig: 10.07. Sinus bradycardia. Acute inferolateral MI with ST elevation in II, III, and aVF. Note the reciprocal changes in I and aVL.

Look for conduction disturbances like Wenckebach or complete heart block. Some clinical clues could include elevated jugular venous pressure or an unexpected drop in blood pressure following nitroglycerin administration.

Posterior Infarction: The posterior infarction usually happens in conjunction with IMI, and is characterized by R waves in V1 to V3, ST depression and upright T waves. It also can occur in association with lateral infarction when the circumflex artery is involved (Fig: 10.08).

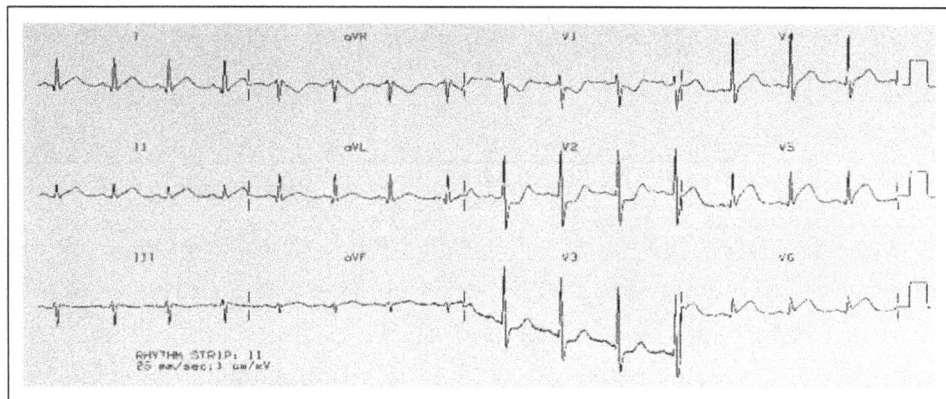

Fig: 10.08. Sinus rhythm with posterior MI with Tall R waves in V1 to V3 along with ST depression. Inferolateral ST elevations are also present.

CHAPTER 10. ISCHEMIA AND INFARCTION

Occasionally, the posterior infarction can be an isolated event, and if we do not pay close attention to the EKG, we could misinterpret the changes in leads V1 to V3 as something else. However, with a classical presentation of chest pain, elevated cardiac enzymes, and these subtle changes, we should be thinking about possible posterior infarction. More than likely the infarction is related to the occlusion of the posterolateral branch of the RCA or one of the distal marginal branches of the circumflex trunk. The amount of myocardial damage is considerably less compared to that of a damage from occlusion of a major branch.

Non-Q Wave Infarction or NSTEMI: This refers to a heterogeneous group of conditions that manifest with elevated cardiac markers like the cardiac enzymes without the evidence for classic ST-segment elevation, Q waves, and loss of R waves.

ST-T Changes: Horizontal ST depression in 2 or more leads suggests subendocardial ischemia. This can be seen in the anterolateral leads or the inferior leads. These ST changes are different from the ones we see with ventricular hypertrophy or BBBs where the ST segments are slightly downsloping with T wave inversions. The Horizontal ST depression is more suggestive of ischemia compared to Up-sloping or down-sloping ST depression.

If these ST-T changes are associated with normal cardiac enzymes, they are presumed to represent subendocardial ischemia, while those associated with elevated cardiac enzymes represent subendocardial infarction (Fig: 10.09). In either case, they represent significant ischemia in a given region and may have a potential for more events down the line. Hence, once the clinical condition stabilizes, it is prudent to perform a nuclear stress test to determine the extent of reversible myocardial ischemia and direct plan accordingly.

CLINICAL EKG INTERPRETATION

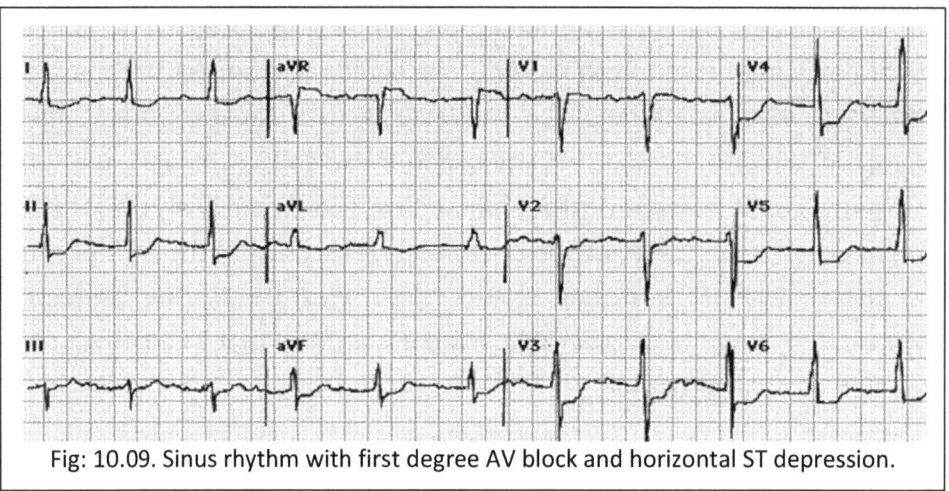

Fig: 10.09. Sinus rhythm with first degree AV block and horizontal ST depression.

T Wave Changes: The T waves normally represent the ventricular repolarization. The changes in T wave morphology also can represent left ventricular strain or ischemia. Usually, we see T wave inversion in the presence of the BBB, which is considered to represent the strain pattern resulting from subendocardial hypoperfusion due to elevated end-diastolic pressure (Fig: 10.10).

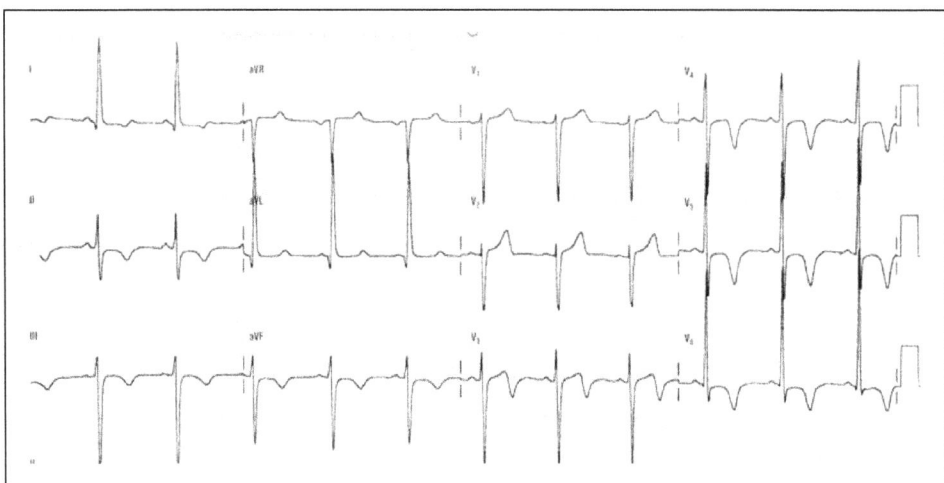

Fig: 10.10. Sinus rhythm with inferolateral T wave inversion. There are voltage criteria for LVH. The ST-T changes represent LVH with strain.

However, it is not uncommon to see symmetrically and deeply inverted T wave in the presence of global left ventricular ischemia. If there is an

CHAPTER 10. ISCHEMIA AND INFARCTION

associated cardiac enzyme elevation, it may represent subendocardial infarction (Fig: 10.11).

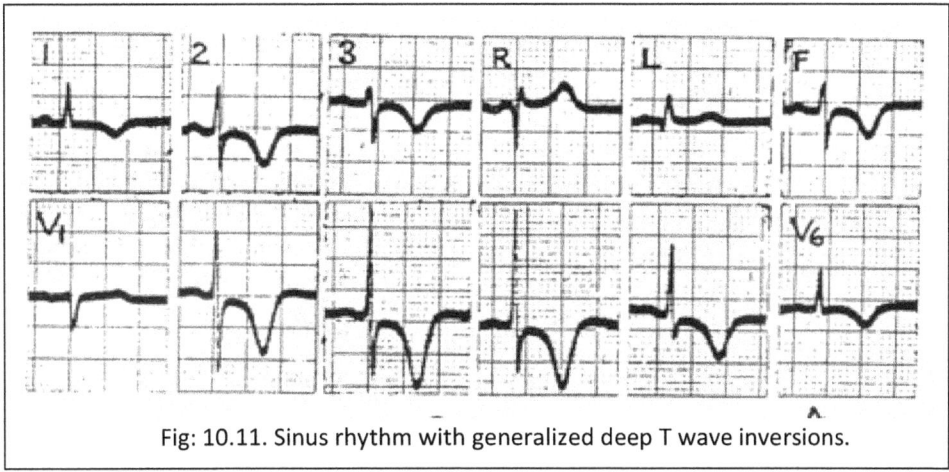

Fig: 10.11. Sinus rhythm with generalized deep T wave inversions.

Occasionally, we may see Giant negative T waves, which may signal cerebrovascular accident or global left ventricular ischemia (Fig: 10.12).

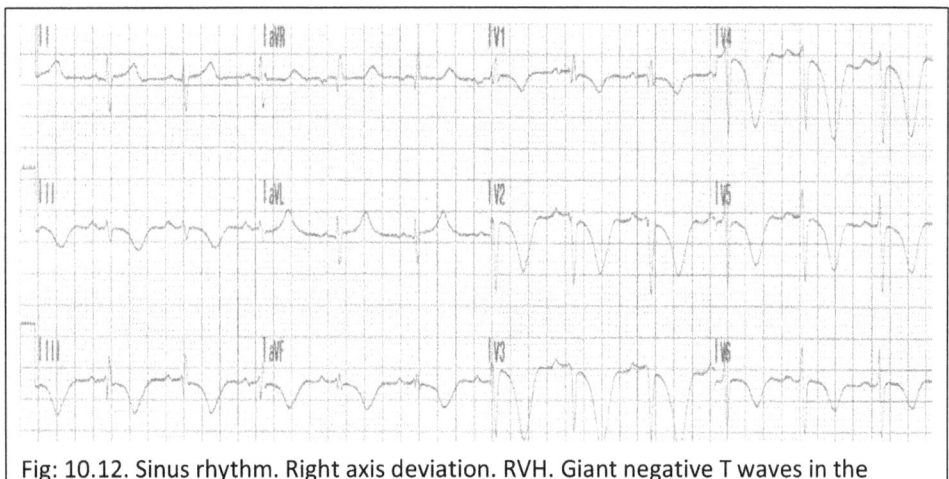

Fig: 10.12. Sinus rhythm. Right axis deviation. RVH. Giant negative T waves in the inferior and anterolateral regions.

More often, we see minor T wave inversions, biphasic T waves, or flat T waves. These are grouped into Nonspecific ST-T changes (Fig: 10.13).

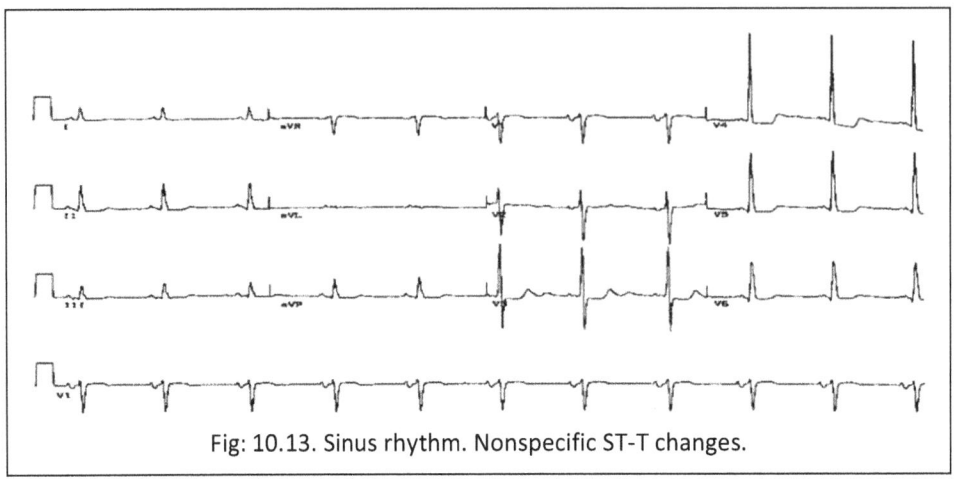
Fig: 10.13. Sinus rhythm. Nonspecific ST-T changes.

Hypothermia: The electrocardiogram features include Osborne Waves (J waves) along with prolongation of the PR, QRS, and QT intervals. These patients are at an increased risk for ventricular premature beats (PVCs). They may have a cardiac arrest due to VT, VF, or asystole (Fig: 10.14).

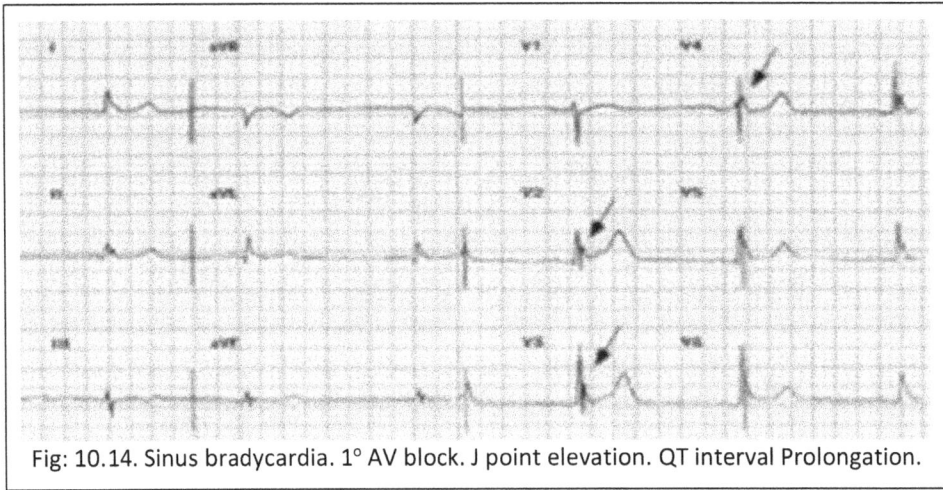
Fig: 10.14. Sinus bradycardia. 1° AV block. J point elevation. QT interval Prolongation.

De Winter ST T waves: The electrocardiogram features include 1-3 mm Upsloping ST depression with upright T waves in the anterior leads, which may suggest acute proximal left anterior descending artery occlusion (Fig:10.15).

CHAPTER 10. ISCHEMIA AND INFARCTION

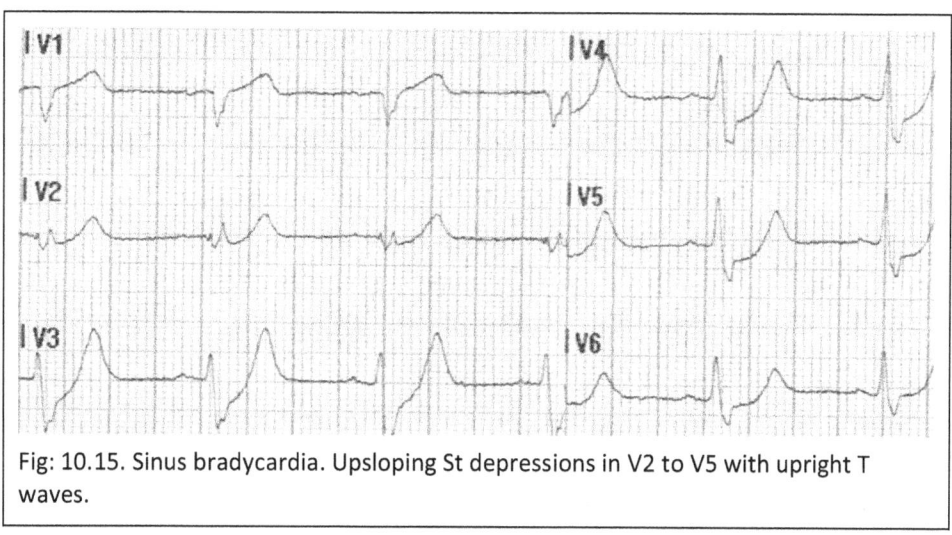

Fig: 10.15. Sinus bradycardia. Upsloping St depressions in V2 to V5 with upright T waves.

Old and New Infarctions: As we focus on an acute ischemic event, we also need to look for other evidence for coronary artery disease such as an old myocardial infarction. For example, when we are dealing with an acute anterior MI, an old inferior wall myocardial infarction can have an overall impact on the patient's recovery, as the new infarct can add insult to the old injury (fig: 10.16).

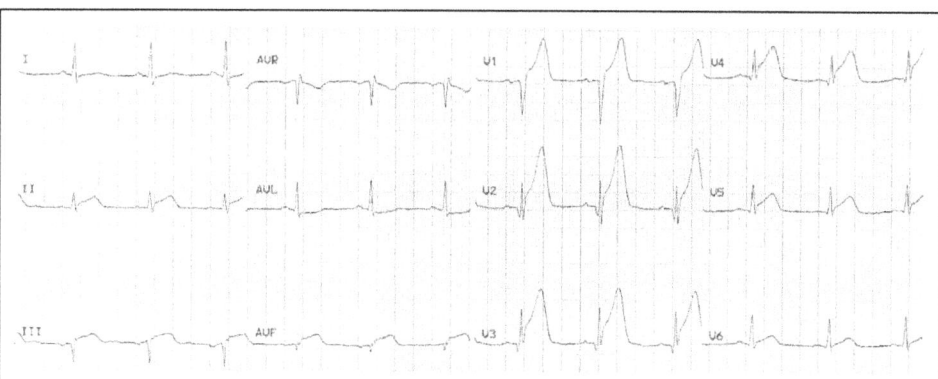

Fig: 10.16. Sinus rhythm. Acute inferior and anterolateral MI. Reciprocal changes are seen in aVL. Notice the presence of Q waves in the inferior leads, even though we see a hyperacute change in the chest leads.

Here is an example of an acute anterior MI in the presence of QS complexes in leads III and aVF. There is also an ST elevation which may suggest recurrent ischemia.

CLINICAL EKG INTERPRETATION

SILENT MYOCARDIAL INFARCTION

As the title indicates the myocardial infarction is silent. The patient may have not noticed any symptoms in the past. However, the electrocardiogram may show clear evidence of an old myocardial infarction. It is more common in diabetics, who may have pain perception problems. We also need to make sure that we are not dealing with lead misplacement. Patients with advanced COPD may have QS complexes as the overexpanded lung tissue may overlap the heart on the left side.

Differential Diagnosis of Acute MI
- Hyperkalemia
- Pericarditis
- LBBB, Anterior ST elevations
- COPD
- WPW
- LAHB

ACLS QUIZ:

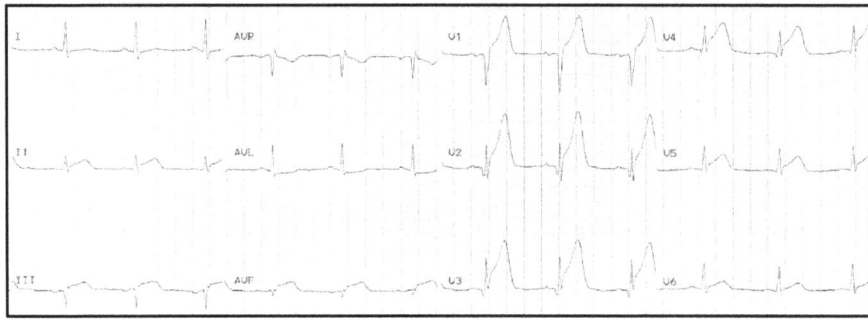

Spot diagnosis

CHAPTER 10. ISCHEMIA AND INFARCTION

NIK'S COMEDY BLOCK (NCB):

Heart Surgery-ICU

One of my patients had heart surgery. He was in the ICU. The nurse taking care of him said, "Mr. Underwood, how are you doing? Your surgery is over. You are doing fine."

"Where am I? Why are all these monitors beeping?"

"Oh! That's just your heart monitor, oxygen monitor, temperature monitor, urine monitor, and mood monitor."

"If I'm fine, why are they all sounding the alarm at the same time? Anyway, what is this place?"

"Mr. Underwood, you are in the ICU."

He said, "I see you too. In fact, I see two of you! Could you please call my doctor?"

The nurse turned to another nurse and said, "Could you please watch my patient."

She told the patient, "Mr. Underwood. I'll bring some tranquilizer; you will be okay. Just relax."

He said, "Just a minute ago you told me I was fine. What changed your mind? What's this tube doing in my chest? And, why is it red?"

"It's called the chest tube. It is draining the blood from your chest cavity."

"Oh God! I had heard the doctors are bloodsuckers. But, I never thought that I would live to see that with my very own eyes."

"Anything else I can do for you, Mr. Underwood?"

"How long I am going to be here?"

"At this rate, not very long!"

"Oh My Lord, I'm coming, I'm coming."

CLINICAL EKG INTERPRETATION

NIK'S COMEDY CLUB:

One day, I was getting ready to do a heart catheterization on a patient. The nurses were taking a little longer to get him ready. I walked up to him and said, "Mr. John, you've been waiting for this test for a long time, haven't you?"

"Yes, Dr. Nik, 72 years! Don't you think that's a long time to be waiting for this one test?"

"I see what you mean," I said.

"Have you done this before?"

"No, you are my first patient."

"What?"

"I, meant today!"

"You better get moving. If you are not ready in 5 minutes, I'm going to put you on the table and start the procedure myself."

ACLS QUIZ:

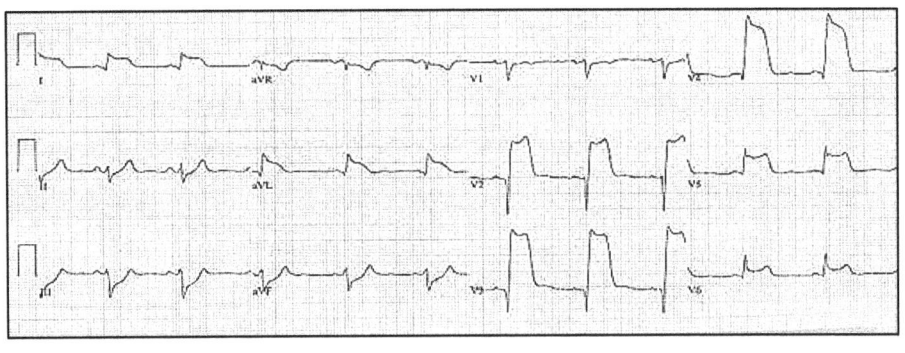

Concerned? _____

Chapter 11 ST Segment Abnormalities

ST Elevation

- ST Elevation with Acute MI
- Normal Variation
- Early Repolarization
- ST Elevation with LBBB
- St Elevation with Pericarditis
- J point Elevation
- Left Ventricular Aneurysm

ST Depression

- Horizontal ST Depression
- Downsloping ST Depression
- Upsloping ST Depression
- Nonspecific ST-T Changes.
  - Reciprocal ST Depression in Acute MI
  - Subendocardial Ischemia v. Infarction

The ST segments can be involved in a variety of conditions, most notably in the setting of an acute myocardial infarction. The ST segment is generally isoelectric and it appears between the QRS complex and the T wave. The point at which the ST segment begins is called the 'J' point. It is not unusual to see 1 mm ST elevation leads V2 and V3 in most electrocardiograms.

ST ELEVATION

Acute Myocardial Infarction: The hallmark of acute myocardial infarction or ischemia is the hyperacute ST elevation. The 'J' point is lifted from the baseline. The ST segments slant upward and blend with the upstroke of the T waves. The ST elevation can range from 2 mm to 10 mm or more. The ST segment elevation is usually localized to a region of the myocardium like the inferior wall, the anterior wall or the lateral wall. Correspondingly, the ST elevation may be seen in II, III, and aVF, or V1 to V4 or I, aVL, and V5-V6. Along with the ST elevation, there is reciprocal ST depression in the opposite leads (Fig: 11.01).

The ST segments may remain elevated for several hours to days. Eventually, they return to the baseline. In rare cases, if the ST segments remain elevated after 4-6 weeks, we should consider a left ventricular aneurysm

The acute ST elevation may sometimes be associated with reciprocal ST depression in the opposite leads. However, when you see ST depression as the primary findings, you do not see a reciprocal ST elevation in the opposite leads. When you do see ST depression in a group of leads check the other leads for any ST-T changes.

Here, the treatment option is between immediate cardiac catheterization and possible PCI for an acute MI versus conservative treatment for subendocardial ischemia or myocardial infarction based on the cardiac enzymes. A patient with ST depression may need more studies before they leave the hospital, but it doesn't warrant an emergency STEMI approach.

This important distinction will help you to identify what is the primary mode of ischemia presentation.

CHAPTER 11. ST SEGMENT ABNORMALITIES

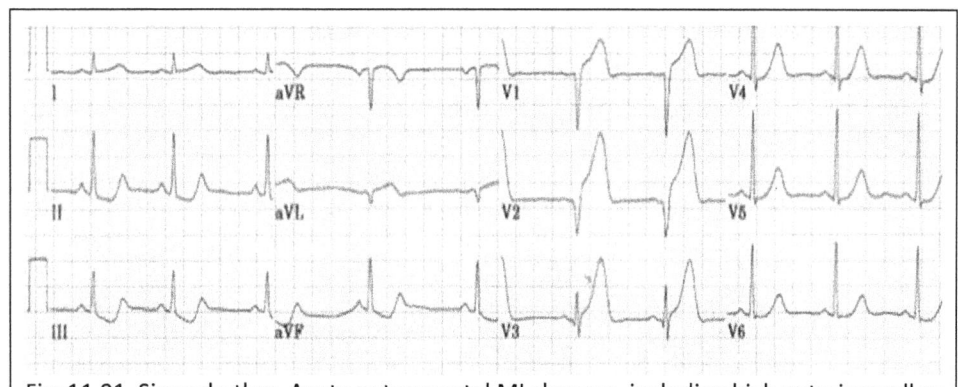

Fig: 11.01. Sinus rhythm. Acute anteroseptal MI changes, including high anterior wall as we see an ST elevation in I and aVL. There are reciprocal changes in leads II, II, and AVF.

Early Repolarization: In young people, we could see a concave ST elevation of 1 mm across the electrocardiogram, which is considered a normal variation or early repolarization.

In early repolarization, the J point is lifted from the baseline. The ST segment is up-sloping and continues as the upstroke of the T waves. The ST elevation can be seen in limb leads and also in the precordial leads (Fig:11.02).

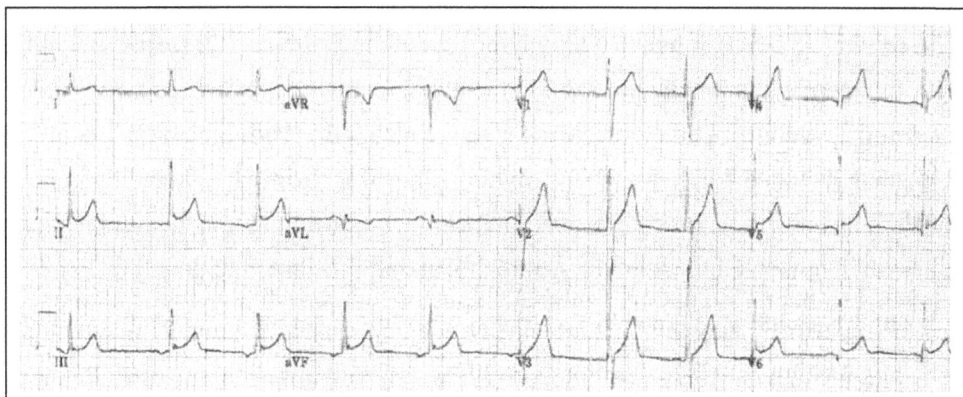

Fig: 11.02. Sinus rhythm. There is ST elevation in leads II, III, and aVF, and to some degree in the chest leads V4, V5, and V6. There is also a slight ST elevation in lead I. The ST segment is concave upward. This is an example of early repolarization.

Pericarditis: Pericarditis causes generalized ST elevation across the entire electrocardiogram. The ST segment elevation can vary from 2 to 10 mm in height. There is an elevation of the J point. The ST segment is concave in nature. The T waves are concordant with the ST segments. There is ST depression in aVR and V1. It is also associated with PR segment depression, which is not the case in early repolarization (Fig: 11.03).

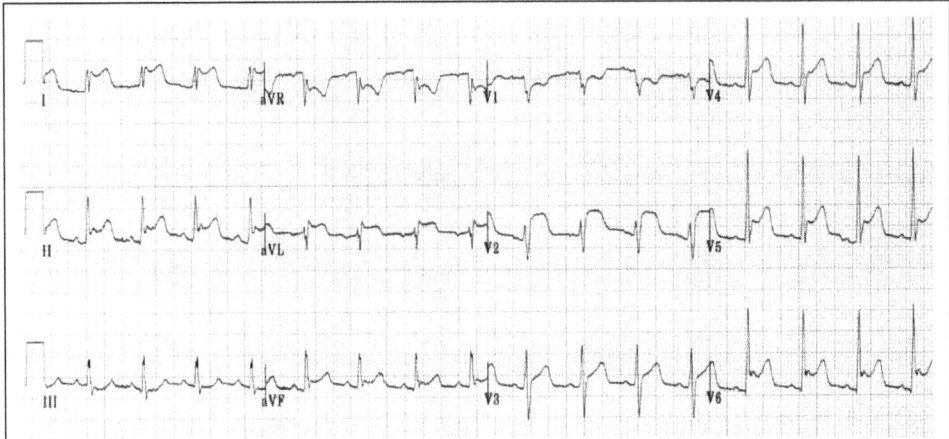

Fig: 11.03. There is a diffuse ST elevation in most leads except aVR and V1. The J point is lifted from the baseline. Note the PR depression, which is another sign of pericarditis. PR depression is not a feature of early repolarization.

The ST-T changes seen in acute pericarditis are due to an inflammation of the epicardial layer of the myocardium. Since pericarditis is generalized, the positive ST-T changes are also generalized and diffuse. Occasionally, when the pericarditis is localized, the ST-T changes may be limited to the involved segment. When the pericarditis is localized, the changes may be indistinguishable from an acute myocardial infarction. However, the course of these ST-T changes are dictated by the underlying pathology. In the case of pericarditis, these changes may persist until the inflammation subsides.

Pericarditis may also resemble the early repolarization seen in young people. However, these patients may be asymptomatic and their previous electrocardiograms may display a similar pattern, whereas in patients with pericarditis the electrocardiogram before and after the pericarditis may be normal. Patients with early repolarization may also have tall T waves in many leads.

As the pericarditis evolves, the ST segments eventually return to baseline along with T wave inversion. After several days, the T waves return to the baseline (Fig:11.04).

CHAPTER 11. ST SEGMENT ABNORMALITIES

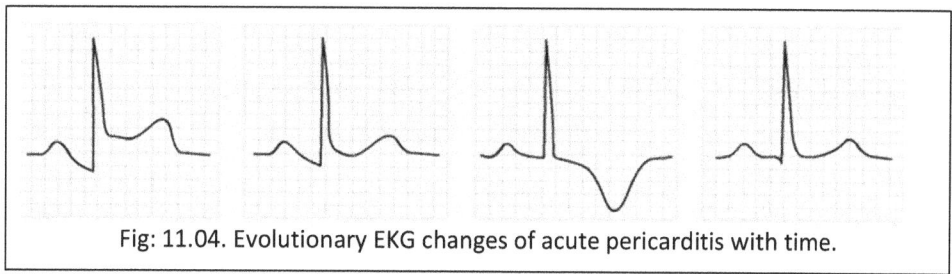

Fig: 11.04. Evolutionary EKG changes of acute pericarditis with time.

However, if there is a development of pericardial effusion, some classic ST-T changes may not be seen. In addition, there may be a loss of QRS voltage due to the fluid around the heart. Another feature that may suggest pericarditis with effusion is the *electrical alternans*.

Pericarditis With Pericardial Effusion
- **Diffuse ST** Segment Elevation
- **Low QRS** Voltage
- **Electrical** Alternans, Where Alternate Beats Have Different Amplitudes

ST DEPRESSION

ST Changes in LBBB: As you can see in the electrocardiograms below, it is not unusual to see an ST-segment elevation in leads V1 to V3 which blends with the T waves. Along with that, you may also see ST depression in I, aVL, and lateral chest leads (Fig: 11.05).

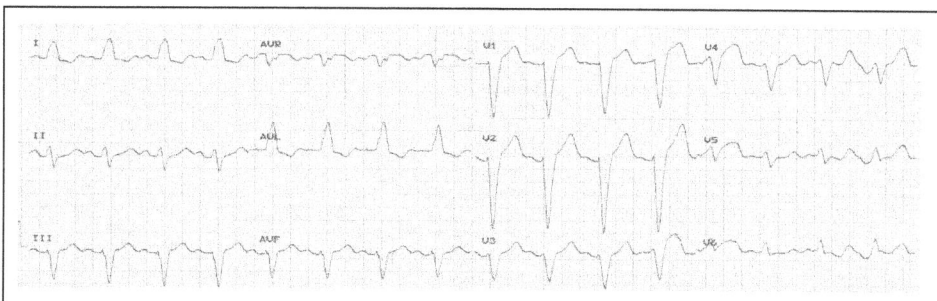

Fig: 11.05. Left bundle branch block is associated with ST-T changes. There is ST elevation noted in V1 to V3, which may vary from 2-5 mm in height. There are also discordant ST-T changes characterized by ST depression and T wave inversion in the leads I, aVL, V4 to V6.

ST Changes in LVH: The electrocardiogram below shows features of left ventricular hypertrophy. Along with left ventricular hypertrophy, we see the so-called strain pattern, characterized by downsloping ST segment with T wave inversion in I, aVL, and V4 to V6. Often we see an ST elevation in leads V2 to V3 (Fig. 11.06).

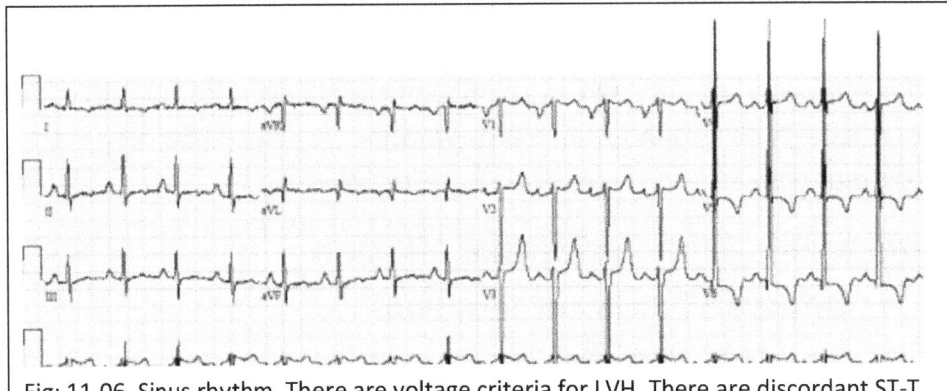

Fig: 11.06. Sinus rhythm. There are voltage criteria for LVH. There are discordant ST-T changes noted in lead I, aVL, V5 and V6. There is also a mild ST elevation in V2 and V3. All these findings are related to the LVH.

Horizontal ST Depression: Horizontal ST depression is a sign of myocardial ischemia. It is often seen in acute coronary syndromes. If the ST segment depression is associated with elevated cardiac enzymes, it represents subendocardial infarction (Fig: 11.07).

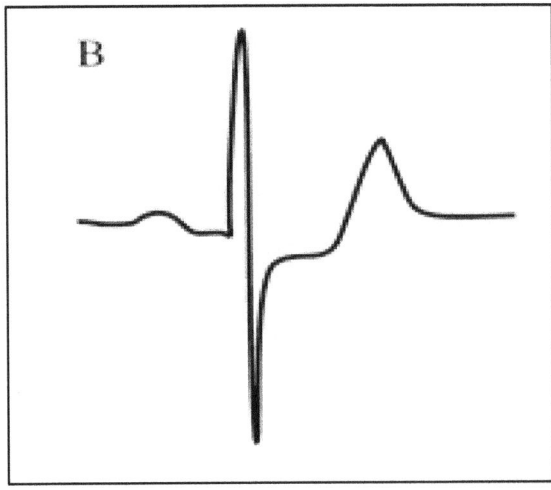

CHAPTER 11. ST SEGMENT ABNORMALITIES

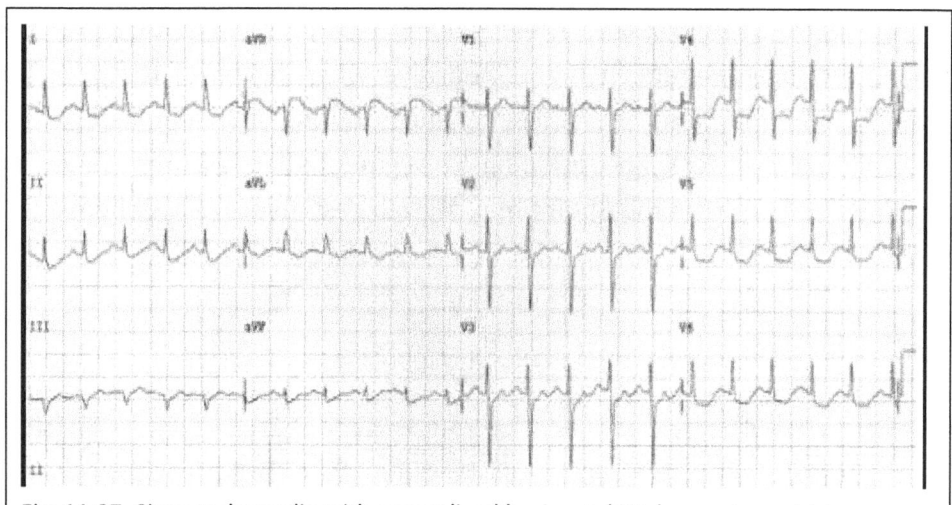

Fig: 11.07. Sinus tachycardia with generalized horizontal ST depression, which may suggest significant global ischemia.

We may also see considerable ST depression (in some cases more than 5 mm) in an SVT with rapid ventricular response (Fig:11.08)

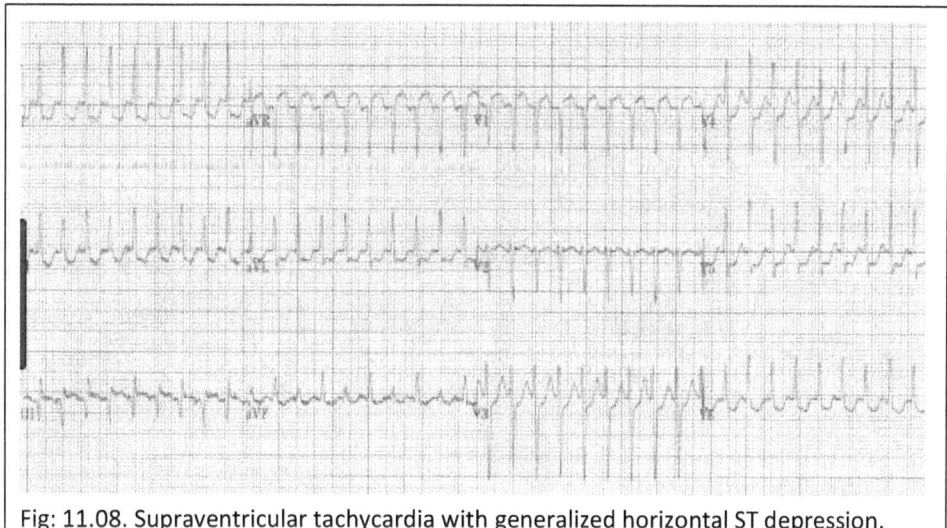

Fig: 11.08. Supraventricular tachycardia with generalized horizontal ST depression, which may suggest significant global ischemia.

CLINICAL EKG INTERPRETATION

Upsloping ST Depression: The upsloping ST depression is also seen often on an electrocardiogram. It is less sensitive when it comes to suggesting ischemia. We may also see similar changes during a treadmill test. In a treadmill exercise test, an upsloping ST segment that is 2 mm below the baseline at 80 ms from the J point may still suggest myocardial ischemia (Fig: 11.09).

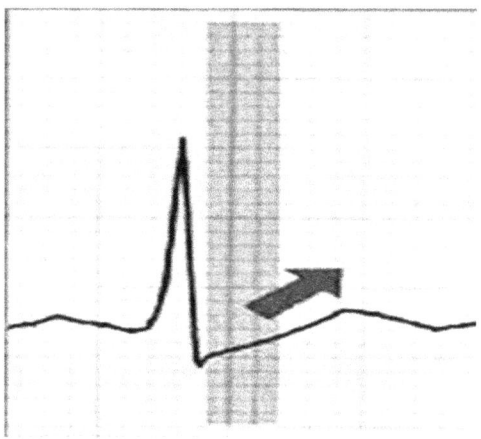

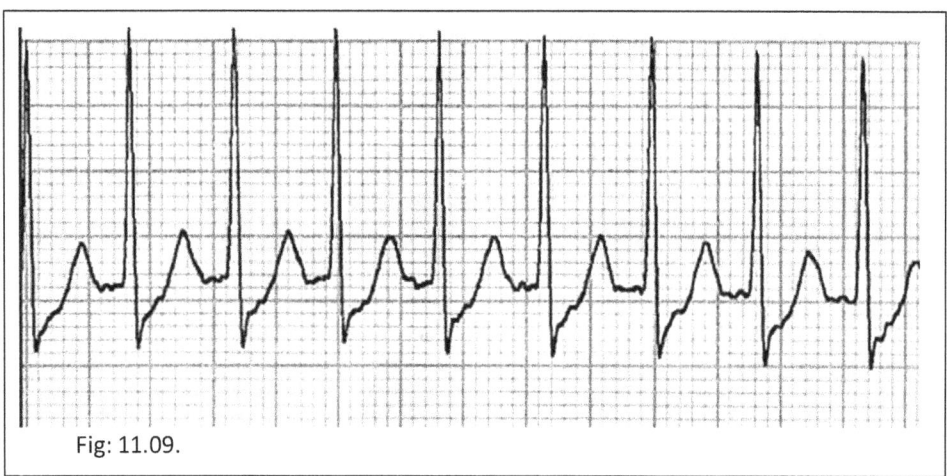

Fig: 11.09.

Downsloping ST Depression: It is frequently seen in the presence of BBB or hypertrophy of the right or the left ventricle. Sometimes, it is referred to as a strain pattern if there is a considerable ST depression associated with the downslope. The T waves are generally inverted. Similar changes are seen in patients with LBBB or RBBB (Fig: 11.10). These ST changes don't change very

CHAPTER 11. ST SEGMENT ABNORMALITIES

much unless there is underlying ischemia or supraventricular tachycardia with a rapid ventricular response. Sometimes you may see more than one type of ST changes: strain pattern in one region and an ischemic pattern at a different location (Fig: 11.11).

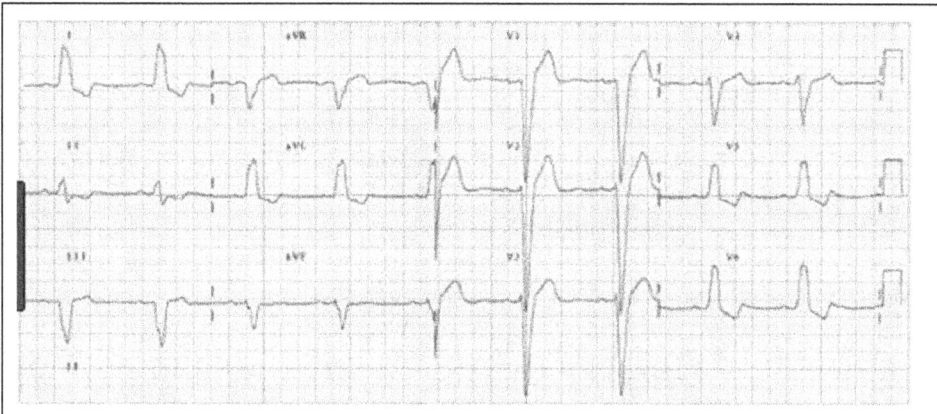

Fig: 11.10. LBBB with downsloping ST segment with biphasic T waves. Also, notice the ST elevation in leads V1, V2, and V3.

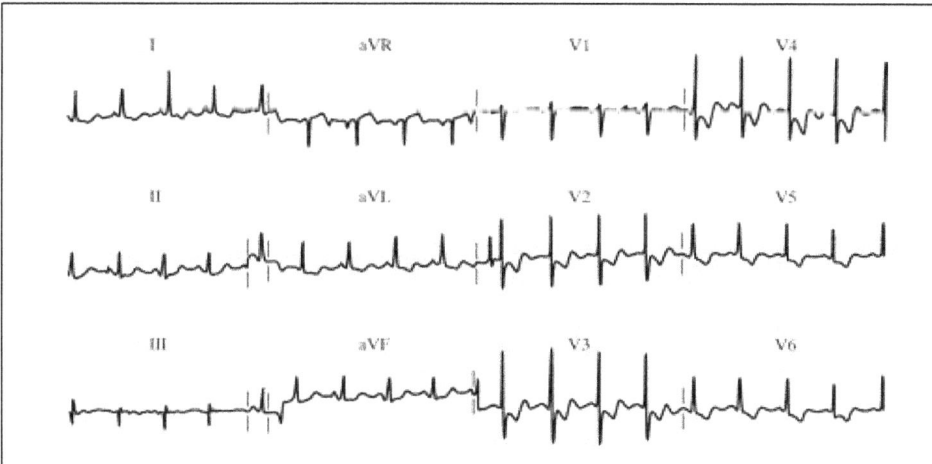

Fig: 11.11. Downsloping ST depression in a patient is chest pain suggestive of ischemia
Ref: https://emj.bmj.com/content/19/2/129

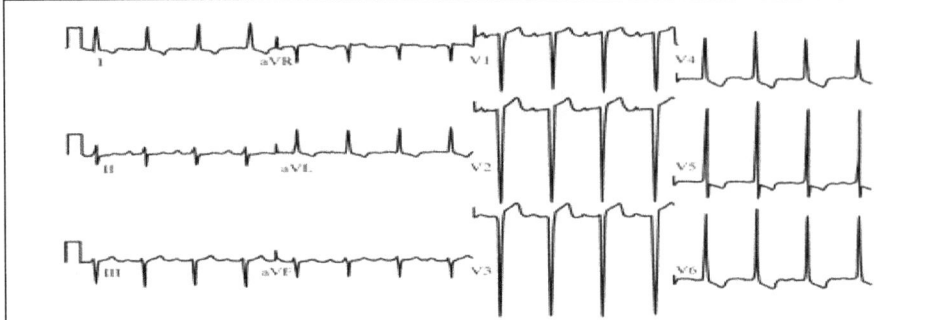

Fig: 11.12. LVH with strain pattern. Notice the downsloping ST segment in the lateral chest leads along with deep QS complexes in V1, V2, and V3. The ST-T changes are discordant to the QRS complexes in V3 to V6.S

Reciprocal ST Depressions: We see this during the phase of an acute myocardial infarction. In anterior MI, the reciprocal changes of ST depression can be noted in the inferior leads (Fig: 11.13). Similarly, with an acute inferior MI, we can see reciprocal ST-T changes in the anterior leads like I and aVL.

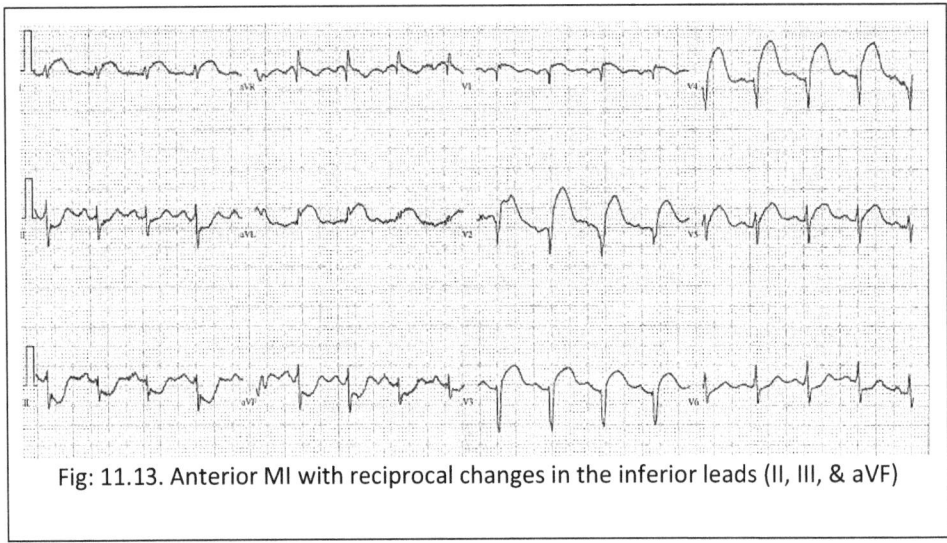

Fig: 11.13. Anterior MI with reciprocal changes in the inferior leads (II, III, & aVF)

In case of a posterior MI, reciprocal ST depression, along with tall R waves can be seen in V1 to V3. This may be the only indirect evidence of isolated posterior Mi, in the absence of inferior wall MI.

Chapter 12 T Wave Abnormalities

- Normal T Wave Variations
- T Wave Changes with BBBs
- Ventricular Ischemia
- Cerebrovascular Accidents
- Tall Peaked T Waves

The T wave represents the ventricular repolarization. It gradually increases in amplitude from the baseline and has a rounded tip, before declining to toward the baseline. Its morphology can vary depending on the leads (Fig: 12.01).

- The T wave is upright in I, II, and V3 to V6
- T waves are inverted in aVR
- T waves are variable in III, aVL, aVF, and V1-V2

The inverted T waves in III, aVL, aVR, and V1 to V2 doesn't represent any cardiac pathology. In women, the T waves may be inverted in V1 to V3.

ACLS QUIZ:

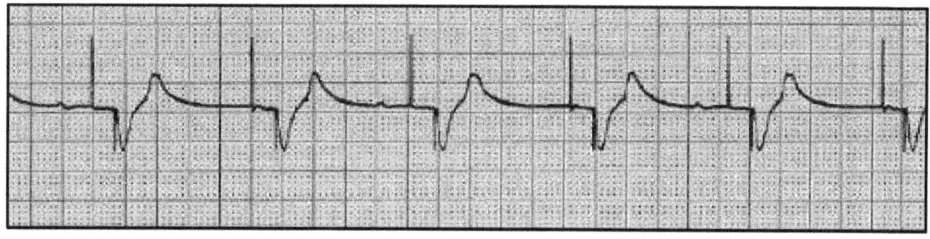

What is this? _____

CLINICAL EKG INTERPRETATION

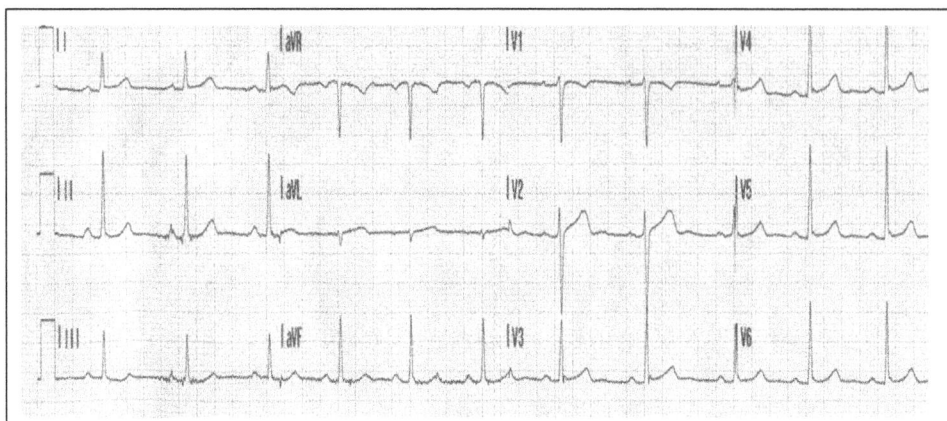

Fig: 12.01. Normal sinus rhythm. The T waves are normally inverted in aVR and V1 or V2. Occasionally they may be inverted in lead III. There is a good R wave progression in the chest leads.

The T waves can be altered in a variety of conditions such as ischemia, acute myocardial infarction, BBB, myocardial hypertrophy, electrolyte abnormalities, body temperature, and cerebrovascular accidents, pulmonary embolus, to juvenile T wave changes.

The ischemic T wave changes often occur in groups of leads that represent an area supplied by a coronary artery or one of its branches. An inferior wall ischemia produces T wave changes in lead II, III, and aVF. Similarly, a LAD territory produces T wave changes in the anterior leads such as I, aVL, V1 to V6. If the T wave changes are occurring in the setting of chest pain and elevated cardiac enzymes, they may represent a Non-Q myocardial infarction. Ischemia T waves are symmetrical and can vary in depth from 2 to 10 mm (Fig: 12.02).

ACLS QUIZ:

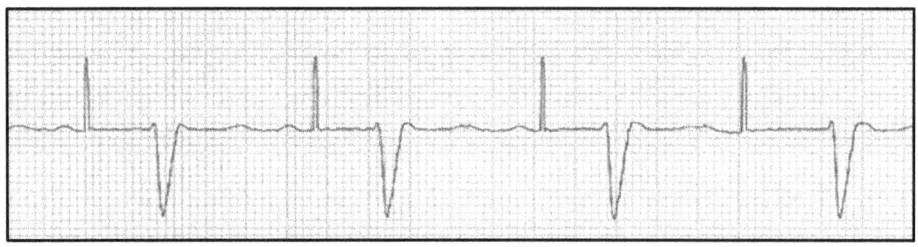

T WAVE ABNORMALITIES

Captured or not? _____

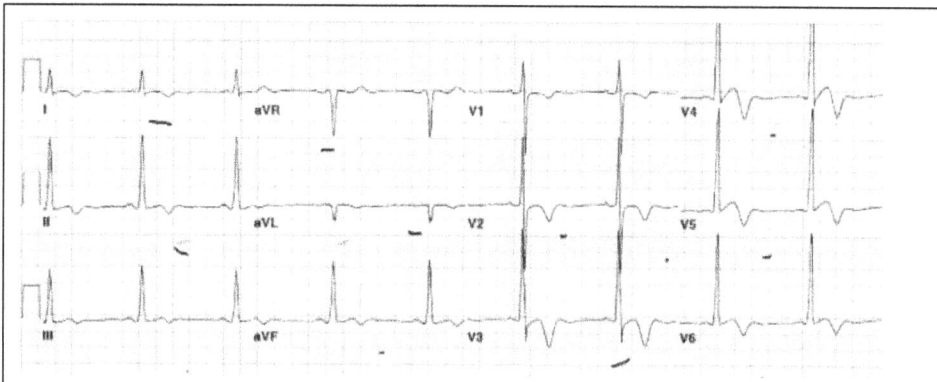

Fig: 12.02. Occasionally, these ischemic T waves may be biphasic in the anterior leads as seen in multiple leads here.

HYPERACUTE T WAVES:

These changes occur in the presence of an acute coronary insufficiency where the ST segment is elevated from the baseline along with the T waves. The ST segment may remain elevated for hours and days while the T waves begin to invert or appear biphasic in nature. Sometimes, the T wave amplitude can exceed the height of the R waves (Fig: 12.03).

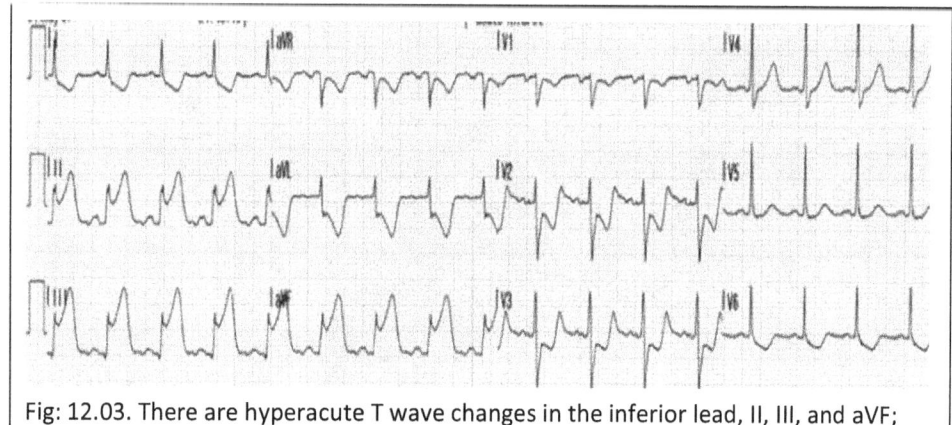

Fig: 12.03. There are hyperacute T wave changes in the inferior lead, II, III, and aVF; with reciprocal changes in leads V1-V3.

If the coronary insufficiency is temporary in cases such as angina, coronary artery spasm (Prinz metal angina), or cocaine-induced spasm, the

ST-T changes may revert to the baseline, once the ischemia resolves spontaneously or with medicines. However, if the ischemia is permanent, 6-8 after hours after the event, there is a development of the Q waves and inversion of the T waves. The T waves don't return to the baseline until the ST segment reaches the baseline. The T waves may remain inverted for several weeks and months following an acute myocardial infarction.

In an old myocardial infarction setting, the T waves may regain their normal upright morphology over several months. If there is a persistent ST elevation due to left ventricular aneurysm, the T waves may remain inverted for months and years.

The T wave inversions can also be seen in acute myocarditis or pericarditis where the epicardium is involved.

BUNDLE BRANCH BLOCKS (BBB) AND ST-T WAVE CHANGES

The T wave inversions noted in BBBs have slightly different morphology. First, they occur in the presence of a BBB. Generally, they are in the opposite direction of the QRS complexes (Fig: 12.04).

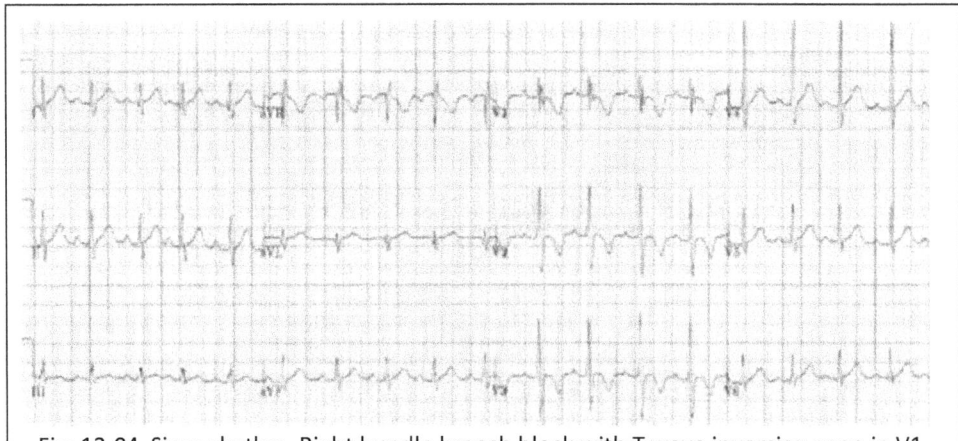

Fig: 12.04. Sinus rhythm. Right bundle branch block with T wave inversion seen in V1, V2, and V3 along with ST depression.

Often, there are varying degrees of down-sloping ST depression, depending upon the degree of the ventricular strain. The T waves are symmetrically inverted in the same leads involving the BBB. Occasionally, the T waves may appear biphasic. Together, the ST-T morphology is related to the BBB and the extent of the ventricular strain. If the strain is severe, there may be significant ST depression, along with the T wave inversion.

Similar changes are also noted in patients with right or left ventricular hypertrophy. Here, we may see other clues related to the ventricular hypertrophy, which is covered in another chapter.

T WAVE CHANGES RELATED TO SERUM POTASSIUM LEVELS

In order to understand the effects of serum potassium levels on the EKG, we need to understand the role of Potassium in the myocardial cell action potential.

Hyperkalemia and T wave Changes: Hyperkalemia has the most profound changes on the electrocardiogram and signals the urgency in recognizing the changes. It also alerts us in initiating prompt treatments to correct the potassium imbalance. Generally, we see this in patients who are on hemodialysis, just before when their dialysis is due. The cardinal EKG findings include:

Hyperkalemia EKG changes (Fig: 12.05)

- **Tall, Peaked T Waves in the Chest Leads**
- **Prolonged PR interval**
- **Flattened P Waves**
- **Widened QRS Complexes**
- **Merging of the QRS With the T waves into a Sine wave & VF if Left Untreated in Patients with Very High Potassium Levels**

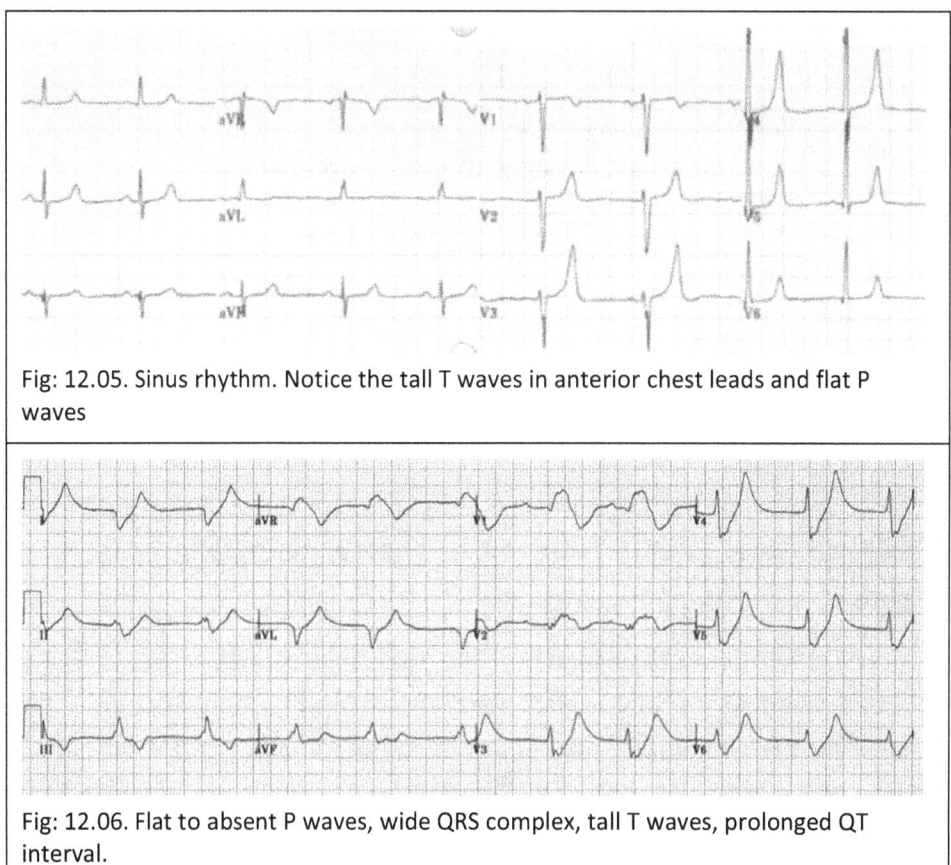

Fig: 12.05. Sinus rhythm. Notice the tall T waves in anterior chest leads and flat P waves

Fig: 12.06. Flat to absent P waves, wide QRS complex, tall T waves, prolonged QT interval.

The more pronounced EKG changes depend upon the serum potassium levels (Fig: 12.07).

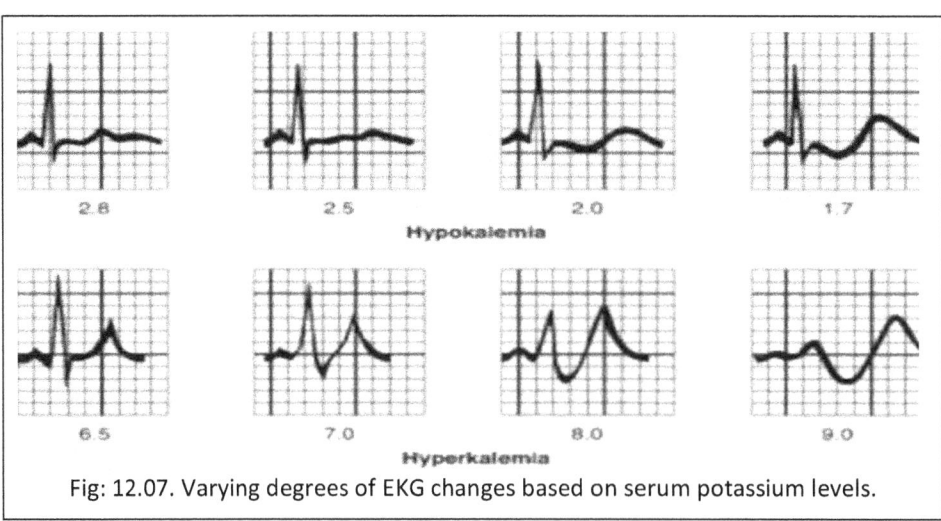

Fig: 12.07. Varying degrees of EKG changes based on serum potassium levels.

T WAVE ABNORMALITIES

- At a serum potassium level of 6.5, there are tall peaked T waves.
- If the serum potassium level is 7.0 or greater, there is a widening of the QRS complex and tall T waves
- As the serum potassium level reaches 8.0, the QRS becomes much wider, the R waves lose their amplitudes, and the T waves become taller.
- When the serum potassium level is 9.0, we begin to see the sine waves where the wide QRS blend with the wide T waves.

The key here is to recognize the earliest manifestations of hyperkalemia on the EKG and try to fix the potassium level before it becomes a life-threatening situation. Hence, monitoring of these high-risk patients during dialysis should include potassium levels and EKGs, and correct the electrolyte imbalances very promptly and diligently.

HYPOKALEMIA AND T WAVE CHANGES

When the serum potassium level drops, it can have the changes reflected on the electrocardiogram. It is common to see variation in serum potassium levels on those who are on diuretics and not receiving supplemental potassium. Hence, check labs during a patient's visit to monitor their electrolytes among others and get an electrocardiogram.

The earliest changes related to low potassium show flattening of the T waves. As the serum potassium drops below 2.5 mEq, there is the appearance of U waves. When the Potassium level is 2.0, we may see a biphasic T wave and as the potassium level drops further, there may be some ST depression along with a biphasic T wave (Fig: 12.08).

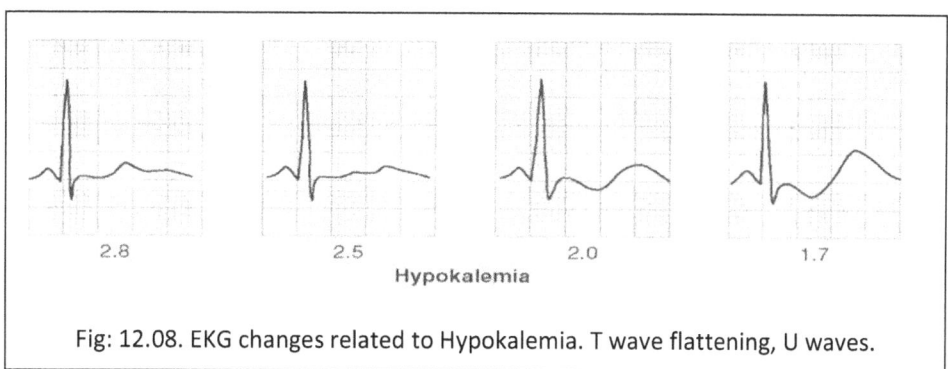

Fig: 12.08. EKG changes related to Hypokalemia. T wave flattening, U waves.

CLINICAL EKG INTERPRETATION

It may be impossible to avoid minor variations in potassium levels. The key to managing these patients is to anticipate and be pro-active in following their lab tests to avoid extreme potassium levels. A correction of 1 mEq deficit in a normal patient requires almost 100 mEq of potassium replacement by IV, by mouth, or by a combination of routes.

GIANT NEGATIVE T WAVES

These changes are seen in patients with cerebrovascular accidents and in patients with global left ventricular ischemia (Fig: 12.09). In either case, it is a grossly abnormal electrocardiogram and signals prompt a workup and management.

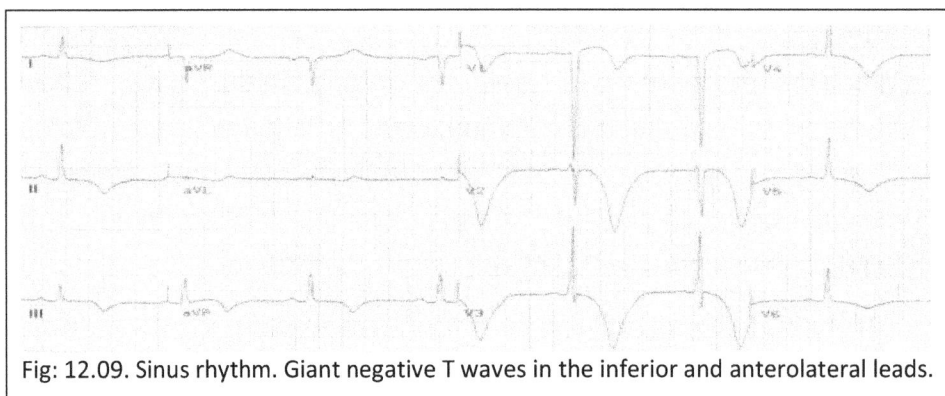

Fig: 12.09. Sinus rhythm. Giant negative T waves in the inferior and anterolateral leads.

The T wave is extremely wide and deeply inverted. The duration can vary from 200 ms to 400 ms or more. Their depth can vary from 5 mm to 20 mm.

ACLS QUIZ:

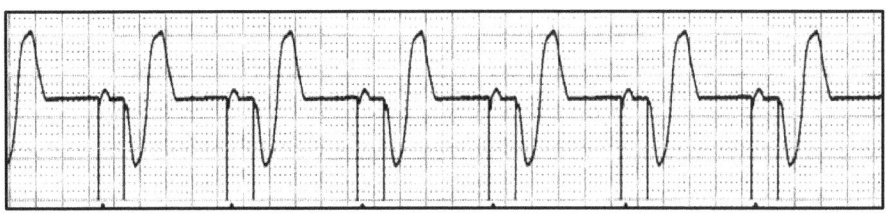

Captured or not? _____

T WAVE ABNORMALITIES

Quiz:

1. What are your findings?

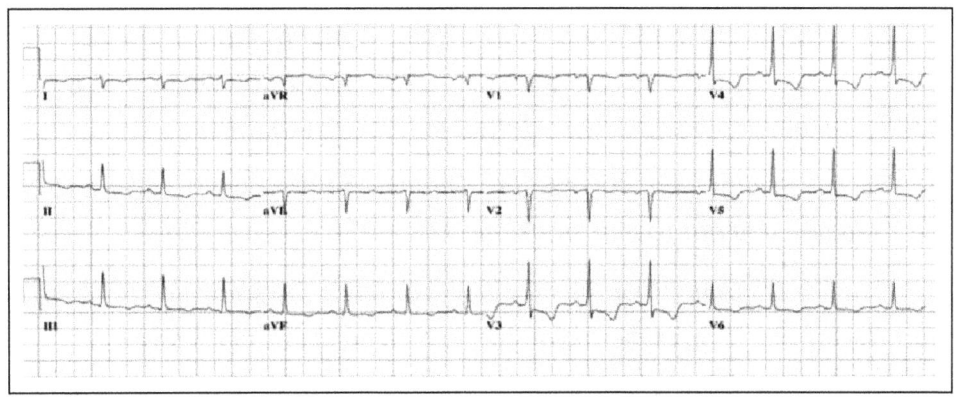

2. What are your findings?

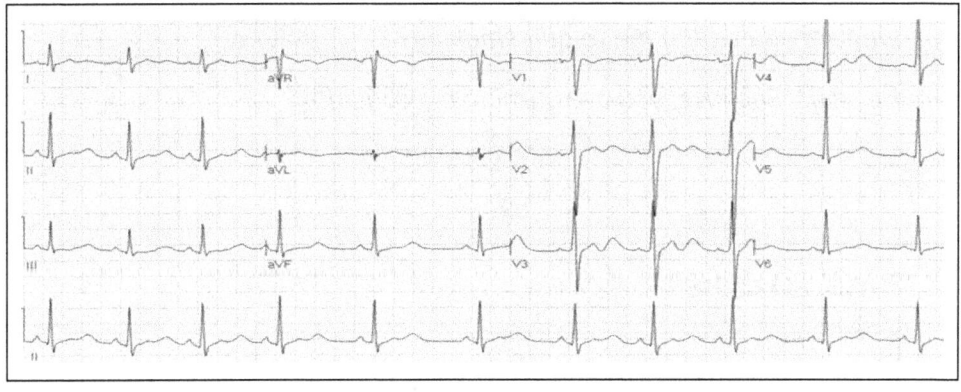

3. What are your findings?

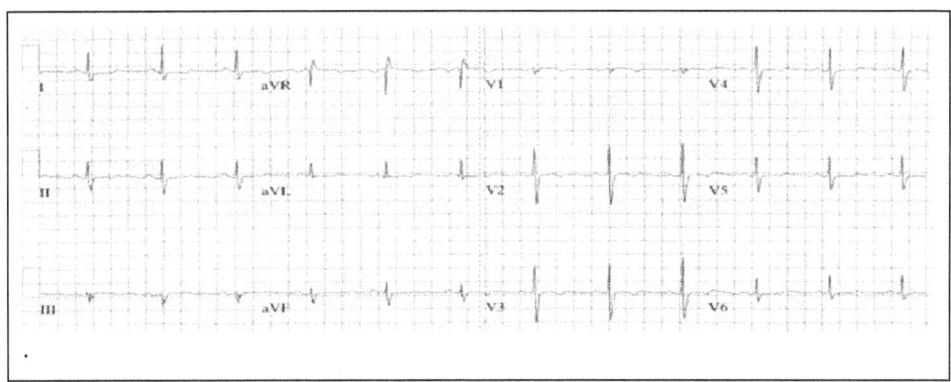

CLINICAL EKG INTERPRETATION

COMIC CLUB BLOCK (CCB)

Lady with a heart attack

This 54-year-old lady had a heart attack. A month later, I saw her in my office. She looked a little bit depressed. Nothing unusual. One-third of heart attack patients get depressed. I referred her to a psychiatrist.

She reluctantly went to see him. The psychiatrist, while talking to her, said, "Ma'am, you got to quit smoking."

"You are a shrink. Why are you worried about my smoking? Besides, my heart doctor didn't refer me to you for a smoking cessation session."

"Ah ah! Didn't your stupid heart doctor tell you that smoking is bad for your heart?"

"I can understand my heart doctor being concerned about my smoking, but, why are you telling me to quit smoking?"

He said, "Because, you are burning my couch!"

*****

BACK TO QUIZ:

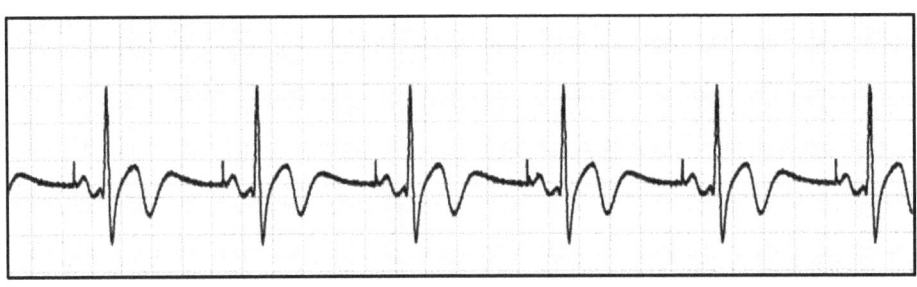

Working or not? _____

Chapter 13 Pacemaker Rhythms

- Indications
- Nomenclature
- Ventricular Pacing
- AV Sequential pacing
- Atrial Sensing and Ventricular Pacing
- Atrial Pacing and Ventricular Pacing

Cardiac pacemakers play a vital role in not only sustaining a cardiac rhythm, but also in enhancing the cardiac function and improving quality of life and long-term survival rates.

Just the recognition of a pacemaker rhythm on an electrocardiogram is not adequate. We need to determine:

- Underlying cardiac condition and rhythm
- Indication for the pacemaker
- What type of pacemaker?
- Is the pacemaker doing its job?
- Is the pacemaker malfunctioning?
- How do you analyze a pacemaker?
- How do you reprogram the pacemaker?

The Underlying Cardiac Condition and Rhythm: The underlying cardiac condition can speak volumes about a patient's cardiac condition and the cardiac reserve. If the underlying rhythm is atrial fibrillation, you know that the patient may have left atrial enlargement and possibly congestive heart failure. It also should draw our attention that the loss of atrial contribution could play a significant role in a patient's symptoms and prognosis.

INDICATIONS FOR PACEMAKERS:

- Symptomatic bradycardia (HR<35/min) or sinus pauses
- Symptomatic CHB or 2nd degree heart block (type 1 or 2)
- Asymptomatic CHB or advanced 2nd degree heart block
- Atrial fib with pauses >= 5 seconds
- Alternating bundle branch block
- After catheter AV nodal ablation
- Severe congestive heart failure with very wide QRS complexes.
- Recurrent VT or V. fib

NBG NOMENCLATURE

1st letter	2nd letter	3rd letter	4th letter
Chamber paced	Chamber senses	Sensing	Rate Response
A: Atria	A: Atria	I: Inhibit	R: rate responsive
V: Ventricle	V: Ventricle	T: Trigger	
D: Dual	D: Dual	D: Dual	
O: None	O: None	O: none	

Example

> VVI: Ventricle paced, ventricle senses, and ventricle inhibited
> DDDR: Dual chamber paced, Dual sensed, inhibited, triggered, and rate responsive

CHAPTER 13. PACEMAKER RHYTHMS

- **CRT**: Cardiac Resynchronization Therapy
- **ICD**: Intra Cardiac Defibrillator

Lower Rate Limit (LRT): This is the lower rate limit at which the pacemaker paces the heart. This rate is usually slower than the steady pacemaker rate. If the actual pacemaker rate is set at 60 bpm, the LRT may be set at 50 bpm to allow time for the heart to activate by its pacemaker cells.

Detect Rate: This is the rate at which the pacemaker detects certain tachyarrhythmias. If the RR rate goes above 170 bpm, it is supposed to do something. This is important for an ICD device to detect a certain rate and QRS morphology and initiate a shock if indicated.

Stimulation: Once a pacemaker detects no activity, it is supposed to send an electrical impulse. The impulse is based on the strength and duration of the current. It is different for the atria and ventricles. The height is called the amplitude, and the duration is called the pulse width. Together they determine the amount of output sent to the tip of the electrode. Remember that the larger the output, the quicker the battery power wears off.

Capture: Capture is the ability of the atria or the ventricles to sense the electrical impulse and generate an action potential of its own. This depends on good contact between the electrode and the myocardium. Hence, if the lead is loose and not touching the myocardium or if the electrode is in an area of the scar, there may be a failure to capture. In this Scenario, you may see an electrical spike but no atrial or ventricular waveforms. Sometimes, increasing the output from the electrode may solve the problem. However, if the issue is related to good contact, the lead should be repositioned in a different place until you get the stimulation with the lowest output. Sometimes, with a scarred ventricle, we may not get the best result. Hence, all pacemakers have an energy safety margin that is 2-3 times the normal threshold. This can be determined when the pacemaker is interrogated as how much output is being used to generate an impulse. This stimulation threshold can vary with metabolic changes, drug effects (class 1c drugs), scar, and or ischemia

Anti-tachycardia: It's a feature by which the pacemaker is used to treat tachyarrhythmias like Ventricular tachycardia, atrial tachycardia, or atrial flutter.

CLINICAL EKG INTERPRETATION

High Energy Shock: this is primarily used by the ICD devices to shock the heart when it senses life-threatening ventricular fibrillation or ventricular tachycardia.

Electromagnetic Impulses (EMI): These are high-frequency wave produced bay many gadgets used in and around the house and in hospital settings. In a hospital setting, devices such as lithotripsy, electroconvulsive shock therapy, radiofrequency ablation, TENs units, and TURP, cause these impulses which can send wrong and unwanted signals to the pacemaker.

Electrocautery and Pacemakers: When using electrocautery, use a bipolar device with a grounding plate >15 cm from the pacemaker. There should be short bursts with at least 10 seconds gap between bursts. Using a magnet also makes the pacemaker function in an asynchronous mode, not responding to these false signals.

MRI and Pacemakers: Older forms of MRI caused high pacing rates resulting in a runaway pacemaker. In addition, the radiofrequency energy may transmit all the way to the cardiac tissue via the electrodes. More modern MRIs and the pacemaker are designed in such a way the pacemakers are MRI compatible. It will say on their pacemaker cards if they are MRI safe. If not, consult with the cardiologist or the company technical staff.

Pacemaker Monitoring and Programming: Today, most people would be able to transmit their pacemaker data using a phone to a central monitoring location where someone can analyze the rhythm and advice. They also can be fully interrogated in a cardiologist office or hospital clinic where several parameters can be reset to suit the situation and optimize the pacemaker function (Fig: 13.01).

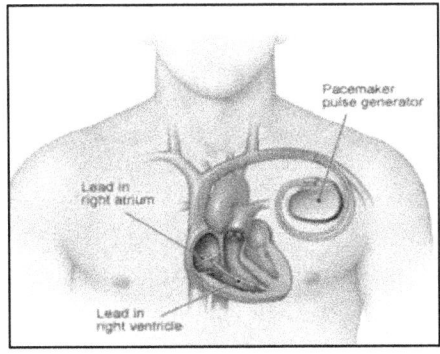 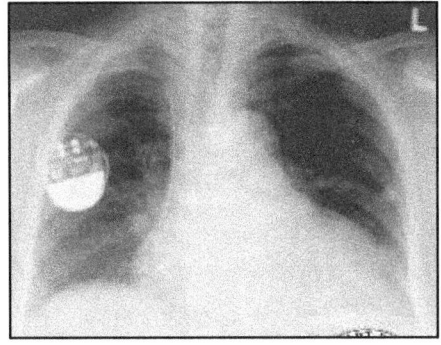

Fig: 13.01 Pacemaker insertion. Chest x-ray showing a pacemaker.

CHAPTER 13. PACEMAKER RHYTHMS

TYPES OF PACEMAKERS

VVI PACEMAKER

It is a single chamber pacemaker with a pacing electrode placed at the right ventricular apex. Some of them are called VVIR, which means these pacemakers are rate responsive. The VVI or VVIR pacemakers are inserted in older patients with chronic atrial fibrillation, who are not very active and just need a steady heart rate so they don't develop very slow ventricular rates with medications used for hypertension or heart disease

Whenever you see a LBBB, always look for hidden pacemaker spikes. Also, check out the atrial rhythm. If it is a sinus, occasionally you may see a fusion beat if there is no complete heart block.

DDD PACEMAKER

The DDD pacemaker is a dual chamber pacemaker with one lead called the atrial electrode, placed at the interatrial septum. The second lead is placed at the RV apex. These two electrodes are usually introduced through the left or the right subclavian vein. The electrodes are connected to a DDD pacemaker battery which is placed underneath the skin and sutured. Many of these pacemakers have a battery life of 10-12 years, they are very durable and safe.

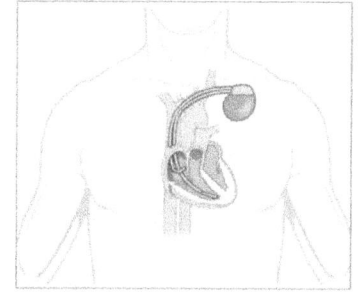

Most modern DDD pacemakers are not only safe around microwaves, but also, they are not affected by MRI studies. Make sure you carry a card from the pacemaker company or from your physician as these are sure to trigger the screening devices at airports.

CLINICAL EKG INTERPRETATION

The pacemaker is able to pace both the atria and ventricles. The main features of DDD pacemaker include (Fig: 13.02):

- Sensing the atria and the ventricular electrical activity.
- Inhibit both the atrial and ventricular output if the inherent rhythm comes in before the next pacer rate.
- Pacing both the atria and the ventricles as needed
- Atrial sensing and ventricular sensing
- It also senses the metabolic demands and increases the heart rate if needed if the rate-responsive feature is built into the pacemaker.

The fact that this pacemaker is capable of so many different functions, it is also prone to malfunction at multiple levels, making the interrogation much more complex compared to the VVI pacemaker.

Any changes in the atrial or ventricular rhythm can change the role and function of this pacemaker. For example, if the patient develops atrial fibrillation, the atrial sensing and pacing mechanisms will be on standby and the pacemaker will function like a VVIR device. Similarly, if there are frequent PVCs, the ventricular lead may not sense the PVCs.

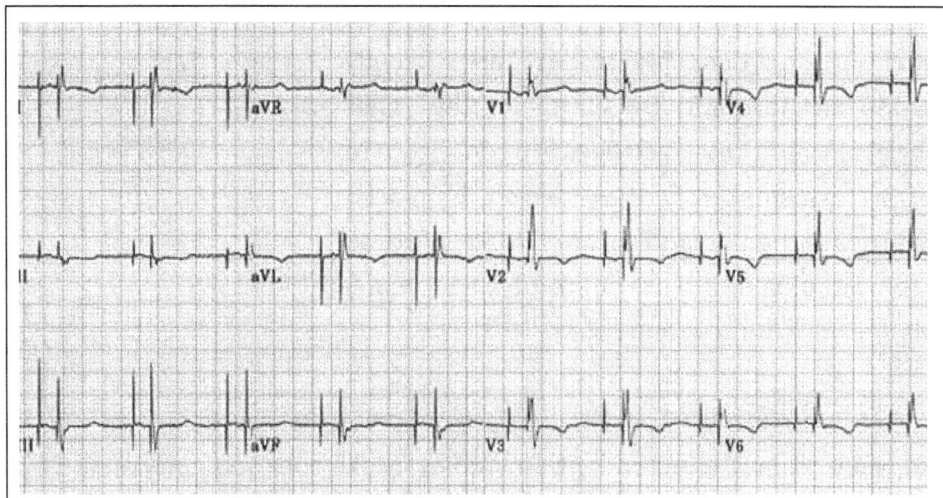

Fig: 13.02. An AV sequential pacemaker with both the atria and the ventricles being paced.

CHAPTER 13. PACEMAKER RHYTHMS

The above electrocardiogram (Fig: 13.02), reveals two spikes, one corresponding to the atrial activation and the other one related to the ventricular activation. At first glance, we can ascertain that the patient is 100% dependent of the DDD pacemaker, as both the atria and the ventricles are being paced.

We can infer the inherent atrial rate is not adequate and hence the atrial pacing. Then the pacemaker waits for the ventricles to kick in at a set PR interval. If the inherent ventricular activation doesn't kick in, the pacemaker will activate the ventricles, as seen in this tracing, and the cycle continues.

All pacemaker patients should be followed by cardiologists and pacemaker interrogation performed ever 3-6 months, as indicated by the pacemaker company guidelines.

Modern pacemakers are so advanced, they not only serve the purpose of pacing the heart and keeping the patients alive; they also store all the history and any events from the time they were inserted.

Hence, reviewing the history will quickly let us know how the pacemaker has behaved during the past several months, how they have responded to any changes in medications, and help in programming the pacemaker for the future challenges. It also will help us to determine the battery life span.

Here are the four possible modes for a DDD pacemaker (Fig: 13.03)
- Atrial pacing and ventricular pacing
- Atrial sensing and ventricular pacing
- Atrial pacing and ventricle sensing
- Atrial sensing and ventricle sensing

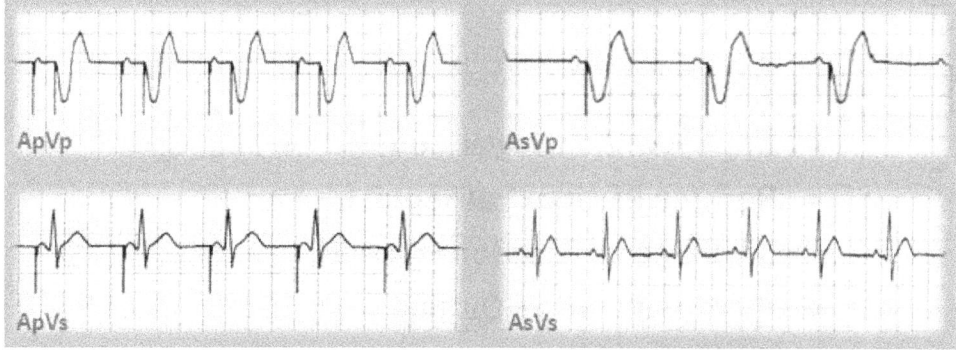

Fig: 13.03 various modes of DDD pacemaker.

Indications: The DDD pacemakers are suited for people with normal atrial activity. It is useful in patients with sinus node and AV node dysfunctions. Pacing the atria may decrease the risk of atrial fibrillation, stroke, pacemaker related syndromes, and improve the quality of life.

If the patient has chronic atrial fibrillation or flutter, it may not be useful as the atrial lead will not be activated. Similarly, in patients with MAT or WPW with a rapid ventricular response, it may be more harmful as they may increase the ventricular rates to a point where patients may begin to have symptoms.

Patients with far-advanced heart failure, with low EF, and QRS complexes greater 140 ms may benefit from Cardiac Resynchronization Therapy (CRT) than from a DDD pacemaker. They may also be beneficial in a patient with carotid sinus syndrome and neurogenic syncope, and symptomatic patient with hypertrophic cardiomyopathies.

CARDIAC RESYNCHRONIZATION THERAPY (CRT):

The main goal here is to provide a steady rhythm and improve the cardiac function and improve the cardiac output in a highly compromised heart failure patient with depressed ejection fractions and very wide QRS complexes. This is accomplished by making both ventricles beat simultaneously to improve the left ventricular filling and increase the left ventricular output. This improves the cardiac output and reduces symptoms of heart failure. It also enhances the quality of life.

Benefits of CRT
- **Improve** Ventricular Contraction Sequence
- **Reduce** Paradoxical Septal Motion
- **Improve** LV Ejection Fraction
- **Increase** Cardiac Output
- **Reduce** Dyspnea, Weakness, and Fatigue

CHAPTER 13. PACEMAKER RHYTHMS

Just as in a dual chamber pacemaker, a lead is placed in the right atrium to activate the atria. The right ventricular pacer lead is placed at the right ventricular apex. This first activates the right ventricle and then the left ventricle. However, a third wire introduced through the coronary sinus is an advance into the left ventricular lateral wall. Thus, both the ventricular pacer wires are activated at the same time simulating a normal sequence of ventricular activation, which increases the left ventricular output and improves the symptoms of heart failure.

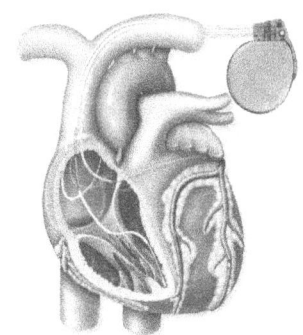

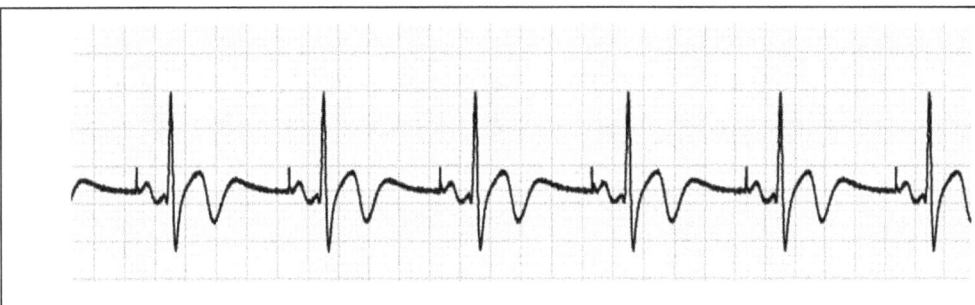

Fig: Fig: 13.04. An AV sequential pacemaker with the atria being paced and the ventricles sensing.

Magnet Mode: When a magnet is placed over a pacemaker, it will shift to magnet mode. This mode varies with the type of pacemaker and the manufacturer. It initiates an asynchronous pacing mode: AOO, VOO, or DOO. It delivers a constant rate, irrespective of the underlying rhythm. This may be useful when using an electric cautery close to a pacemaker as the cautery can create muscle tremors that can confuse the pacemaker.

The asynchronous mode also carries a risk of R on T phenomenon and set off more dangerous ventricular arrhythmias. However, if the same magnet is applied to an ICD device, it turns off the defibrillation function.

IMPLANTABLE CARDIAC DEFIBRILLATOR (ICD)

This is a special dual chamber pacemaker with defibrillation capabilities. It has a lead in the atrium and a lead in the right ventricular apex. For the most part, it functions as a pacemaker. In case it senses V. tach or V. Fib, it delivers s shock through the ventricular electrode to defibrillate the ventricle.

It also has anti-tachycardia pacing mode where one of the chambers can be paced at a very high rate to break atrial or ventricular tachycardias.

For those patients who do not need back-up pacing or ATP, there are simpler devices that can be placed beneath the skin without the need for an electrode.

Problems Related to Pacemakers:
- **Lead** Misplacement
- **Improper** Sensing
- **Improper** Pacing
- **Failure to** Capture
- **Low Battery** Power
- **Inadequate** Rate Response
- **Runaway** Pacemaker
- **Pacemaker** Site Infection

The capture problems can arise if the lead is not in good contact with the muscle or if the lead is placed close to a scar tissue, which doesn't generate an electrical impulse nor can it transmit an electrical impulse.

CHAPTER 13. PACEMAKER RHYTHMS

Pacemaker EKG QUIZ

EKG 13.1

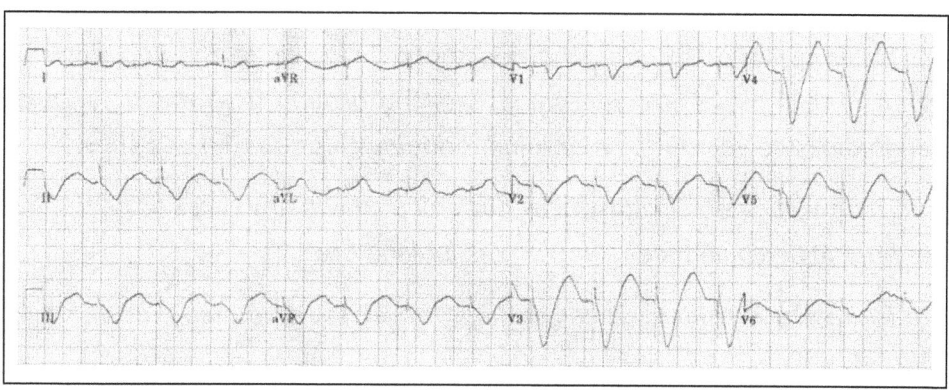

EKG 13.2

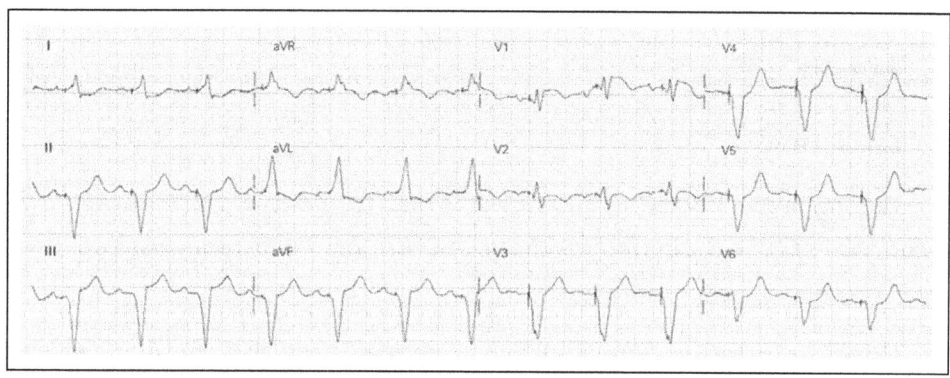

EKG 13.3

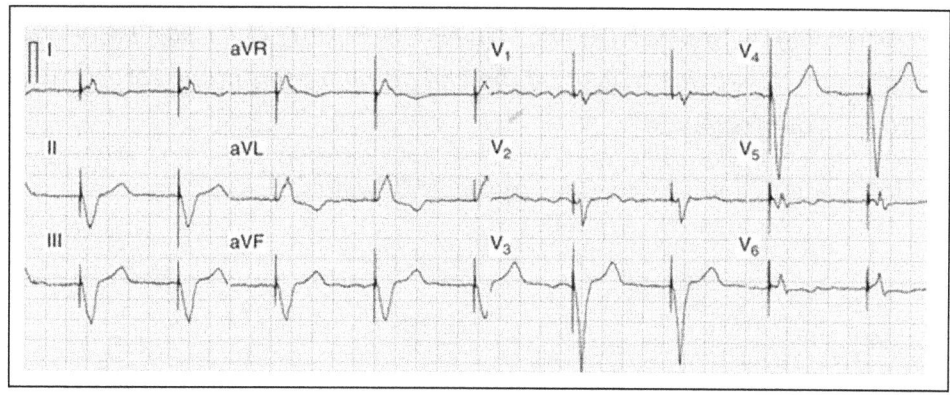

Email to drniknikam@gmail.com with a page reference for keys

NIK'S COMEDY CLIPS (NCC)

Dog show

This man takes his dog to a dog show. The guys at the dog show say, "What is this? What are you doing, walking around with this ugly looking mongoloid? Are you out of your mind, bringing this dog to a dog show?"

The owner said, "I know, he is not going to win any races or prizes. But I was hoping he could meet some better-looking dogs."

That's the way I feel whenever I drag myself to a wedding reception or a Gala.

When I see people at a distance, looking at me and making ugly faces, I just use my telephoto camera, capture their frustrations/expressions put them on social media, and wait for their reaction.

******

Larry, I am. . .

When I was in Toastmasters Club, I had to make a presentation. I had spent a lot of time preparing for that presentation. I was really excited. It was my first major speech.

When I started my presentation, I noticed that half the audience was sleeping while the other half was snoring, except for Larry, who was in the front row. He was wide awake. He was listening to everything I was saying.

At the end of my presentation, I walked up to Larry and said, "Larry I want to thank you for staying awake till the end of my presentation. Later, I would like to get your feedback."

Larry said, "Don't thank me, I'm the next speaker."

Chapter 14 Miscellaneous Conditions

- Preoperative EKG Evaluation
- Stress Test
- Low voltage
- Electrical Alternans
- Hyperkalemia
- Hypokalemia
- Hypercalcemia
- Hypocalcemia
- Hypomagnesemia
- Hypothermia
- Cardiac Transplant
- Hyperthyroidism
- Muscle Tremors

PREOPERATIVE EKG EVALUATION:

Thousands of people undergo preop EKG and in a vast majority of the cases, they are glanced at by the anesthesiologist before the patient is taken for surgery. In fact, some patients have been taken to surgery in the presence of significant myocardial ischemia or infarction, because no one really looked at the EKG properly.

CLINICAL EKG INTERPRETATION

Ideally, the preoperative electrocardiogram should be done 2-3 days prior to the surgery to allow adequate time for the interpreting physician to read the EKG and communicate the results to the surgeon and the anesthesiologist involved.

Several points need attention before deciding that a patient is cleared for surgery.
- What is the rate and rhythm? If the patient has a sinus tachycardia at 120 bpm, is this just anxiety or is there some underlying pathology for the sinus tachycardia? Remember, that sinus tachycardia is not normal and is always secondary to something. It is your mission to find out what is that "something".
- If the patient has atrial fibrillation, flutter, or MAT, is the rate controlled (<100bpm)? What medicines they are taking and those medicines should be started as soon as feasible after the surgery.
- Should you hold antiarrhythmic drugs on the day of surgery?
- Is there any evidence of ischemia or significant ST-T changes that need a specialist's attention?
- Heat blocks. Anything more than a 1degree heart block needs attention. Does this patient have advanced heart block or bifascicular block or trifascicular block? The stress of surgery can lead to complete heart block during or immediately following surgery.
- Does this patient have a pacemaker or a defibrillator? Do you plan on using an electric cautery near the pacemaker site? If the patient has any type of pacing device, the pacemaker device has to be thoroughly interrogated and adjusted for the type of the surgical procedure. Sometimes, you may have to make the pacemaker fixed by using a magnet. Occasionally, the ICD device has to be turned off its recognition of tachyarrhythmias based on the nature of the surgery and any interference that may simulate a VT. Hence, these patients must be evaluated by a qualified cardiologist before the surgery and they should be readily available if needed during or immediately following the surgery.
- Cardiovascular medicines should be started as soon as the clinical condition permits

CHAPTER 14. MISCELLANEOUS ABNORMALITIES

- It is not uncommon for patients to develop an acute myocardial infarction in the peri-operative period. If there are signs of an acute MI, these patients must be treated like a STEMI and taken to the catheterization lab if possible, to deal with the medical emergency. When these patients undergo percutaneous intervention, they will be placed on strong blood thinners that can complicate perioperative recovery. Hence, it is of paramount importance to evaluate patients with a previous cardiac history or those who have abnormal ischemic changes on the EKG. They may need complete cardiac evaluation, including an echocardiogram and a stress test to access their risk before h surgery.

- Watch for development of tachyarrhythmias after the surgery. The tachycardia can be related to a variety of factors such as pain, fever, anemia, sympathetic excess, and anesthetic agents, all of which can precipitate a tachyarrhythmia or make an existing one worse. Any new onset PACs and PVCs should be aggressively treated as they may be premonitory symptoms of a tachyarrhythmia coming in due course. Hence, pay attention to electrolytes and fluid balance in the perioperative period.

STRESS TEST

The main purpose of the treadmill testing is to determine if the patient has stress-induced ischemic changes on the electrocardiogram. The patient is connected to a 12 lead EKG machine and exercised on a treadmill or a bicycle until a target heart rate is reached. At the same time, the patient is carefully monitored for the physical capacity, symptoms, or any electrocardiographic changes.

Target Heart Rate: The target heart rate is determined by the age and the maximum heart rate. The maximum heart rate is calculated by subtracting the patient's age by 220. For example, if the patient age is 60 years, the target heart rate is (220-60) = 160 bpm. When we exercise patient on a treadmill, we use 85% of the target heart rate as the endpoint.

Target Heart Rate: (220-Age in years) X 0.85 = 85% PMHR

CLINICAL EKG INTERPRETATION

Many types of stressors are available for those who cannot exercise on a treadmill. We could use chemical stressors like dobutamine infusion and adenosine injection as a bolus and combined with either echocardiography or nuclear scan to get a better understanding of stress-induced ischemia.

When the patient is on a treadmill, we monitor the heart rate, heart rhythm, symptoms of fatigue, chest pain, shortness of breath, or weakness. Hence, we may have several endpoints, not just the predicted maximum heart rate. We may terminate the stress test if the patient:

- Develops chest pain with more than 2 mm horizontal ST depression in multiple leads.
- Has hypotension with weakness and dizziness
- Has frequent multifocal PVCs
- Is not able to continue because of leg fatigue or weakness.
- Develops symptomatic SVT or VT, V. Fib.
- Is uncomfortable.

The main ST-T changes we look for in a treadmill exercise test are focused on ST-T segments.

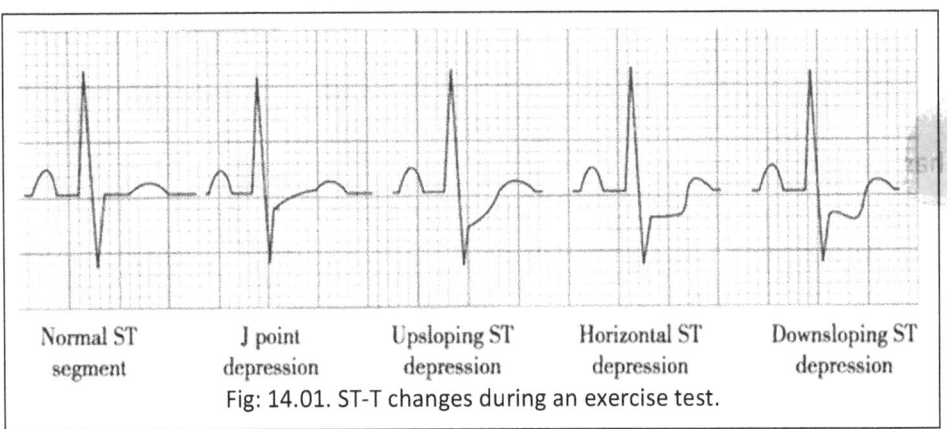

Fig: 14.01. ST-T changes during an exercise test.

The most diagnostic change would involve horizontal or downsloping ST depression of more than 1.5 mm in any leads during peak exercise. The time it takes to return to the baseline also dictates the amount of ischemia or the degree of coronary occlusion resulting in reduce myocardial perfusion.

CHAPTER 14. MISCELLANEOUS ABNORMALITIES

The upsloping ST depression is less diagnostic unless the ST segment at 80 ms from the J point is still more than 1.5 mm depressed from the baseline.

Similarly, a drop in blood pressure during exercise may be a sign of global ischemia that deserves prompt attention.

Dobutamine Exercise Test: The concept of dobutamine exercise is based on the fact that with increasing heart rate there is increasing myocardial oxygen demand. The areas with reduced blood circulation will show signs of ischemia. This is useful in patients who cannot exercise due to arthritis or any other conditions. However, dobutamine may cause palpitations and sometimes precipitate ventricular arrhythmias. We look for the same type of ST-T changes during dobutamine stress as we do when we exercise a patient on a treadmill test. We often combine dobutamine with a nuclear scan or an echocardiogram for a better evaluation of exercise induce ischemia.

Adenosine Exercise Test: This is generally used in conjunction with the nuclear scans to look for evidence of reversible myocardial ischemia. This is based on the concept that adenosine is a powerful coronary vasodilator. It can increase coronary flow by 4-6 folds. When it dilates the coronaries, the branches with critical occlusion may not dilate as briskly as the normal segments. As a result, these areas are hypoperfused compared to the normal segments. Thus, comparing the rest and stress-induced images, we will be able to identify areas with decreased myocardial perfusion. The adenosine may slightly increase the heart rate, but not enough to reach the 85% of the PMHR. Often, we combine hand and leg exercises in bed along with adenosine injection to increase the heart rate that greatly enhances the reliability of the test results.

Here, the main focus is on the nuclear scans for perfusion mismatch and not so much on the classic electrocardiographic changes we expect to see in patients on a treadmill. It also doesn't tell us about the patient's physical fitness and their exercise capacity.

CLINICAL EKG INTERPRETATION

LOW VOLTAGE EKG

Low voltage in an electrocardiogram can result in low R wave amplitudes in multiple leads. If the R wave amplitude in the limb leads in less than 5 mm (0.5 mV), and if the R wave amplitude is less than 10 mm (1.0 mV) in the chest leads, the electrocardiogram is supposed to represent low voltage. There are many causes of low voltage electrocardiograms.

Hence, a thorough history and physical examination is necessary to exclude cardiac and non-cardiac causes for low voltage.

Common Causes of Low Voltage on the EKG
- **Hypothyroidism**
- **Pericardial** Effusion
- **Pneumothorax**
- **Infiltrative** Heart Diseases such as **Amyloid** Heart Disease
- **Lead** Misplacements
- **Improper** Voltage or Gain Standardization
- **Digitalis** Effect

Along with low QRS voltage, we may also see low amplitude T waves or flat T waves (Fig: 14.02). It can occur in just limb leads without similar changes in the precordial leads (voltage discordance). It can vary depending on the distance between the recording electrode and the heart structure. Hence, it is not uncommon to see an increased voltage in precordial leads in very thin people, while the voltage may be decreased in obese individuals, or in patients with severe emphysema, large pleural, or pericardial effusion.

CHAPTER 14. MISCELLANEOUS ABNORMALITIES

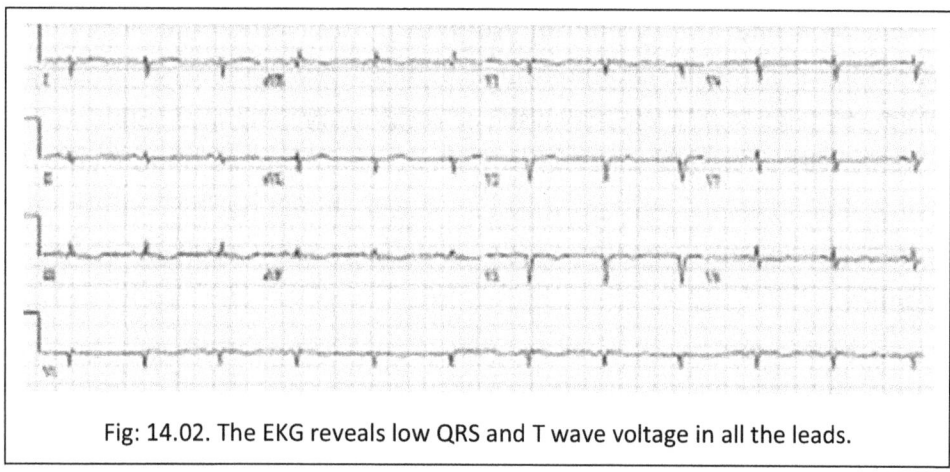

Fig: 14.02. The EKG reveals low QRS and T wave voltage in all the leads.

Look at the voltage gain marker to make sure it is representing 10 mm. If for some reason, the voltage gain is reduced by half, the voltage on the surface electrocardiogram may be low.

ELECTRICAL ALTERNANS

Electrical alternans is where the P, QRS, and T wave voltages vary with alternate beats. This is most commonly seen in patients with pericardial effusion where a swinging heart can be at varying distances from the chest wall. It is most often seen in the precordial leads.

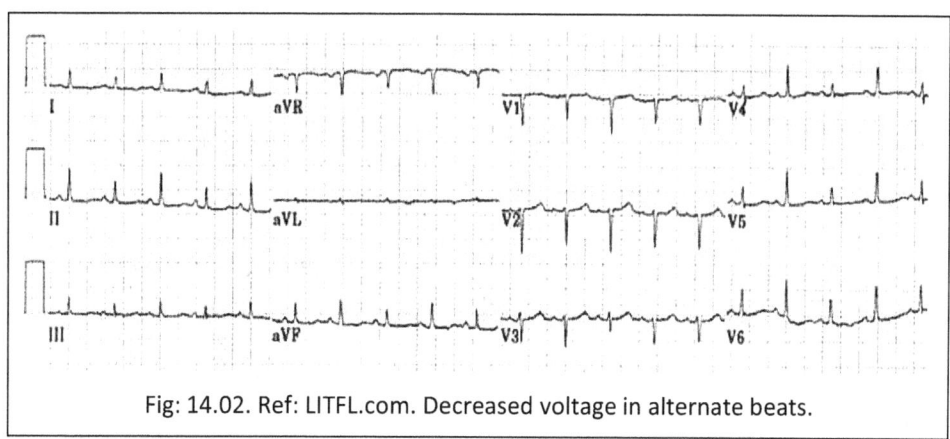

Fig: 14.02. Ref: LITFL.com. Decreased voltage in alternate beats.

CLINICAL EKG INTERPRETATION

Electrical alternans is different from the pulses alternans, which refers to the pulse pressure and volume changes noted in alternate beats as recorded on a graph (Fig: 14.03). We may also see respiratory variations superimposed on that. This is commonly seen in patients with cardiac tamponade. The electrical and pulses alternans may co-exist. It should not be confused with alternations in pulse pressure seen in patients with atrial or ventricular bigeminy.

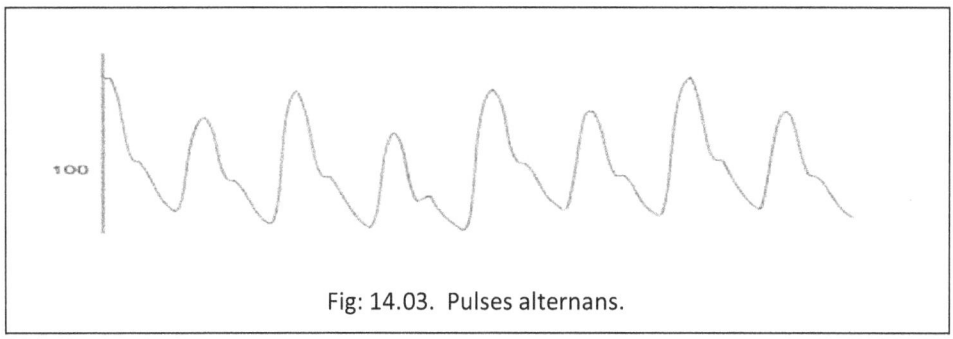

Fig: 14.03. Pulses alternans.

HYPERKALEMIA

It produces the most dramatic changes on the electrocardiogram, which should be apparent at first glance. It is a medical emergency and the electrocardiogram may be the first sign of hyperkalemia. Most often, it happens in the presence of renal failure and those patients who are on dialysis. It also can occur in patients who are receiving potassium-sparing diuretics.

The electrophysiologic effects of hyperkalemia are directly related to both the absolute plasma potassium and its rate of rise.

Rising extracellular potassium reduces excitability of the pacemaker cells and the myocardium. As the serum potassium level rises, it suppresses the impulse generation and propagation through the conducting system.

The characteristic electrocardiographic finding in patients with hyperkalemia if the tall peaked T waves in the anterolateral chest leads. As the serum potassium level goes up the electrocardiographic changes become more dramatic (Fig:14.04).

CHAPTER 14. MISCELLANEOUS ABNORMALITIES

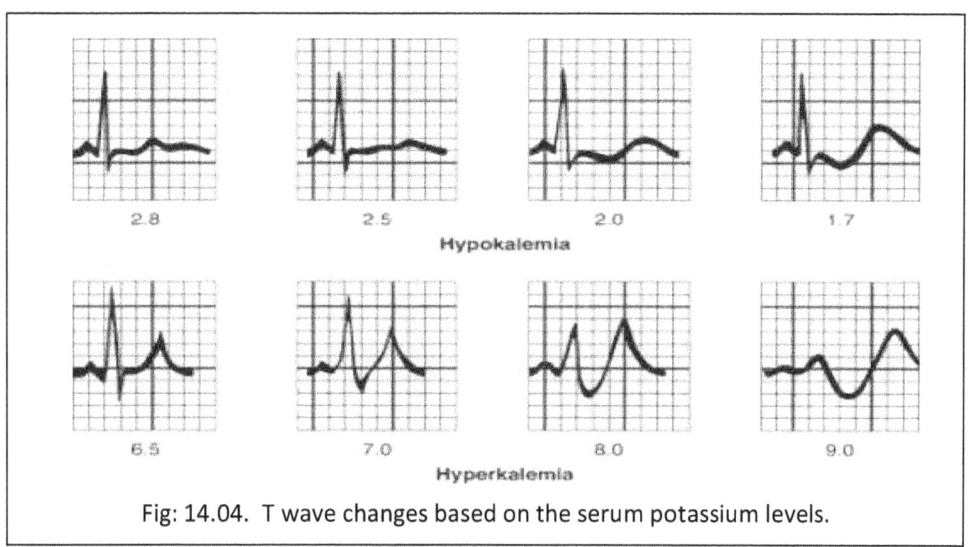

Fig: 14.04. T wave changes based on the serum potassium levels.

As the serum potassium level goes up above 7 mEq/L, the T waves become tall and peaked like tents. Their heights may reach anywhere from 5 mm to 20 mm. The ST segment may blend with the upstroke of the T waves. The P waves become flat and the PR interval is prolonged (Fig: 14.05).

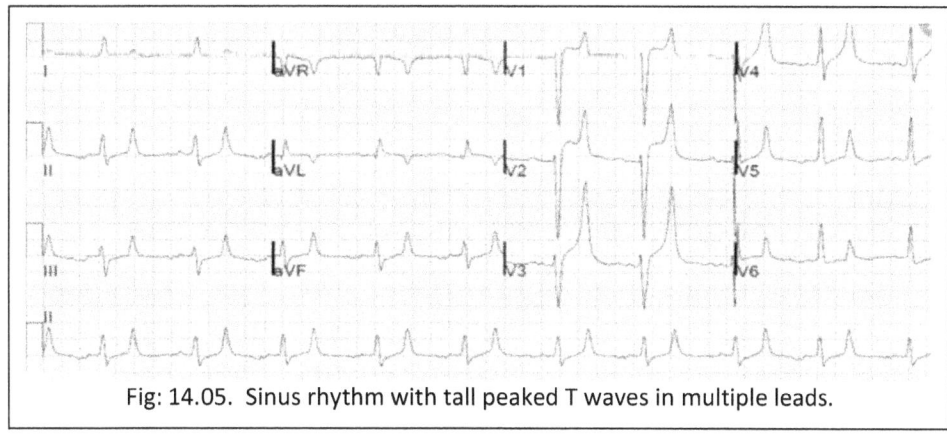

Fig: 14.05. Sinus rhythm with tall peaked T waves in multiple leads.

As the serum potassium level reaches 8 mEq/L, the QRS begins to widen markedly, with a slurred upstroke of the ST-T segment (Fig: 14.06). Beyond a serum level of 9 mEq/L, there is a loss of R waves and the electrocardiogram will begin to look like a wide QRS slow tachycardia. The QRS also appears like a sine wave. The P waves will disappear. The same pattern may be seen in all the leads.

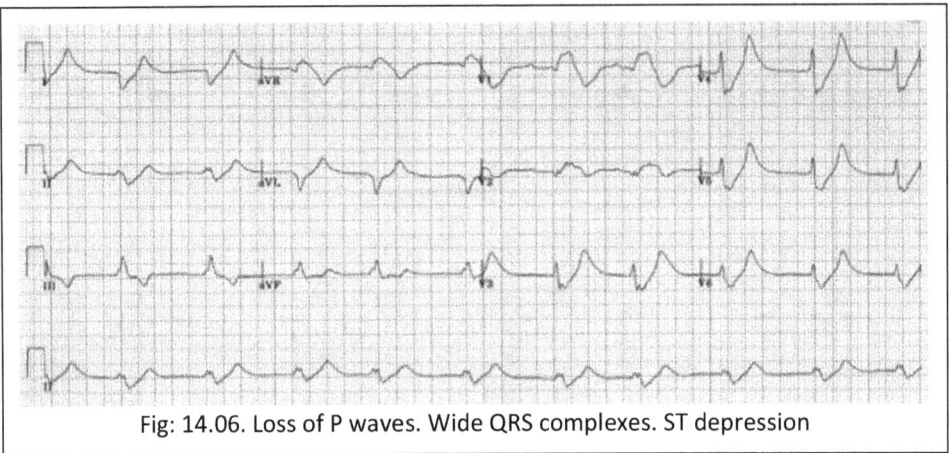

Fig: 14.06. Loss of P waves. Wide QRS complexes. ST depression

If left untreated, it may progress to ventricular fibrillation and asystole. This is a medical emergency and these patients should be admitted to the intensive care unit and immediate measures are taken to lower the serum potassium level below 5 mEq.

Treatment of Hyperkalemia: Hyperkalemia is a medical emergency and these patients need to be in the intensive care unit. The treatment of hyperkalemia should begin in the emergency departments. The immediate goal should be to reduce the serum potassium level close to normal as quickly as possible

The following options are available for treating hyperkalemia:

Calcium Gluconate 10 mL of 10% solution given as an IV bolus over 1-3 minutes for potassium levels > 6.5 mEq/L. Calcium chloride helps to stabilize the cell membrane and accelerate impulse conduction.

Insulin: It facilitates the intracellular movement of potassium in the skeletal muscles. The dose is 10 units of regular insulin combined with 25 g of 5% glucose in 50 mL given intravenously over 10 minutes.

Sodium Bicarbonate: It shifts potassium intracellularly, but is not considered the first choice. It is given as an IV bolus of 1ml/Kg of sodium bicarbonate. It may take several hours for the sodium bicarbonate to reduce

CHAPTER 14. MISCELLANEOUS ABNORMALITIES

the serum potassium level. It should be used with caution in patients with heart or kidney failure as it increases the sodium load.

Beta$_2$ Agonist: Albuterol stimulates Na+K+-ATPase thus promoting intracellular potassium movement. However, it requires larger doses like 10 to 20 mg and the amount of a drop-in serum potassium level could only range from 0.3 to 0.6 mEq/L over 30 minutes. At these dose levels, it also could stimulate Beta$_1$receptors which can lead to tachycardia.

Diuretic: Loop diuretics work within 15 to 60 minutes and promote potassium loss through increased diuresis. It works best in patients with an expanded volume or those who are fluid overloaded.

Cation Exchange Polymer: Sodium polystyrene sulfonate (SPS) is given in a dose of 15 to 30 g by mouth or as an enema along with sorbitol to increase potassium loss through the gut. Because of its high sodium content, it should be used with caution in patients with heart or kidney failure. It may take more than 2 hours to reduce the serum potassium level.

Hemodialysis: It is the preferred choice if the oral agents fail to reduce the potassium level in 60 minutes. It may take three hours to reduce the serum potassium level by 2 mEq/L.

Patiromer: It is an oral potassium binding polymer useful in treating mild hyperkalemia in an outpatient setting. It may be useful in patients who have kidney disease and need ACE inhibitors, ARBs, or aldosterone inhibitors. The dose ranges from 8.4 g to 25.2 g given once daily. The powder should be mixed with water and taken immediately.

Table 1. Summary of Approved Therapy Options for Hyperkalemia

Medication	Recommended Doses for Hyperkalemia	Route of Administration	Onset of Action
Calcium	10 mL calcium chloride or calcium gluconate (10%)	IV	Immediate 1-3 min
Insulin (short-acting)	10 units	IV	20 min
Albuterol	10-20 mg	Inhalation	30 min
Furosemide	40-80 mg	IV	15 min
Sodium polystyrene sulfonate (available sorbitol-free)	15-60 g / 30-50 g	Oral / Rectal	>2 h
Patiromer[a]	8.4-25.2 g daily	Oral	7 h

[a] Should not be used as an emergency treatment for life-threatening hyperkalemia because of its delayed onset of action. Source: References 11-14, 16, 19.

HYPOKALEMIA

Hypokalemia occurs more commonly in those patients who are on long-term loop diuretics without potassium replacements. It also can happen in patients with severe diarrhea or in patients who are receiving a vigorous colon prep.

Hypokalemia is defined as a serum potassium level below 3.5 mmol/L. A patient is supposed to have moderate hypokalemia when the serum potassium level is <3.0 mmol/L and severe hypokalemia when the serum potassium level is <2.5 mmol/L.

Hypokalemia EKG changes
- Increased Height and Width of the P Waves
- PR Prolongation
- Flattened and Inverted T waves
- ST Depression
- Prominent U waves
- Fusion of T and U Waves May Make QT Interval Look prolonged
- Frequent PACs and PVCs
- Atrial Flutter or Fib.
- Ventricular Arrhythmias

CHAPTER 14. MISCELLANEOUS ABNORMALITIES

Often the low potassium is associated with low magnesium levels. Hence, all patients with low potassium should have serum magnesium levels. Both must be corrected before we can see an improvement in the ectopic activities.

> **Hypokalemia EKG Changes -Differential Diagnosis**
> - **Hypothyroidism**
> - **Pericardial Effusion**
> - **Pneumothorax**
> - **Infiltrative Heart Diseases Such as Amyloid Heart Disease**
> - **Lead Misplacements**
> - **Improper Voltage or Gain Standardization**
> - **Digitalis Effect**

Potassium Replacement: It can be replaced by IV or by mouth depending upon the serum potassium level and ectopic activity.

We can give up to 40 mEq potassium by mouth every 6-8 hours. Intravenous potassium can be given as a 20 mEq potassium in 100 mL of normal saline over an hour. Make sure the potassium is given through a large vein as it irritates the veins and causes burning. We could inject 10-20 mg of Lidocaine into the vein and it may alleviate the burning. Sometimes, smaller veins may undergo sclerosis following potassium infusion. It takes 100 mEq of external potassium to bring the potassium level from 2.5 to 3.5 mEq/L. It may take almost 24 hours to correct a severe potassium deficit.

However, in patients with renal insufficiency, extra precaution should be taken while administering large doses of potassium by mouth or through the intravenous route. It is better to give 20 mEq IV infusion weight a couple hours, check the serum level and make the next decision based on the recent potassium level.

CLINICAL EKG INTERPRETATION

CALCIUM AND EKG CHANGES

Calcium is an important element in the myocardial action potential. Hence, changes in calcium levels can not only reflect changes on the surface electrocardiogram but also have an effect on myocardial function. However, when we measure calcium levels, we should also include ionized calcium levels and the serum albumin level. It is the ionized calcium that has direct interaction in the action potential. The Osborn waves are related to transmural voltage gradient during the early part of ventricular repolarization.

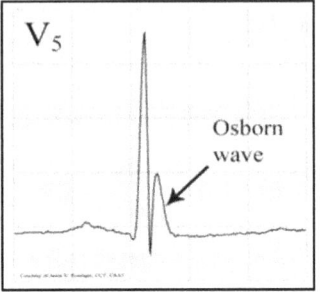

Hypocalcemia: < 8.5 mg/dL (Fig: 14.07)	Hypercalcemia: >10.5 mg/dL (Fig: 14.08)
Prolonged ST segment	Shortened ST segment
Prolonged QT interval	Shortened QT interval
Torsades de Pointe	

Hypercalcemia causes shortening of the ST segment leading to short QT interval (Fig: 14.07). Digoxin is the only other agent that causes the short QT interval. The ST segment has a scooping upward slope, as it blends into the T wave upstroke. Cardiac arrhythmias are rare, although AV block, sinus arrest, and ventricular tachycardia have been seen in patients with hypercalcemia.

ACLS QUIZ:

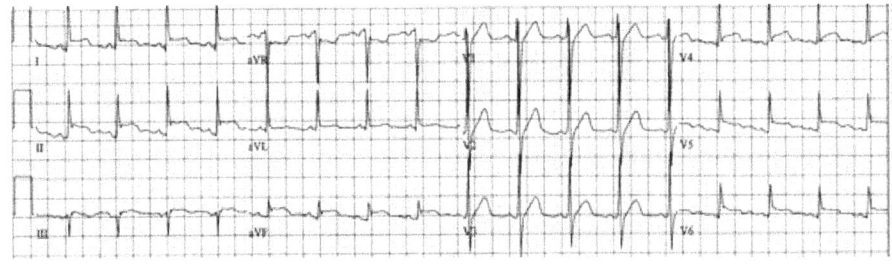

What do you see? _____

HYPERCALCEMIA EKG

CHAPTER 14. MISCELLANEOUS ABNORMALITIES

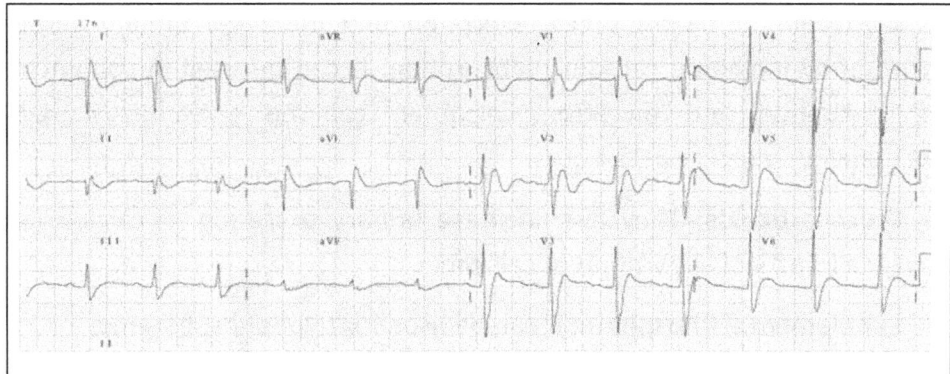

Fig: 14.07. An EKG from a patient with hypercalcemia. Note the short ST and QT intervals. Osborn waves are also present.

HYPOCALCEMIA EKG

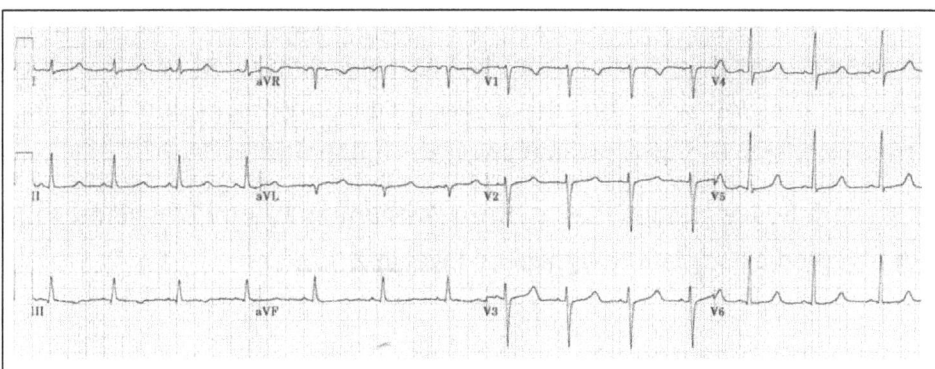

Fig: 14.08. An EKG from a patient with hypocalcemia. Note the long ST and QT intervals.
Ref: https://litfl.com/hypocalcaemia-ecg-library/

Treatment of Hypercalcemia:

A hypercalcemic crisis is where the serum calcium rises above 14 mg/dL.

Hydration and Forced Diuresis: Loop diuretics decrease the absorption of calcium by the kidney. Hydration is important to counteract dehydration and increase diuresis. Some patients may need as much as 2000 mL of fluids per hour. It may take 24 hours to reduce the serum calcium by 1-3 mg/dL.

Calcitonin: It blocks bone resorption and increases urinary calcium excretion by inhibiting calcium reabsorption. It can be used in conjunction with hydration and diuretics. Calcitonin can be given as 4 IU/Kg subcutaneously, every 6-12 hours.

Glucocorticoids: They also increase urinary excretion of calcium and decrease intestinal absorption of calcium.

Supplemental Phosphate: It can be used for hypophosphatemia.

If all measures fail, try dialysis. Follow serum calcium levels every 8 hours.

HYPOMAGNESEMIA AND EKG CHANGES

Magnesium levels below 1.0 mmol/L (Normal 0.8 to 1.0 mmol/L) have been associated with frequent atrial and ventricular ectopic beats. Often, it occurs in combination with hypokalemia, which can contribute to some arrhythmias. Low magnesium levels can also lead to prolonged QT_c intervals. If a patient presents with Torsades de Pointe and low magnesium level, it can be treated with 2 G of magnesium given as an IV bolus.

Generally, we can give 1-2 g of magnesium in 100 ml of saline over an hour followed by a repeat magnesium level in 2-4 hours.

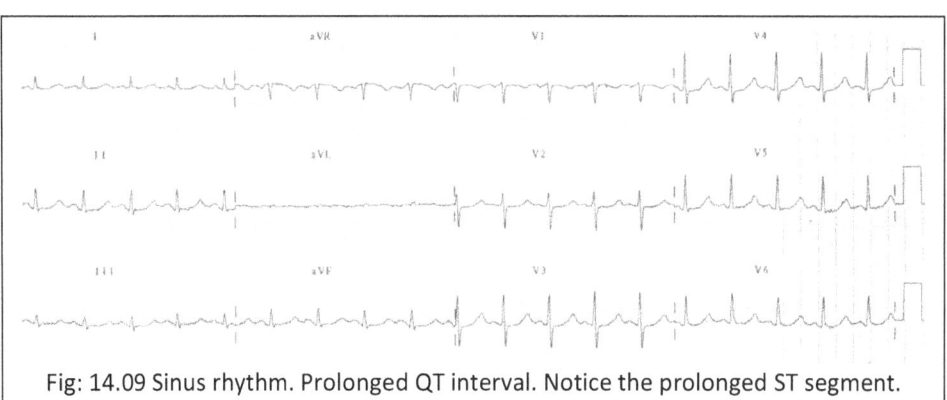

Fig: 14.09 Sinus rhythm. Prolonged QT interval. Notice the prolonged ST segment.

CHAPTER 14. MISCELLANEOUS ABNORMALITIES

CARDIAC TRANSPLANT

When a cardiac transplant is done, part of the recipient's atrial muscle is left behind. The atria from the donor's heart are attached to the host's atrial muscle. As a result, we may see two distinct atrial activities, one from the host and the other from the donor heart (Fig: 10.10). The transplanted heart is denervated and doesn't respond to the autonomic nervous system signals. Atrial arrhythmias and conduction disturbances are common. The rate of the donor's heart is greater as it is not controlled by the autonomic system. Right bundle branch block occurs in more than 50% of the patients.

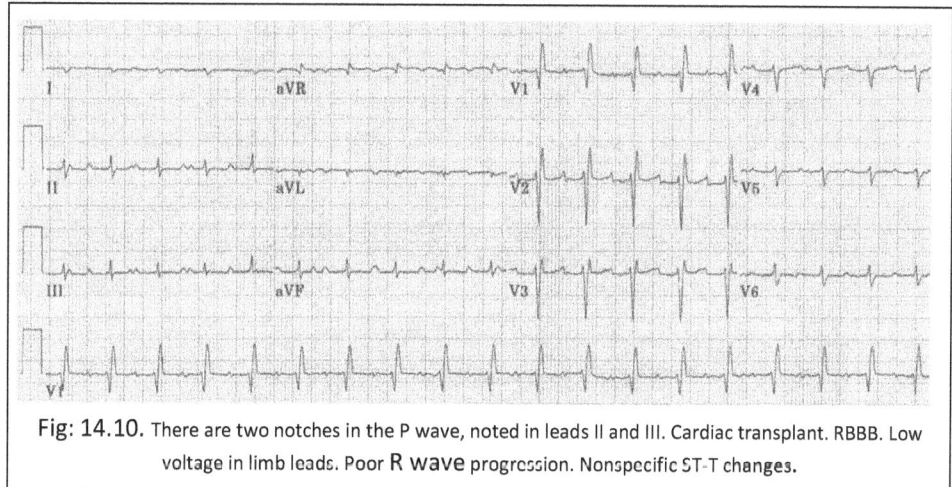

Fig: 14.10. There are two notches in the P wave, noted in leads II and III. Cardiac transplant. RBBB. Low voltage in limb leads. Poor R wave progression. Nonspecific ST-T changes.

HYPOTHERMIA

Hypothermia is a condition where the body temperature drops below 35°C or 91° F and has a profound effect on bodily functions, and if not recognized and treated promptly, it could be fatal. Based on the body temperature it is considered Mild: 32°-35° C, Moderate: 29°-32° C, or Severe: <29° C

Hypothermia can be accidental like when people get stranded in freezing weather with no proper gear or it can be induced like during cardiac surgery when the body temperature is reduced to decrease the metabolism and oxygen requirements.

CLINICAL EKG INTERPRETATION

Hypothermia EKG Changes: (Fig: 14.11)

- It is characterized by a Notch on the QRS complex - Osborne waves
- The P Waves May be Flat Along with the T Waves.
- Low Voltage.
- Prolongation of PR, QRS, QT,
- Sinus Bradycardia, Junctional Bradycardia, Atrial Fibrillation
- High-grade AV Blocks
- Muscle Shakes on the Surface EKG
- Ventricular Ectopic Beats, VT, or VF

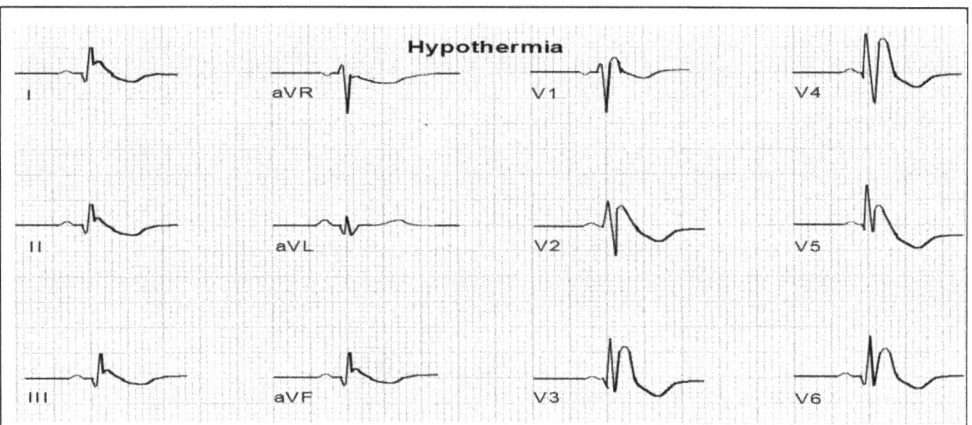

Fig: 14.11. Notice the elevation of the J point and Osborne waves. Also, notice the Osborne wave continuing as the ST segment along with T wave inversion.

It is seen in 85% of the people with a core body temperature of <35° C. Similar changes may be seen in patients with hypercalcemia. The electrocardiographic changes are thought to be related to outward potassium current leading to repolarization abnormality. The J waves are usually seen in lead II and V2-V6. It may also be noted in patients coming off cardioplegia during cardiac surgery

CHAPTER 14. MISCELLANEOUS ABNORMALITIES

LONG QT SYNDROME

Long QT syndrome is characterized by prolongation of the QT interval. Note the broad T waves with a possible notch which may represent U waves (Fig:14.12). These patients are at increased risk for Torsades de Pointes. They may also have syncope and susceptible to sudden death. These patients are best candidates for ICD implantation and beta blockers.

Multiple medications, including antiarrhythmics and tricyclic antidepressants, can prolong the QT intervals. While measuring the QT interval, we need to take the longest QT interval measured either in limb leads or chest leads. Computer measurements should always be validated by visual inspection or manual measurement.

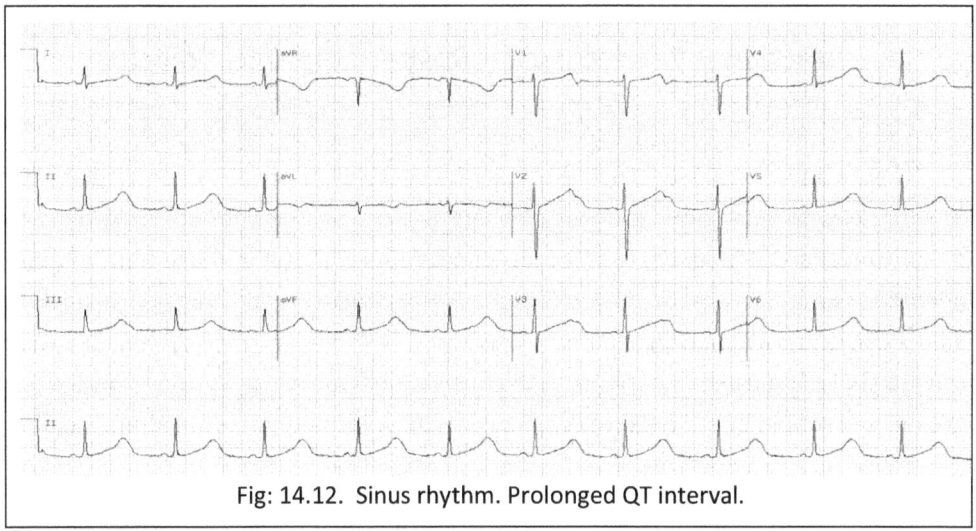

Fig: 14.12. Sinus rhythm. Prolonged QT interval.

DIGITALIS EFFECT

The role of digoxin in modern practice is becoming less and less important, partly due to better drugs available for heart failure treatment and partly due to, its significant side effects, especially in a patient with compromised renal function.

Keep in mind the following side effects and electrocardiographic changes that are unique to digitalis, which is called the "Digitalis Effect."

CLINICAL EKG INTERPRETATION

Digitalis Toxicity (Fig: 14. 13)
- **J Point Depression and ST Downsloping, Blending with Biphasic T Waves**
- **Sino-Atrial block**
- **Sinus Bradycardia or Pauses**
- **1°, 2°, and 3° Heart Blocks**
- **Bundle Branch Blocks**
- **Short QT intervals**

- **Unifocal or Multifocal PVCs**
- **V. Tach, Flutter, or Fibrillation**
- **Paroxysmal Atrial Tachycardia with Block**
- **Junctional Tachycardia – Suspect Digitalis Toxicity**

It may one of the few drugs that may be useful in controlling ventricular rates in patients with atrial fibrillation when there is a contraindication for beta-blockers or calcium channel blockers use. It may also be useful in the management of acute decompensation of chronic heart failure. Always measure the digoxin levels and adjust the dosage based on the renal function. The lowest digoxin dose that can do the job should be used. In patients with chronic renal failure or for those on dialysis, the digoxin should be reduced to 0.125 mg orally or intravenously on alternate days.

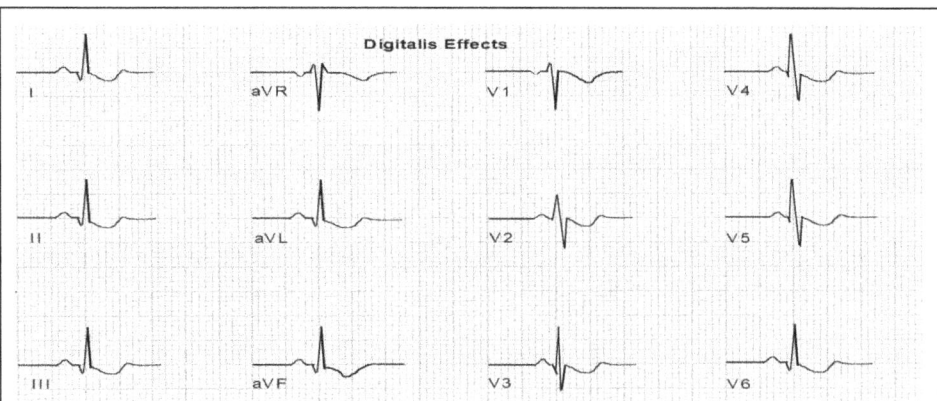

Fig: 14.13. Notice the downsloping ST segment, which blends into the inverted T wave with a biphasic morphology.

CHAPTER 14. MISCELLANEOUS ABNORMALITIES

KARTAGENER'S SYNDROME

This syndrome is characterized by chronic sinusitis with dextrocardia. If you record right chest leads, mark them so they are not confusing. Also, note the progression of the QRS complex as you move from the right sternal border to the right axillary line. It will also have extreme right taxis at the impulse travels from left to the right side (Fig: 14.14).

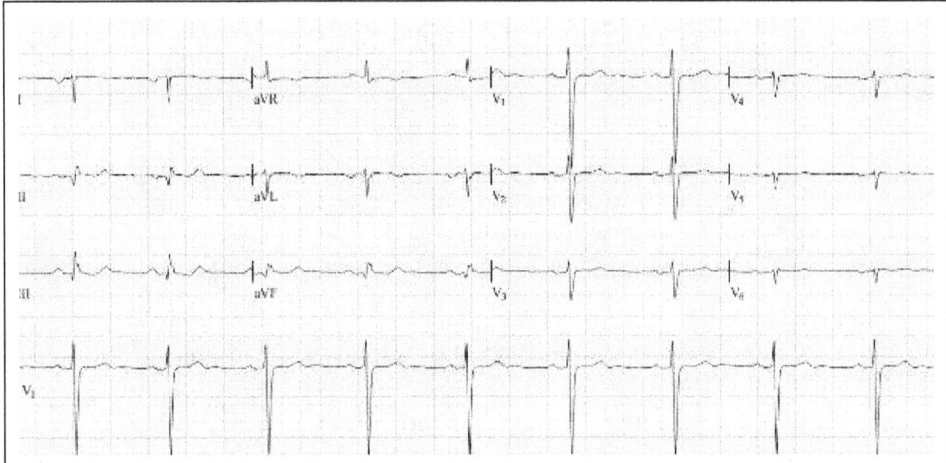

Fig: 14.14. Sinus rhythm. Note the extreme right axis deviation as the impulse travels from the left to the right side. Also, notice the R Waves in the lateral chest leads which are diminished.

TETRALOGY OF FALLOT EKG

It is characterized by extreme right axis deviation, right ventricular hypertrophy, ST-T changes leads V1, V2, deep S waves in the lateral chest leads, Peaked P waves in II, III, and aVF

ACLS QUIZ:

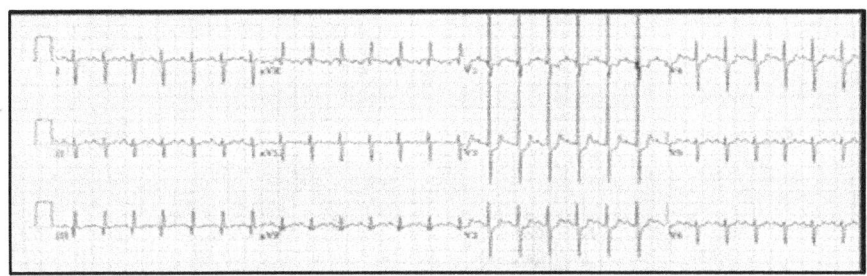

CLINICAL EKG INTERPRETATION

What are the findings? _____

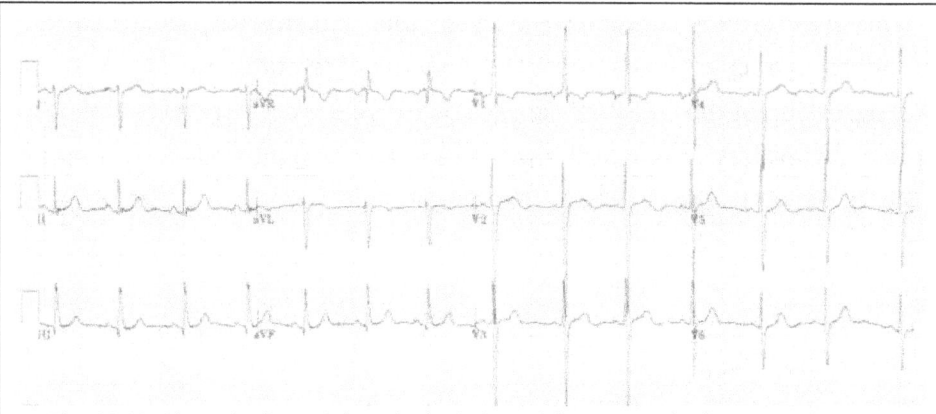

Fig: 14.15. Sinus rhythm. Right axis deviation, right ventricular hypertrophy, ST-T changes leads V1, V2, deep S waves in the lateral chest leads, Peaked P waves in II, III, and aVF.

ARTIFACTS

They may look like muscle tremors, a short run of atrial fibrillation or flutter. Always, look at the rhythm before and after the artifacts. March the QRS complexes and see if they remain same through the artifacts. It is common to see muscle tremors in patients with Parkinson's disease and when the room temperature is cold and the patient is shivering. Don't blame the patient. Get a blanket and over the patient.

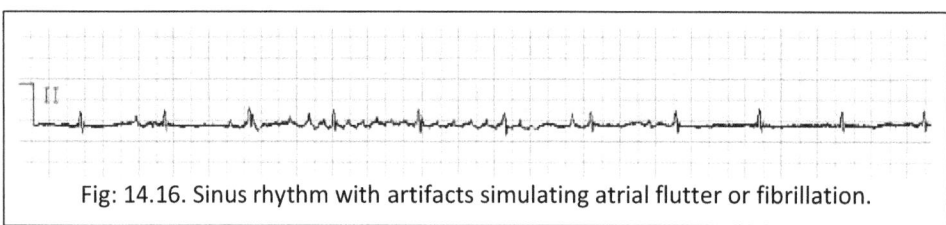

Fig: 14.16. Sinus rhythm with artifacts simulating atrial flutter or fibrillation.

SIXTY CYCLE INTERFERENCE

If there is a lot of noise in the electrical connections, it can create a 60-cycle interference. Try to switch the outlet and see if it works. If your machine has a battery backup, try pulling the cord from the outlet while recording the

CHAPTER 14. MISCELLANEOUS ABNORMALITIES

electrocardiogram. As a last resort, get a new technician! There is nothing wrong with the machine!

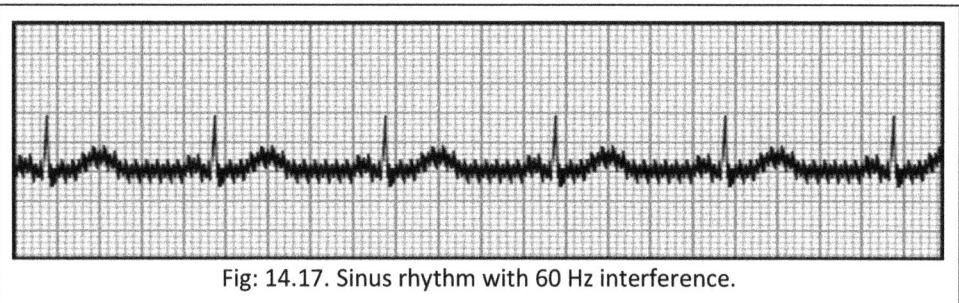

Fig: 14.17. Sinus rhythm with 60 Hz interference.

PROMINENT U WAVES

The U waves are thought to be related to afterdepolarizations in the ventricles. They can trigger automaticity and precipitate arrhythmias, including Torsades de Pointes. The usual U wave is in the same direction as the T wave and about 30% of its height. They are most often seen in V2 and V3. The upstroke is more rapid compared to the downstroke, and that is opposite of T wave progression (Fig: 14.18).

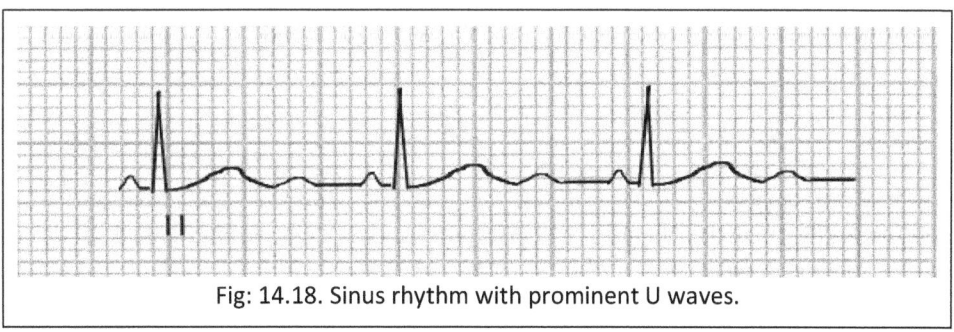

Fig: 14.18. Sinus rhythm with prominent U waves.

Negative or "inverted" U waves are usually associated with Ischemic heart disease. It is often associated with left main or LAD disease. They may be seen in:

- Myocardial infarction (in leads with pathologic Q waves)
- During an episode of acute ischemia (angina or exercise-induced ischemia)

CLINICAL EKG INTERPRETATION

- During coronary artery spasm (Prinz metal's angina)

They may be seen in a variety of conditions like:

> **Differential Diagnosis of U Wave Abnormalities:**
>
> - **Sinus bradycardia**
> - **Hypokalemia**
> - **Hypothermia**
> - **Quinidine and Other types 1A Antiarrhythmics**
> - **CNS Disease with Long QT**
> - **LVH (Right Precordial Leads with Deep S Waves)**
> - **Mitral Valve Prolapse (Some Cases MVP)**
> - **Hyperthyroidism**

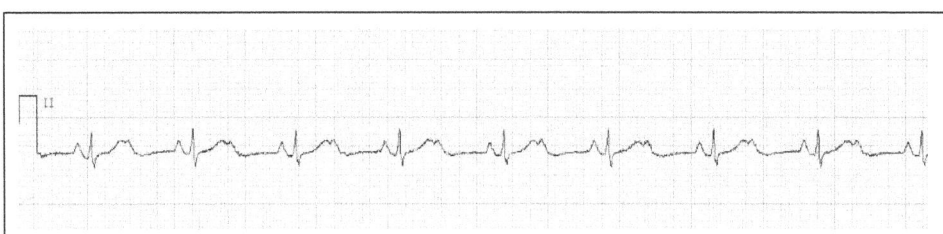

Fig: 14.19. Sinus with 2: 1 AV block. Note the notch on the T waves. PACs would come earlier than the previous PP interval.

Epstein's Anomaly: It is associated with giant (~Himalayan~) P waves, but with a right ventricular conduction delay (often with wide, atypical qR complexes in V1-V3) (Fig: 14.20).

CHAPTER 14. MISCELLANEOUS ABNORMALITIES

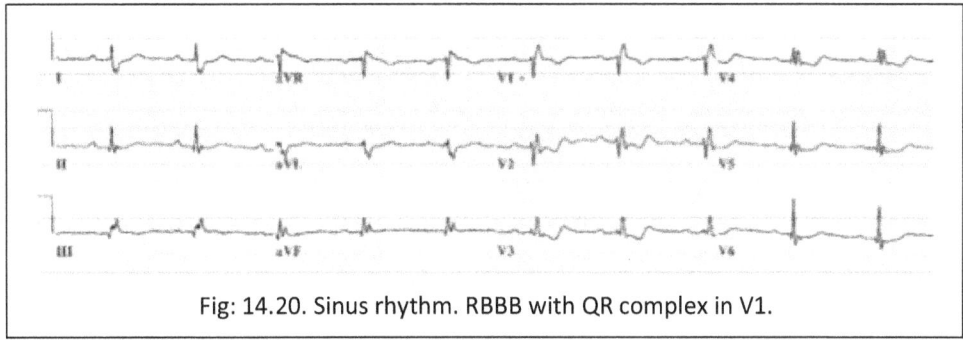

Fig: 14.20. Sinus rhythm. RBBB with QR complex in V1.

Infiltrative Cardiomyopathy: Diffusely low voltage may be a clue to cardiac amyloid, especially in the setting of clinical evidence of restrictive cardiomyopathy.

DEXTROCARDIA

This is a condition where the heart is located on the right side of the chest, instead of on the normal left side. The atria are on the left sternal border, while the ventricles extend toward the right axillary lines.

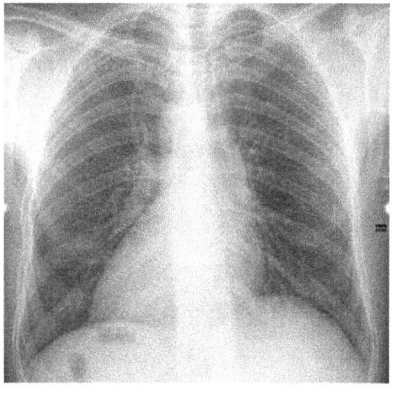

The chest X-ray shows the anatomical orientation of the heart in the mediastinum. The normal right heart border is located to the left of the sternum and the apex of the heart is resting on the right hemidiaphragm just above the liver. Similarly, the position of the superior and inferior vena cave is shifted to the left side. The aortic notch is on the right side.

The electrocardiogram will display a mirror image of the normal electrocardiogram:

- Lead I will look like aVR.
- Lead aVL will look like lead I
- There is a progressive loss of R waves from V1 to V6.
- rS or qS complexes across the chest leads

CLINICAL EKG INTERPRETATION

- However, if we were to place the chest leads to the right of the sternum, we will notice the normal progression of the R waves.
- You may also see negative T waves in multiple leads

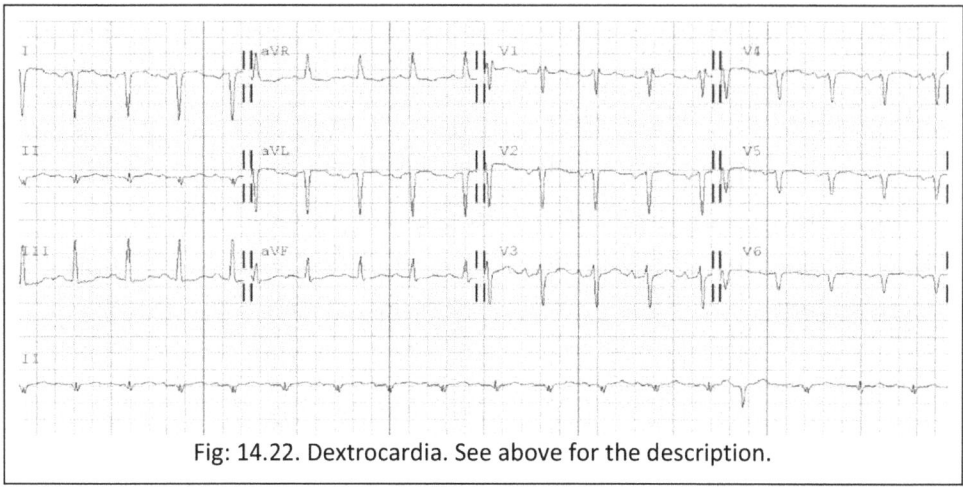

Fig: 14.22. Dextrocardia. See above for the description.

MUSCLE TREMORS

Muscle tremors and shivering can cause dramatic changes on the electrocardiogram. You may have noticed them while performing an electrocardiogram in the post-operative room immediately after surgery when the body temperature may be low or the patient is shivering.

Certain neurological conditions such as Parkinson's tremors can have a classic effect on an electrocardiogram that can mimic atrial flutter or ventricular flutter. When you see large rhythmic, undulating waves that that doesn't fall into any specific pattern like a flutter, look for clues that can unravel the mystery.
- Find a lead where these undulating waves are least visible
- Look for QRS deflections
- Measure the RR intervals and see if they are regular
- Look for any pause in the undulating waves that can reveal the underlying atrial mechanism

CHAPTER 14. MISCELLANEOUS ABNORMALITIES

- If you can see a normal underlying rhythm behind all this noise, give yourself a pat in the back
- Ask your colleagues to interpret the EKG and collect all the differential diagnoses you can

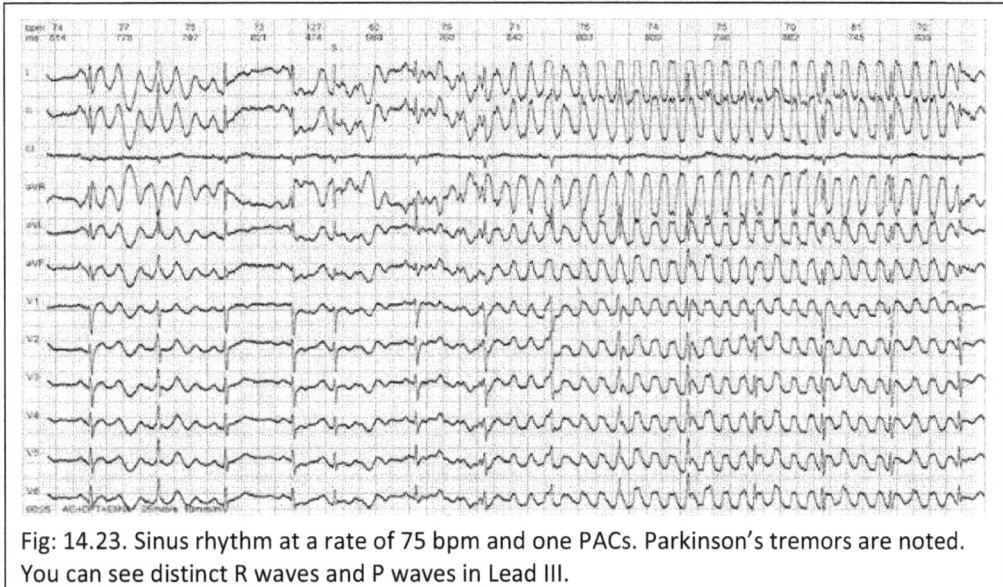

Fig: 14.23. Sinus rhythm at a rate of 75 bpm and one PACs. Parkinson's tremors are noted. You can see distinct R waves and P waves in Lead III.

If you have access to an electrocardiogram machine, try experimenting with one of your co-workers. Have that person mimic the Parkinson's tremors in the hands or legs and document the changes on the electrocardiogram. Take turns and see who can do better.

CLINICAL EKG INTERPRETATION

MISTERY EKG

What is your diagnosis?

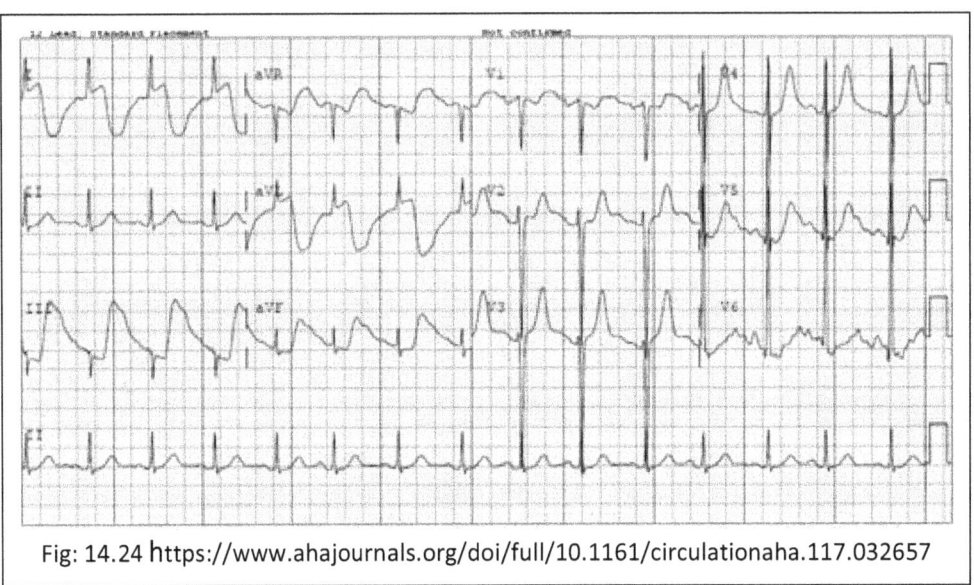

Fig: 14.24 https://www.ahajournals.org/doi/full/10.1161/circulationaha.117.032657

This is an electrocardiogram from a 32-year-old renal patient with an AV fistula in the left arm. Notice the ST elevation and deep T wave inversion in leads I and aVL. This is an artifact produced by the superficial arterial pulse as the changes march along the QRS complexes. There are also reciprocal changes in the leads III and aVF. However, if you place the left arm lead away from the AV fistula site, these changes disappear (Fig: 14.25).

Whenever you see bizarre wide swings in the waveforms, always look for a lead that has the least changes and try to unravel the mystery from there. Then, try to find out what might be causing the mystery changes. Next challenge your friends and co-workers.

CHAPTER 14. MISCELLANEOUS ABNORMALITIES

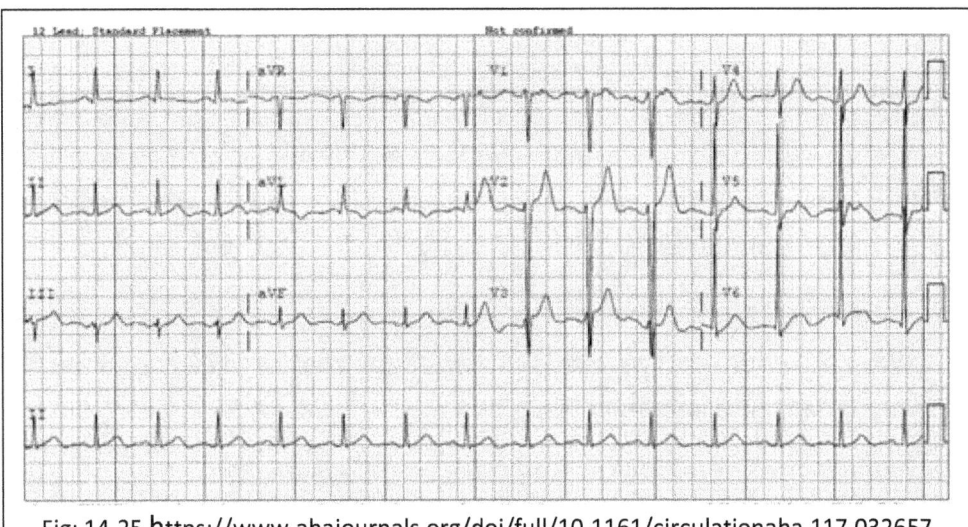

Fig: 14.25 https://www.ahajournals.org/doi/full/10.1161/circulationaha.117.032657

COMIC CLUB BLOCK

Shrink hospital

The psychiatrist was making rounds in the hospital. He sees one of his patients listening to the wall. The shrink walks up to him and says, "Hey! Walter, what are you doing?

"Suh, doc, listen!" Says Walter."

Now, this board-certified shrink listens to the wall for five minutes, he tells Walter, "I don't hear anything."

Walters says, "Ah ah! Doc, it's been like that all day long."

Interestingly, both the patient and the shrink serve time behind locked doors in a psychiatric hospital. Except one of them has a remote hope of getting out alive, when his insurance expires. Amen!

Chapter 15 Cardiac Monitoring

Cardiac monitoring for extended periods of time is required in some patients to determine the frequency and the nature of the tachyarrhythmias or other symptoms. The indications for extended cardiac monitoring may include:

- Evaluation of symptoms of palpitations, weakness, or dizziness.
- Estimate the frequency and duration of tachyarrhythmias or bradyarrhythmia's in a patient.
- Access the efficiency of treatment in suppressing a given arrhythmia with procedures or medicines.
- Monitor patients with pacemakers and other devices.

There are various types of devices available depending upon the needs of a patient.

- Continuous ambulatory EKG (24-48 Hours)
- Event Recorders: Triggered by the patient
- Looping recorder
- Post symptom recorder
- Implantable loop recorders (up to 3-year battery life)

There are event monitors that can work anywhere from 2 weeks to 2-3 years. These are called the event recorders and the patients may be able to trigger them when they experience symptoms.

All these reordering devices serve one purpose – correlate the patient' symptoms to any electrocardiographic changes we may or may not notice on the electrocardiogram. Then, we can decide what to do with those findings.

COMEDY TIME

A sixteen years old young lady, Kelly, asks her dad Brendan, "Daddy can I borrow your car for the weekend. We are planning to go to Galveston.

Brendan said, "Hold on, Hold on, young lady. You just got your driver's license a week ago. You want to borrow my Mercedes Benz car, and then go to Galveston? Did I get that right?"

"Yep!"

Brendan, "And, who is this 'we'?" Asked.

Kelly, "Oh! That's Josh and I!"

"Who is Josh?" Brendan asked.

"He is in my choir group. He is HS senior."

"There is no way I'm going to give you my car so you can go with a stranger, that too out of town. You know, you need to have an adult with you in the car when you drive?"

Kelly said, "Don't worry dad, Josh is 21."

Brendan asked, "He is 21 and he still an HS senior? There is no way that you are taking my car."

Kelly replied, "That's all right dad. That's your baby, I understand. You have the right to make your decisions."

"You better believe it!"

Kelly said, "I just want you to know that 25 to 30 years from now, I decide which nursing home you go to!"

Brendan asked, "Wow! Not bad. Did Josh tell you to say that?"

"I am telling you," replied Kelly.

"Make sure you return before 9 pm. Stay safe, and no texting while driving'!" As he reluctantly handed the keys.

EKG

Multiple Choice Questions

1-100

CLINICAL EKG INTERPRETATION

1 EKG findings in pericardial effusion include all except

   A. PR depression
   B. Low QRS voltage
   C. Electrical alternans
   D. Short QT interval
   E. ST elevation

2 Low voltage is defined as the QRS amplitude < _____ in the limb leads and <_____ in the chest leads

   A. 6, 12
   B. 5, 16
   C. 10, 5
   D. 5, 10

3 An EKG reveals atrial flutter with 2:1 conduction. Which ventricular rate most likely match the rhythm?

   A. 90 bpm
   B. 200 bpm
   C. 300 bpm
   D. 145 bpm

4 Right axis deviation is seen in all these conditions except.

   A. Right ventricular hypertrophy
   B. Left posterior hemiblock
   C. Lead reversal
   D. Pulmonic stenosis
   E. Right bundle branch block

5 Repolarization abnormalities related to LBBB are often seen in

   A. II, III & aVF
   B. aVR and V1
   C. V4 to V6
   D. None of the above

EKG MCQ QUIZ 1- 100

6. A condition that can mimic RVH include all except
   A. WPW
   B. RBBB
   C. Posterior MI
   D. Chronic COPD
   E. All of the above

7. ST elevation and Q waves in II, III, aVF represent MI involving the
   A. High anterior MI
   B. Inferoposterior MI
   C. Anteroseptal MI
   D. Inferior MI
   E. Anterolateral MI

8. Causes of ST elevation include all except
   A. Acute MI
   B. Early repolarization
   C. Pericarditis
   D. LV aneurysm
   E. Subendocardial ischemia

9. The electrical system of the heart consist of
   A. Sinus Node
   B. Purkinje fibers
   C. Bundle of His
   D. Coronary sinus
   E. Bundle branches

10. Phase zero of the action potential results from:
   A. The influx of potassium into the cells
   B. Efflux of calcium into the cells
   C. Influx of Magnesium
   D. Movement of sodium into the cells

CLINICAL EKG INTERPRETATION

11. ST elevation and Q waves in I aVL represent MI involving the

    A. High anterior MI
    B. Inferoposterior MI
    C. Anteroseptal MI
    D. Inferior MI
    E. Anterolateral MI

12. The sinus rate varies from:
    A. 60-100
    B. 120-200
    C. 40-60
    D. 200-300

13. The RR interval covers 5 big boxes or 25 small boxes. The heart rate is
    A. 100 bpm
    B. 75 bpm
    C. 50 bpm
    D. 80 bpm
    E. 60 bpm

14. The QRS duration represents the
    A. Ventricular relaxation
    B. Ventricular excitation
    C. Atrial contraction
    D. Part of the ventricular depolarization

15. The upper limit of the corrected QT interval in men is
    A. 450 sec
    B. 440 mm
    C. 510 ms
    D. 445 ms
    E. 475 ms

16. ST depression is seen in the following conditions except

EKG MCQ QUIZ 1- 100

   A. LVH
   B. LBBB
   C. Pericarditis
   D. Subendocardial ischemia
   E. Positive stress test

17. Each small box on the electrocardiographic paper represents
    A. 20 sec
    B. 50 ms
    C. 25 ms
    D. 40 ms
    E. 1 sec

18. ST elevation and Q waves in V1, V2, V3, and V4 represent MI involving the
    A. High anterior MI
    B. Inferoposterior MI
    C. Anteroseptal MI
    D. Right ventricular MI
    E. Anterolateral MI

19. Chest lead V1 is placed on the
    A. 2nd right intercostal space
    B. 4th left intercostal space
    C. 6th right intercostal space
    D. 4th right intercostal space

20. A 12-lead EKG has:
    A. 3 precordial leads, 3 augmented leads, and 3 chest leads
    B. 6 limb leads, 6 chest leads, and 3 augmented leads
    C. 3 leads, 3 augmented leads, and 6 chest leads
    D. 4 leads, 4 augmented leads, and 4 chest leads

21. Chest lead V6 is placed in the
    A. Midaxillary line, left 4th intercostal space
    B. The anterior axillary line, left 3rd intercostal space
    C. Midaxillary line, left 5th intercostal space

CLINICAL EKG INTERPRETATION

D. Midclavicular line, left 5th intercostal space

22. The adrenergic response includes the following except

A. Sweating
B. The rise in blood pressure
C. Flushing
D. Increase in contractility
E. Reduced AV conduction

23. ST elevation and Q waves in leads I, aVL, V5, and V6 represent MI involving the

A. High anterior wall
B. Inferoposterior wall
C. Inferior wall
D. Subendocardium
E. Anterolateral MI

24. The parasympathetic response includes

A. Prolongation of the sinus node impulse cycle
B. Acts on norepinephrine receptors located on the cells
C. Acetylcholine is the main chemical mediator
D. Drop in blood pressure
E. Slows AV nodal conduction

25. The normal electrical axis of the heart is between

A. +90° and +180°
B. −90° and −30°
C. −30° and +90°
D. +180° and −90°
E. +90° and +180°

26. The Wenckebach heart block is characterized by

A. Progressive prolongation of the PP interval
B. Progressive shortening of the RR interval
C. Constant RR intervals
D. Progressive shortening of the PR intervals
E. All of the above

EKG MCQ QUIZ 1- 100

27. All of the EKG findings may be seen in patients with mitral stenosis except
    A. Left atrial enlargement
    B. LBBB
    C. Right ventricular hypertrophy
    D. Opening snap
    E. Right atrial enlargement

28. Patients with LBBB may have
    A. Wide fixed splitting of the S2
    B. Paradoxical wide splitting of the S2
    C. Soft S1
    D. Mid-systolic click
    E. Wide splitting of the S2

29. EKGs of patients with renal failure can show all except
    A. LVH with strain
    B. Tall T waves
    C. Short QT interval
    D. Low voltage
    E. Slow wide QRS rhythm

30. ST depression and tall R waves in V1, V2, and V3 are seen in
    A. High anterior MI
    B. Posterior MI
    C. Anteroseptal MI
    D. Anterolateral MI
    E. Inferior MI

31. Patients with aortic stenosis may have all these EKG features except
    A. LVH
    B. Left atrial enlargement
    C. RBBB
    D. PVCs
    E. Strain pattern

32. Patients with COPD may have the following EKG features except
    A. Right axis deviation
    B. Biatrial enlargement
    C. Poor R wave progression across the anterior leads
    D. Right atrial enlargement
    E. Low voltage

CLINICAL EKG INTERPRETATION

33. Symmetrical deep T wave inversion in the chest leads represents
    A. High anterior MI
    B. Ventricular ischemia
    C. Anteroseptal MI
    D. Subendocardial MI
    E. Anteroposterior MI

34. Complete heart block EKG features include all except
    A. AV dissociated
    B. Atrial and ventricular rates are different
    C. There is no relationship between the atrial and ventricular beats
    D. Sometimes fusion beats can be seen
    E. The QRS complex can be narrow or wide

35. ST elevation can be seen in the following conditions except
    A. Acute MI
    B. Pericarditis
    C. LBBB
    D. Angina attack
    E. LV strain pattern

36. All of the following features are true of RBBB except
    A. RSr" in V1
    B. Slurred terminal S wave in multiple leads
    C. Concordant ST-T changes
    D. A QRS duration of >120 ms
    E. Right axis deviation

37. All of the following are true of LBBB except
    A. Wide notched QRS in leads I, aVL, V5, and V6
    B. Discordant ST-T changes
    C. Right axis deviation
    D. May be difficult to diagnose acute MI in the presence of LBBB
    E. ST elevation in V2 and V3

38. All of the following are true of left axis deviation except
    A. QRS frontal axis between –45 and –90 degrees
    B. Deep S waves in III, AVF
    C. QRS duration is less than 110 ms
    D. S wave height is greater than the R wave in lead II
    E. May be associated with left posterior hemiblock

EKG MCQ QUIZ 1- 100

39. All the features are true of Brugada syndrome except
    A. Evidence of RBBB
    B. Prone for runs of ventricular tachycardia
    C. Left atrial enlargement
    D. Terminal slurring of the S waves in V1 and V2
    E. The QRS duration of >120 ms

40. All the points regarding the EKG graph are true except
    A. Each small square represents 40 ms time on the horizontal line
    B. Each small square along the vertical line represents 0.1 mV
    C. Each small square along the vertical line represents 1.0 mV
    D. One second is represented by 25 smaller boxes or 5 big boxes
    E. Each big box represents 200 ms

41. LVH is characterized by the following features except
    A. Increase voltage in the lateral chest leads
    B. An R wave of >20 mm in aVL
    C. Seep S waves in V2 and V3
    D. Concordant ST-T depression
    E. Left atrial enlargement

42. The QRS complex represents all the following except
    A. Septal activation
    B. Left ventricular activation
    C. Right bundle branch
    D. Atrial depolarization
    E. Right ventricular depolarization

43. Pericarditis can be associated with these features except
    A. ST elevation in multiple leads
    B. The ST segments display concave surface facing down
    C. There is J joint elevation
    D. The ST changes may last for 2-4 weeks
    E. Pleuritic chest pain

44. Differential diagnosis of atrial fibrillation includes all except
    A. Atrial flutter with viable ventricular
    B. Atrial tachycardia with variable conduction
    C. Multifocal atrial tachycardia
    D. WPW with tachycardia
    E. Torsades de Pointe

CLINICAL EKG INTERPRETATION

45. Complete heart block may be characterized by all except
    A. Slow heart rate
    B. The atria and ventricles beating separately
    C. The QRS can be narrow or wide
    D. Hypotension
    E. Fusion beats

46. Tall R waves in V1, V2, and V3 may be seen in all except
    A. RVH
    B. RBB
    C. Posterior MI
    D. WPW syndrome
    E. LBBB

47. A vasovagal attack is characterized by all except
    A. Bradycardia
    B. Sinus pauses
    C. Dizziness
    D. Ventricular rhythm
    E. Hypotension

48. Atypical atrial flutter may have the following features except
    A. Narrow QRS tachycardia
    B. Clockwise conduction through the accessory pathway
    C. Sawtooth appearance in leads II, III, and aVF
    D. Variable AV conduction: 2:1, 3:1, 4:1, etc.
    E. Rounded bimodal waves in leads II, III, and aVF

49. Drug of choice for treatment of WPW tachycardia is
    A. Adenosine
    B. Beta-blockers
    C. IV calcium channel blockers
    D. Procainamide IV or PO
    E. Digoxin IV

50. Elective cardioversion is recommended for all except
    A. Atrial fib with a very rapid ventricular response
    B. Atrial flutter
    C. PAT

D. Ventricular flutter
E. Torsades de Pointe

51. Elective cardioversion is recommended for all except
    A. Atrial fib with a very rapid ventricular response
    B. Atrial flutter
    C. PAT
    D. Ventricular tachycardia
    E. Torsades de Pointe

52. Drugs recommended for SVT include all except
    A. Adenosine
    B. Esmolol
    C. Verapamil
    D. Lidocaine
    E. Ibutilide

53. Ventricular tachycardia is characterized by the following except
    A. Wide QRS complexes
    B. 150 to 200 bpm
    C. AV dissociation
    D. Occasional 2:1 conduction
    E. Fusion beats

54. EKG changes during hypothermia include all except
    A. Bradycardia
    B. Osborn waves
    C. Short PR interval
    D. Muscle tremor on the baseline
    E. Prolonged QT interval

55. Ventricular tachycardia is characterized by the following except
    A. Wide QRS complexes
    B. 150 to 200 bpm
    C. AV dissociation
    D. Occasional 2:1 conduction
    E. Fusion beats

56. Horizontal 3 mm ST depression in V2 to V6 represents
    A. High anterior MI

B. Subendocardial ischemia or infarction
C. Anteroseptal MI
D. Posterior MI
E. Inferolateral MI

57. The characteristic changes seen in cerebrovascular accident can include
    A. ST elevation across the chest leads
    B. ST depression in the inferior leads
    C. Q waves in the anteroseptal leads
    D. Short QT interval
    E. Giant negative T waves in multiple chest leads

58. EKG change diagnostic of stress-induced reversible ischemia is
    A. Upsloping ST depression of less than 1 mm at 80 ms from the J point
    B. T wave inversion in multiple leads
    C. Atrial fib
    D. Horizontal reversible ST depression of more than 2 mm in the chest leads
    E. Hypertension

59. Sleep disorder EKG changes can include
    A. Sinus pauses
    B. First- and second-degree heart blocks
    C. PACs and PVCs
    D. Osborn waves
    E. Sinus arrhythmia

60. The right coronary artery occlusion may result in MI involving
    A. Lateral wall
    B. High anterior wall
    C. Posterolateral papillary muscle
    D. Inferior wall
    E. Right ventricular wall

61. Circumflex coronary artery occlusion can involve all except
    A. Lateral wall
    B. High anterior wall
    C. Posterolateral wall
    D. Inferior wall
    E. AV node

62. Prominent U waves are seen in the following conditions except

EKG MCQ QUIZ 1- 100

   A. Hypothyroidism
   B. Hypothermia
   C. Hypercalcemia
   D. Hypokalemia
   E. Antiarrhythmics

63. Atrial sensing and ventricular pacing means
   A. There are two electrodes, one in the atrium and one in the ventricle
   B. It is pacing both the atria and the ventricles
   C. It is recognizing the atrial activity and pacing the ventricles as needed
   D. Pacemaker malfunction
   E. Atrial lead displacement

64. All of these are features of a DDD pacemaker except
   A. Dual-chamber sensing
   B. RV and LV pacing
   C. Sensing atria and pacing ventricles
   D. Dual chamber trigger or inhibit
   E. Dual-chamber pacing

65. All of these relate to a CRT pacemaker except
   A. It is a cardiac resynchronization therapy device
   B. It has pacer wires in the atrium, right, and left ventricles
   C. It simulates normal ventricular contractions by pacing both ventricles simultaneously
   D. It has pacer wires in the atrium, right ventricle, and coronary sinus
   E. It is used in patients with heart failure and wide QRS complexes (>120 ms)

66. What does the QRS segment on the EKG represent?
   A. Atrial activation
   B. Ventricular depolarization
   C. Resting membrane potential
   D. Ventricular repolarization
   E. AV conduction

67. Paroxysmal atrial tachycardia includes the following features except
   A. Narrow QRS tachycardia at a rate of 160 to 220 bpm
   B. Constant PP and RR intervals
   C. May present with 1:1, 2:1 conduction
   D. Fusion beats
   E. May be associated with ST depression and T wave inversion

CLINICAL EKG INTERPRETATION

68. What does the ST segment on the EKG represent?
    A. Atrial repolarization
    B. Ventricular depolarization
    C. Resting membrane potential
    D. An early part of the ventricular repolarization
    E. The phrase "0" of the action potential

69. Pulmonary embolus EKG features may include the following except
    A. Sinus tachycardia
    B. S waves in lead I
    C. Q waves in lead III
    D. T wave inversion aVL
    E. RBBB

70. What does the T wave on the EKG represent?
    A. Atrial repolarization
    B. Ventricular depolarization
    C. Resting membrane potential
    D. Ventricular repolarization
    E. The phrase "2" of the action potential

71. The R-R interval on the EKG represents
    A. Rest and relaxation interval
    B. Ventricular depolarization
    C. Two cardiac cycles
    D. One cycle of action potential
    E. Resting membrane potential interval

72. Multifocal tachycardia features include the following except
    A. Heart rate >100 bpm
    B. Varying P wave morphology
    C. Adenosine is the treatment of choice
    D. Seen in patients with COPD and CHF
    E. Easily mistaken for atrial fibrillation

73. A PVC falling on _____ can precipitate a serious ventricular arrhythmia. This is known as the _____ on _____ phenomenon.
    A. T, R, R
    B. R, T, R
    C. T, T, R
    D. T, R, T

EKG MCQ QUIZ 1- 100

74. You notice a deep S wave in lead I and R wave aVF. What is the axis?
    A. Normal axis
    B. Left superior axis
    C. Right axis deviation
    D. Indeterminate axis
    E. Horizontal axis

75. Digitalis toxicity and subendocardial infarction have what in common?
    A. ST elevation
    B. PR prolongation
    C. Prolonged QT interval
    D. ST depression

76. Pathological Q waves include all these features except
    A. Seen in groups of leads
    B. They are more than 40 ms in duration
    C. Maybe as deep as 25% of the R wave
    D. Reciprocal change in other leads
    E. Some q waves may disappear after 1- 18 months

77. The low QRS voltage may be seen in patients with
    A. Pneumothorax
    B. Large pericardial effusion
    C. Hypothyroidism
    D. Hyperkalemia
    E. Infiltrative heart disease

78. Which lead records a positive deflection when the impulse is moving from the head to the toe?
    A. Lead I
    B. V1 and V2
    C. aVR
    D. aVF

79. Left atrial enlargement includes all these features except
    A. Negative P wave of >40 ms in V1
    B. The P wave of >1 mm deep in lead V1
    C. A biphasic P wave in leads II, III, and aVF.
    D. Negative P wave in lead I

80. The normal duration of the QRS complex is
    A. Less than 120 ms

CLINICAL EKG INTERPRETATION

B. Greater than 120 ms
C. 0.2 sec
D. 0.14 sec

81. If the R-R interval covers 4 large boxes or 20 small boxes the heart rate is
    A. 100 bpm
    B. 60 bpm
    C. 80 bpm
    D. 40 bpm
    E. 75 bpm

82. The sinus node is located in the
    A. Left atrium
    B. Interatrial septum
    C. Near coronary sinus
    D. Right atrium near superior vena cava
    E. Right AV groove

83. The beta blockers actions include all except
    A. Slow the heart rate
    B. Increase the PR intervals
    C. Reduce LV contractility
    D. Shorten the QRS duration
    E. May cause hypotension

84. All these conditions may require an electric shock except
    A. V. fib
    B. V. tach
    C. Atrial flutter with rapid ventricular rate and hypotension
    D. Asystole
    E. Atrial fib with RVR and dizziness

85. How many leads do you attach to a patient to get a 12-lead EKG?
    A. 8 Leads
    B. 12 lead for a 12 lead EKG
    C. 6 leads as the augmented leads use the limb leads
    D. 10 leads

EKG MCQ QUIZ 1- 100

86. A rapid and irregular atrial rate greater than 340 bpm is called
    A. Atrial flutter with block
    B. Multifocal atrial tachycardia
    C. Atrial fib
    D. Artifacts
    E. Parkinson's disease

87. The time taken for a sinus node impulse to reach the AV node and activate the ventricles is known as
    A. P wave
    B. PR interval
    C. QRS duration
    D. TP interval
    E. Baseline interval

88. Hypertrophic cardiomyopathy features include all except
    A. Narrow and deep Q waves in II, II, and aVF
    B. Increase voltage in all precordial leads.
    C. T wave inversion in I, aVL
    D. LBBB
    E. T wave inversion in V1 and V2

89. All these conditions may require an electric shock except
    A. V. fib
    B. V. tach
    C. Atrial flutter with a rapid ventricular rate and hypotension
    D. Asystole
    E. Atrial fibrillation with RVR and dizziness

90. How many leads do you attach to a patient to get a chest leads EKG?
    A. 6 Leads
    B. 12 lead for a 12 lead EKG
    C. 6 leads as the augmented leads use the limb leads
    D. 10 leads

91. All these features are seen in patients with hyperkalemia except
    A. Wide QRS complexes
    B. PR prolongation

CLINICAL EKG INTERPRETATION

   C. Short QT interval
   D. Flat P waves
   E. Tall peaked T waves in anterior chest leads

92. The characteristic EKG finding in hypercalcemia include
    A. Tall T waves
    B. Prominent U waves
    C. Short QT interval
    D. Low voltage in limb leads
    E. ST depression

93. One EKG finding that may be a clue to ischemia or infarction in LBBB is
    A. ST elevation in the anterior leads
    B. St depression in the lateral chest leads
    C. Long QT interval
    D. Concordant ST-T changes
    E. A QRS duration of >140 ms

94. The following EKG changes may be seen in mitral stenosis except
    A. Left atrial enlargement
    B. Right atrial enlargement
    C. Right ventricular hypertrophy
    D. Left ventricular hypertrophy
    E. Right axis deviation

95. Differential diagnosis of atrial fib at 260 bpm with WPW include all except
    A. Atrial flutter with a rapid rate and QRS aberration
    B. Ventricular tachycardia
    C. MAT with BBB
    D. PAT
    E. Torsades de Pointe

96. What type of pacemaker will be suited for a sedentary elderly patient with atrial fib and heart block?
    A. DOO
    B. VVI
    C. DDDR
    D. CRT

97. Narrow QRS tachycardia at a rate of 165 per minute is seen in all except
    A. Atrial tachycardia
    B. Flutter with 2:1 conduction
    C. Atrial fib

D. Accelerated Junctional rhythm

98. A DDD pacemaker has the following features except
   A. Atrial sensing and ventricular sensing
   B. Atrial pacing and ventricular pacing
   C. Atrial sensing and ventricular pacing
   D. Defibrillation capabilities
   E. Atrial inhibited and ventricular pacing

99. During a stress test, the following findings are ominous signs except
   A. Horizontal ST depression of 3 mm in the chest leads
   B. ST elevation
   C. Upsloping ST depression of less than 1mm at 80 sec from the J point
   D. Hypotension
   E. Frequent PVCs and short runs of V. tach

100. Synchronized cardioversion is useful in the following except
   A. Atrial fib with RVR and hypotension
   B. Atrial flutter with RVR and hypotension
   C. Torsades de Pointe
   D. Symptomatic PAT not responsive to adenosine

CLINICAL EKG INTERPRETATION

1. D. The short QT interval is not a feature of pericarditis or pericardial effusion
2. 5, 10. Read the instructions carefully as 10,5 and 5,10 can be confusing.
3. D. The atrial flutter rate is between 240 and 340. With a 2:1 conduction, the right answer is D.
4. X
5. C. Since we see wide QRS in leads V4 to V6, we see repolarization changes in the same leads as discordant ST-T changes. St depression and T wave inversions.
6. E. Yes, all these conditions can produce tall R waves in V1 and V2.
7. D. Leads II, III, and aVF represent the inferior wall. If there were additional changes in V1 and V2, they may represent inferoposterior MI. High anterior MI involves leads I and aVL. Anteroseptal MI involves leads V1 to V4. Anterolateral MI involve leads V2 to V6. However, you need to be aware that different sources use different definitions for the same thing. Familiarize yourself with how your board examiners define these regions and stick to that. After all, you want to pass the exam. From a practical standpoint, if you are seeing an STEMI patient, the more important question is what is the extent of the MI and the most likely culprit artery involved. You can determine that as soon as you do the initial angiograms. The seminal point is how quickly you can re-establish flow in a totally occluded coronary artery. But, when you are in an exam hall focus on what your examiner expects you to answer.
8. E. Subendocardial ischemia causes ST depression. The most significant is the horizontal ST depression, followed by down-sloping ST depression. The up-sloping ST depression is less reliable. However, If the ST depression is more than 2 mm it is significant. If the same changes are associated with chest pain and positive cardiac enzymes, it is supposed to represent subendocardial infarction. Note that subendocardial infarction should be more thoroughly evaluated for reversible ischemia after the patient settles. The incidence of further

cardiac events is high in the ensuing three months following the current episode.

9. D. The coronary sinus is the large vein behind the heart in the AV groove that drains the venous blood from the heart to the right atrium. The coronary sinus is not part of the electrical system of the heart. It is important to know that anatomy of the heart very well.

10. D. You need to know the various phases of an action potential and the different elements involved in multiple phases. As you recall, phase 4 is the resting membrane potential and phase 0 results from the sudden influx of sodium into the myocardial cells. That is followed by a plateau brought on by efflux of potassium out of the cells—Phase 1. Next, phase 2 results in sustained potential resulting from movement of calcium into the cells and potassium out of the cells. Phase 3 results from a continued leak of potassium out of the cells.

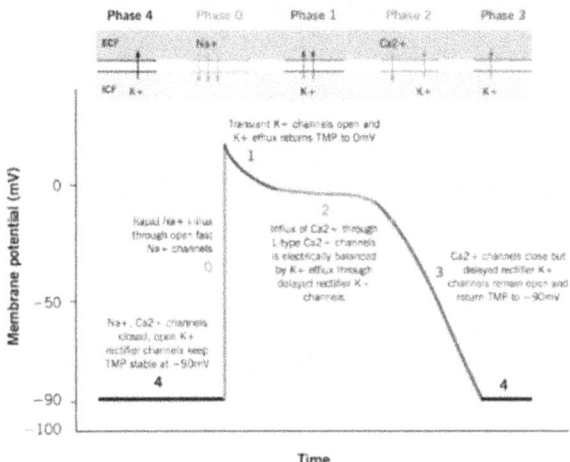

11. A. High anterior wall. Some other authorities may use different terminology. This region is usually supplied by the proximal diagonal branches of the LAD.

12. A. The sinus rate varies from 60 to 100 bpm. Sinus tachycardia varies from 100 to 160 bpm. Atrial tachycardia varies from 160 to 225 bpm.

CLINICAL EKG INTERPRETATION

13. E. Note that 5 big boxes or 25 small boxes represent 1 second. So, if the heart is beating every second, the heart rate is 60 bpm.
14. D. If you notice the action potential, QRS represents part of the action potential, as the action potential also involves the ventricular repolarization.

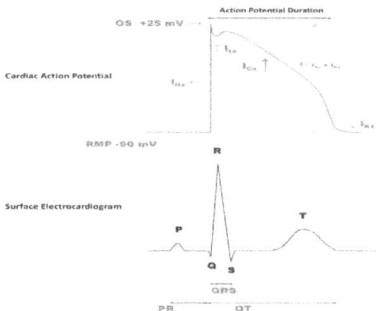

15. B. Note there is a difference between QTC and QT interval. QTC represents the QT interval corrected for the heart rate. Hence, pay attention to small prints.
16. C. Pericarditis usually causes ST elevation. It is seen in multiple leads. There is J point elevation with a concave ST segment, which is different from the ST elevation associated with an acute MI.
17. D. The smallest box on the EKG represents 40 ms, based on that fact that the paper is running at 25 mm/sec (1000 ms/25 = 40 ms).
18. C. Look at the earlier description about the location of the MI based on the leads showing the changes.

19. D. It is very important to familiarize yourself with the exact position of the placement of chest leads. You also need to be aware of the body habitus as very obese people's hearts may be situated high up in the chest and horizontally, while thin and tall people's hearts may be located much lower and sitting vertically. Hence, if you are dealing with a thin and tall person, the EKG may show QS complexes in the usual chest lead positions. In such cases, placing the leads one intercostal space below the recommended places may give a more realistic EKG. Similarly, in women with large breasts there is a tendency to place the leads above the breast level, which also can produce QS complexes across the chest leads. If that happens, take time to place the chest leads underneath the breast so you get a better R wave progression across the chest leads.
20. C. When you are taking a test and do not expect such a basic question, you may be likely to rush and choose a wrong answer. Simply read the question and pick the answer that is correct. Similar number combinations could be deceiving.
21. C. The V6 electrode is placed in the mid-auxiliary line in the 5th ICS.
22. E. An adrenergic response is the fight of the "fight or flight" response. It is a sympathetic response that speeds up everything. Actually, the adrenergic response speeds up the AV conduction and increases the heart rate.
23. E. Anterolateral MI. See the previous description.
24. B. Parasympathetic response slows the heart rate and causes sinus pauses. Its chemical mediator is acetylcholine. The usual vagal response causes vasodilatation in the legs and bradycardia that can lead to a drop in blood pressure. It also slows the AV conduction.

CLINICAL EKG INTERPRETATION

25. C. The normal electrical axis is between −30 and +90 degrees.

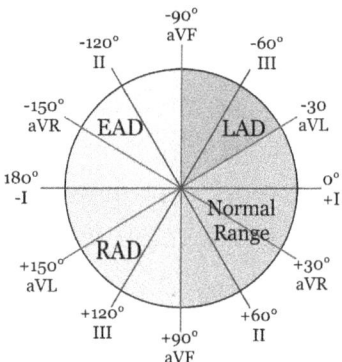

26. D. Again, the terminology may be confusing and, in a rush, you may think you are choosing the right answer. The hallmark of Wenckebach is a progressive prolongation of the PR interval, not the RR interval.

27. B. Mitral stenosis doesn't affect the left ventricle. It affects all the structures in line behind it.

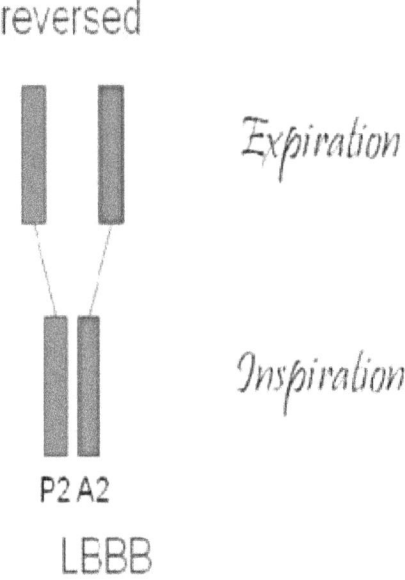

28. B. There is reversed splitting of the second sound.
29. D. Renal failure patients may have LVH and hyperkalemia.

EKG MCQ QUIZ 1- 100

30. B. Posterior MI. These are actually mirror images of hyperacute changes in the posterior wall.
31. C. Aortic stenosis patients may have LVH, LAE, PVCs, and LV strain pattern. RBBB is a feature of aortic stenosis. Yes, you can find a case with an RBBB, but they are looking for the most appropriate answer given the choices. So, it is better to be more logical than smart.
32. B. Biatrial enlargement is not a feature of COPD.
33. B. Generalized symmetrical T wave inversion is a cardinal sign of global ventricular ischemia. Another condition in which we may come across T wave inversion would be in patients with cerebrovascular accidents, when there are giant negative T waves seen in multiple leads.
34. D. Complete heart block (CHB) has an independent atrial and an independent ventricular rhythm. The ventricular rhythm is slower and it can be from the lower junction, bundle branch, or the ventricle. There is no correlation between the atria and the ventricles. AV dissociation is the cardinal finding in CHB. Since there is no electrical connection between the atria and the ventricles you do not see a fusion beat. If you do see a fusion beat, then you have a high-grade AV block which is one grade lower than CHB.
35. E. LV strain pattern involves down-sloping ST depression with T deep T wave inversion.
36. E. Left axis deviation is not a common feature of RBBB. However, in real practice we have often seen RBBB with LAHB. This falls in the category of a bifascicular block, which simply means there is more advanced involvement of the conduction system. Note that beta blockers and calcium channel blockers are contraindicated in a patient with bifascicular blocks. To this, if you add prolonged PR interval it would become a trifascicular block. Patients with a bifascicular or a trifascicular block are at an increased risk for development of CHB.

CLINICAL EKG INTERPRETATION

37. C. Yes, we do see 2-5 mm ST elevation in V2 to V4 in the presence of complete LBBB. These ST changes are indicative of ischemia or infarction. Next time you see an LBBB look for these ST changes and you will find them.
38. E. Left posterior hemiblock doesn't cause left axis deviation.
39. C. Brugada syndrome is associated with RBBB pattern with terminal slurring of the S waves in the anterior leads. These patients are prone to ventricular arrhythmias. Left atrial enablement is not a feature of Brugada syndrome.
40. C. You need to familiarize yourself with the EKG paper. The paper speed is 1 sec or 1000 msec. There are 25 small squares and each square is 40 ms. Vertically the axis represents the electrical voltage. 10 mm = 10 mV. Voltage criteria are used to recognize the chamber enlargement of hypertrophy while the time criteria help us accurately measure the heart rate and intervals.
41. D. Look at the Estes criteria in the book for LVH. An important feature of LVH or LBBB is the discordant ST-T changes. That means the ST-T changes are in the opposite direction of the major QRS deflection.

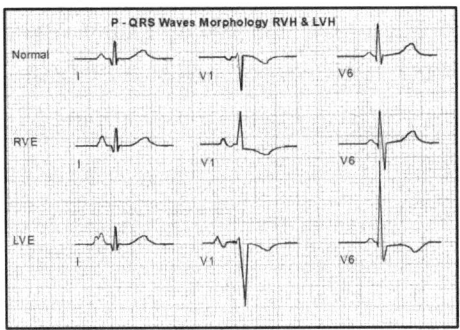

42. D. The P wave represents the atrial electrical activity, while the QRS represents the ventricular electrical activity.
43. B. You need to learn to read each word and see if they are placed deliberately to confuse you. In pericarditis and early repolarization, the ST segments are concave facing up.
44. E. Trades are a wide QRS ventricular flutter with shifting axis.

EKG MCQ QUIZ 1- 100

45. Fusion beats more or less exclude CHB. If any atrial impulses can reach the ventricles, then you do not have a complete heart block (CHB. There may be high-grade AV block, but not a CHB.
46. E. LBBB cause the classic deep rS or QS complexes in leads V1, V2, and V3.
47. D. Vasovagal attack. It is the common flight mechanism of the "fight or flight" response to stress. Vagal stimulation acts on the cardiovascular system by slowing the heart rate, sinus pauses sometimes, and vasodilation in the legs drops the blood pressure leading to dizziness or syncope. Chose the most suitable answer.
48. E. Typical atrial flutter has the saw tooth appearance.
49. D. Remember the drug of choice is P like to WPW and not A, B, C, or D.
50. E. Synchronized cardioversion delivers the shock on the QRS, but cardioversion is not the choice for Torsades. It needs a DC shock.
51. C. If the patient is not stable, DC cardioversion.
52. E. You need drugs that block the AV conduction to reduce the rate and break the circuit. Drugs like lidocaine may increase the AV conduction and may, in fact, increase the ventricular rate.
53. D. You see 2:1 or 3:1 conduction with atrial arrhythmias as the ventricular conduction could be 2:1 or 3:1.
54. C. Hypothermia slows the metabolism and everything slows down, including the PR, QRS, and the QT intervals.
55. A. Read every word and see if they match.
56. B. ST depression represents subendocardial ischemia or infarction. If the cardiac enzymes are positive, it is called subendocardial infarction. Transmural MI causes hyperacute ST elevations.
57. E. These giant negative T waves are classic EKG changes seen in patients with cerebrovascular accidents. Generalized symmetrical T wave inversions of lesser depth are seen in patients with ventricular ischemia. And, of course, you see tall T waves in hyperkalemia. Read through the chapter on T wave abnormalities, which covers all the T wave morphologies.

CLINICAL EKG INTERPRETATION

58. D. This is a lesson on diagnostic EKG changes during an exercise test. Horizontal ST depression of 2 or more mm during peak exercise is diagnostic of reversible ischemia. It is almost 97% accurate in men but is only 60% accurate in women. Also, the time it takes to return to the baseline also signifies the degree of coronary stenosis. Upsloping ST depression is less reliable unless it is 2 mm down 80 ms after the J point. Downsloping ST depression is also significant. Note that if the patient has baseline ST-T changes related to LVH or LBBB, the EKG changes become less reliable. Still, you may get some good insight into the patient's physical capacity.
59. D. Sleep apnea can mimic a lot of arrhythmias. Osborne waves are seen in patients with hypothermia and hypercalcemia.
60. B. The right coronary artery supplies the sinus node, the AV node, the right ventricles, and the lower third of the interventricular septum. In 15% of the patients the lateral wall through the postero-lateral branch. Generally, the circumflex marginals supply the lateral and postero-lateral walls. In 30% of the patients, it can supply the LV apex. So, depending upon the location of the occlusion, it can cause inferolateral MI, inferior MI, IMI with right ventricular involvement, or conduction disturbances related to the AV node or SA node. A high anterior wall in supplied by the diagonal branches of the LAD.
61. B. See previous explanation.
62. C. Anything that slows the action potential or prolongs its cycle can lead to the appearance of the U waves. Most often, you see U waves when the heart rates are slower. Hypercalcemia shortens the action potential and the cycle length.

EKG MCQ QUIZ 1- 100

63. C. This is a lesson in dual-chamber pacing and how the pacemaker works in various modes. Please refer to the chapter on pacemakers for a more detailed explanation. Atrial sensing means the pacemaker recognizes the atrial activity and suppresses the atrial pacing mechanism. Ventricular pacing refers to the function when the pacemaker doesn't see a ventricular impulse after a certain PR interval and sends the impulse to activate the ventricles. In other words, it paces the ventricle. This pacemaker atrial lead works well only in patients with atrial activity. It may not work in patients with atrial flutter or fibrillation. It may not pace the atria.

64. B. This pacemaker paces only the RA and RV. It doesn't pace the LV. You have both ventricular pacing in CRT or cardiac resynchronization therapy where an electrode is placed in the LV lateral wall through the coronary sinus. This is used in patients with far advanced heart failure and very wide WRS complexes.

65. B. See previous explanation. It paces the left ventricle but the pacer wire is now in the left ventricle.

66. B. Refresh your knowledge on action potential in correlation with EKG as you may see some question on board exams.

67. D. Fusion beats are not a feature of PAT unless as a PVC fusion with a supraventricular beat. Fusion beats generally mean a supraventricular beat fusing with a VT beat.

68. D. Review the chapter on action potential.

69. E. The cardinal features of an acute pulmonary embolus include S1Q3T3. Not that you are going not to confirm your PE diagnosis based on this combo, but it may help you to score a point on your board exams.

70. B. Ventricular repolarization. The electrolyte movements rapidly drop the intracellular voltage until it reaches the baseline or the resting membrane potential.

71. D. Note that one action potential cycle has phases 4, 0, 1, 2, 3. Most people may think the action potential cycle represents only electrical depolarization.

CLINICAL EKG INTERPRETATION

72. C. Adenosine may slow the ventricular rate but it has no effect on the atrial excitation, which is the mechanism by which multifocal tachycardia arises. Treatment of COPD, hypoxia, and pulmonary infection may help improve this rhythm or even restore sinus rhythm.
73. A. Remember the R on T phenomenon. This is the period during which the ventricle is most vulnerable for serious ventricular arrhythmias.
74. C. Right axis deviation
75. D. Read the chapter on digitalis toxicity as you may get one or two questions on board exams. Downsloping ST depression, J point depression, and T wave insertion are classic digitalis effect features. PAT with 2:1 conduction is the favorite question of digitalis toxicity.
76. D. Q waves don't produce reciprocal changes. The reciprocal changes we have seen in acute MI involve the ST-T segments of the opposite leads. With IMI you see those changes in leads 1 and aVL. With anterior MI you see reciprocal changes in leads II, III, and aVF. With posterior MI you see changes in the anterior leads.
77. D. Low QRS can be related to the intrinsic heart disease or conditions that create a barrier from the heart to the chest leads. Even though very high potassium levels can make the QRS wide and create a sine wave, that is not the most suitable answer among the choices.
78. D. Review chapter 1 for details.
79. D. Negative P wave in lead I may represent lead misplacement or an ectopic atrial rhythm. First look for right and left arm lead misplacement. Here, the P waves will be upright in aVR. Dextrocardia also can cause a negative P wave and you may see this on your board exams.
80. A. Always pay attention to switches between sec and ms meant to confuse you.
81. E. You need to familiarize yourself with the EKG paper graph inside and out and up and down. You have fewer than 60 seconds to answer your board questions.
82. D. Anatomy of the normal electrical system and the accessory pathways are essential for understating EKGs and arrhythmias.

EKG MCQ QUIZ 1- 100

83. H. Beta blockers don't shorten the QRS duration. Most common situations where you see QRS shortening include hypercalcemia and digitalis effect.
84. D. Asystole? There is nothing to shock. Some may argue that asystole may represent very fine fib but you have to choose the answer that can get you a point.
85. D. Ten leads for 12-lead electrocardiograms, which also includes a ground electrode to the right leg. Is this important? If it happens to be on your exam, the answer is "Yes!" One point can make a difference.
86. C. The very basic question here and there to give you some rest.
87. B. It represents the atrial activation and the time needed to transfer the AV node and activate the ventricles.
88. D.
89. F. Require or not, require can be like a curveball.
90. E. Number game. You need to perform EKG yourself to remember this. You also need to know where exactly each lead needs to be placed.
91. C.
92. C. Read up on hypercalcemia. They may include an EKG that may have more than one electrolyte effect on the EKG or, better yet, an electrolyte and an ischemic effect.
93. D. You usually see discordant ST-T changes in LVH or LBBB in the leads with maximum QRS deflections.
94. D. Mitral valve stenosis doesn't affect the left ventricular size.
95. D. PAT has a regular tachycardia with a rate ranging from 16 to 220 bpm.
96. B. A simple ventricular pacer.
97. I. The accelerated junctional rhythm rate is between 60 and 100 bpm.
98. I. Only ICD has defibrillation capabilities. ICD also could have all the features of a DDD pacemaker.
99. C. See the chapter on EKG changes during stress testing.
100. Torsades de Ponte. This is a life-threatening ventricular arrhythmia. This needs a DC shock with maximum power.

CLINICAL EKG INTERPRETATION

*****

COMEDY RELIEF!

What Do You Mean Who Is This?

The phone rang at my house the other day. I picked up the phone and said, "Nik's residence. Who is this?"

"What do you mean who is this? This is your daughter, who left for college, just two weeks ago! I can't believe this!" said a crying lady at the other end.

"Hold it! Hold it, miss! Really, who is this?"

"This is your daughter, what do you mean who is this?" she asked in a demanding voice.

"Boy, you sure sound different this time!"

"I know, I need more money this time!" she said.

"I don't have any money!"

"You are lying through your teeth. I just checked your bank account online before making this call."

"No, that's not for you," I said.

"Well, I just called to let you know that I was transferring the money to my account."

"No, you are not!"

"I already did it."

"It is two in the morning, what the hell are you doing?!" I yelled.

"Homework!" She replied

"What, checking on my bank account?"

"Yes, that's homework too. I'm sitting at home and doing my work, and that's considered homework!"

EKG MCQ QUIZ 1- 100

In the Indian community, our kids are on our payroll all their lives. When we can't handle it anymore, they take over the checkbook, the house, the car, and the cell phone and put us in the outhouse.

*****

CLINICAL EKG INTERPRETATION

Cardiology Board EKG QUIZ

All the points on the answer keys are covered in this quiz, along with references to the corresponding chapters in the book for an in-depth explanation.

CLINICAL EKG INTERPRETATION

Tip: Look at the EKG from top to bottom, from bottom to the top, and then from side to side.

- What is the rate and rhythm?
- What are the intervals—PR, QRS, ST, QT?
- Is there any roadblock? More than one?
- What are the P and QRS morphology?
- Are the Ps still married to the QRSs?
- Where are the ST and T waves? Are they screaming with pain?
- Are the Ts tall, flat, or face down?
- Are the QRSs getting too tall or too fat?
- Now, check everything you see on the answer sheet, not just one major item like LVH!
- Appearances are deceptive on purpose!
- Are there uninvited guests at the table? PACs and PVCs?
- Who is running behind who and why? Are they drunk?
- What are those spikes and how many are there? What are they doing? Look for malfunction!
- Did someone say stroke?
- Can you spell metabolic in alphabet soup?
- What's that P-ig doing on the T mount?
- Bradycardia is not, until proved otherwise? 2:1 block?
- Did you miss S1, Q3, T3?
- MI in patients with a pacemaker and LBBB?
- Concordant and discordant ST-T changes!
- Short QT_C—hypercalcemia and digoxin
- ST up and PR down? Pericarditis and not MI!

EKG INTERPRETATIONS QUIZ 1-50

EKG 1

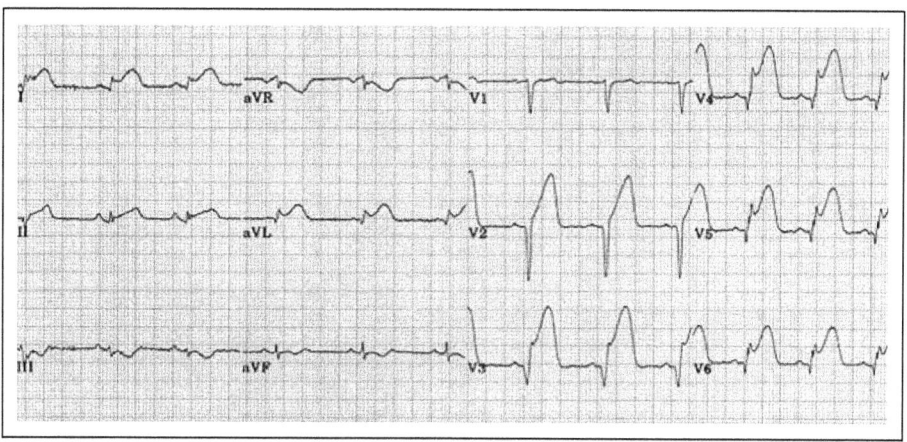

EKG 2

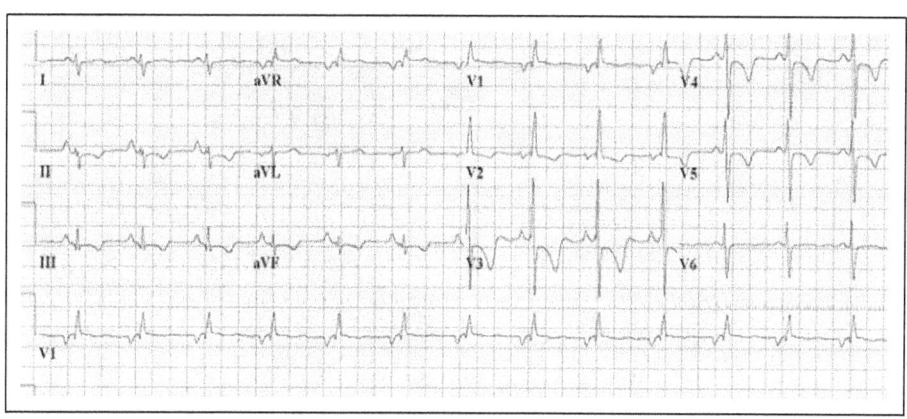

EKG 3

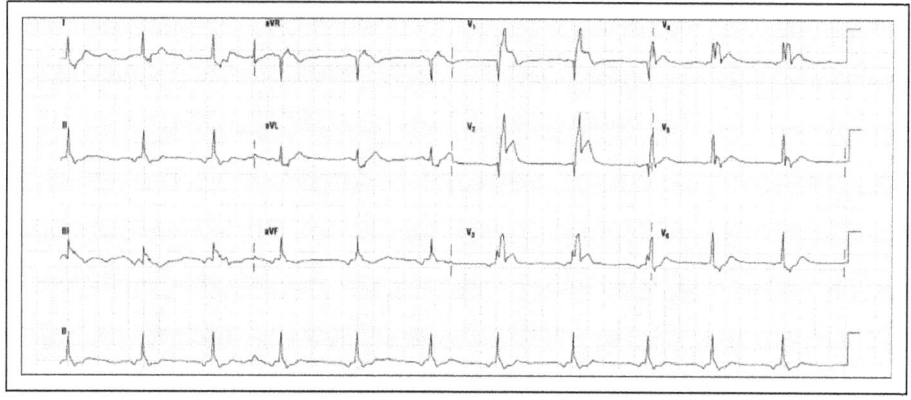

CLINICAL EKG INTERPRETATION

EKG 4

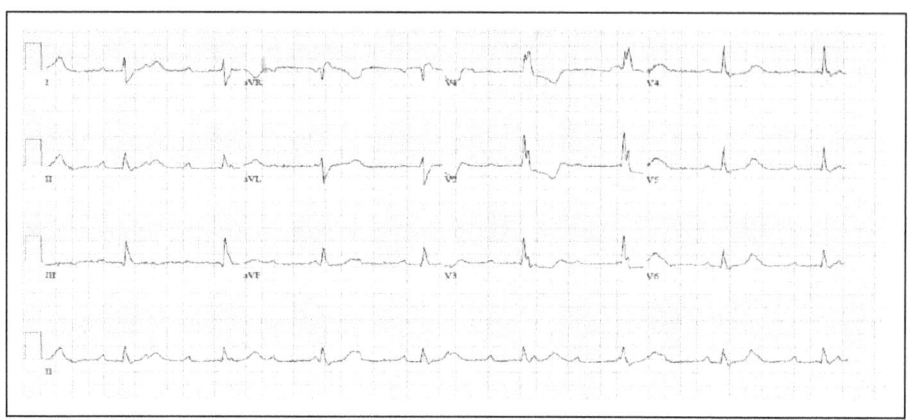

EKG 5

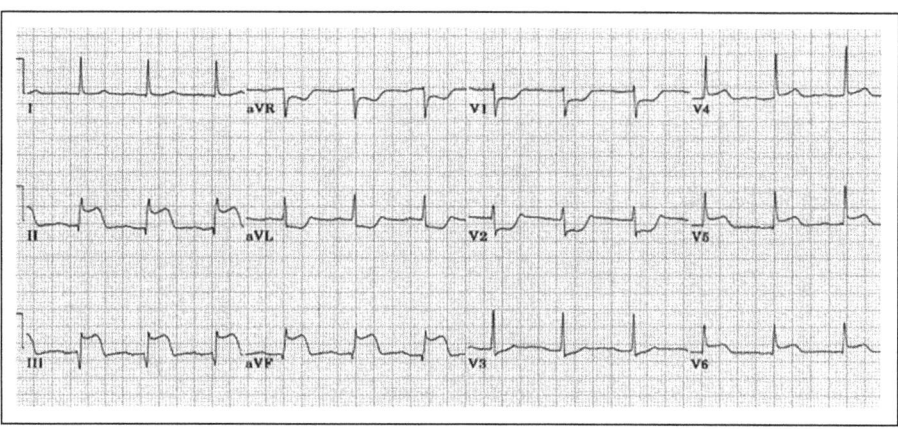

EKG 6

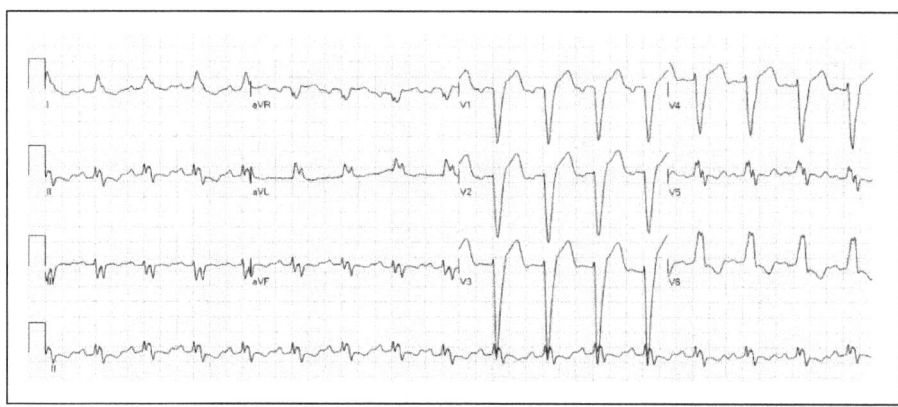

EKG INTERPRETATIONS QUIZ 1-50

EKG 7

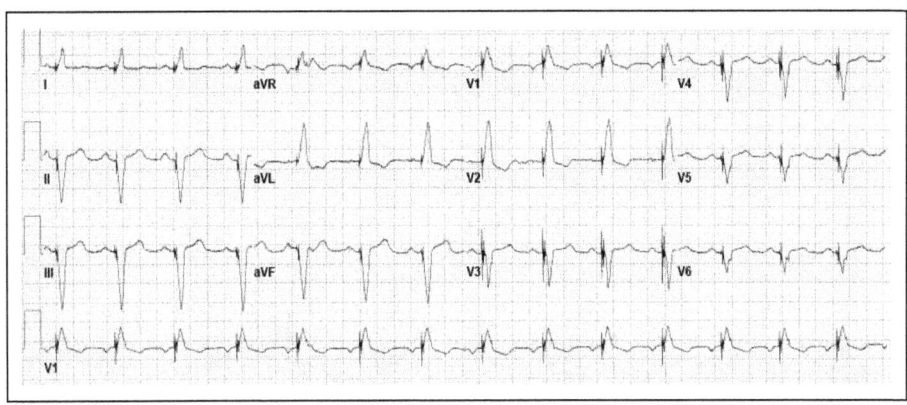

EKG 8

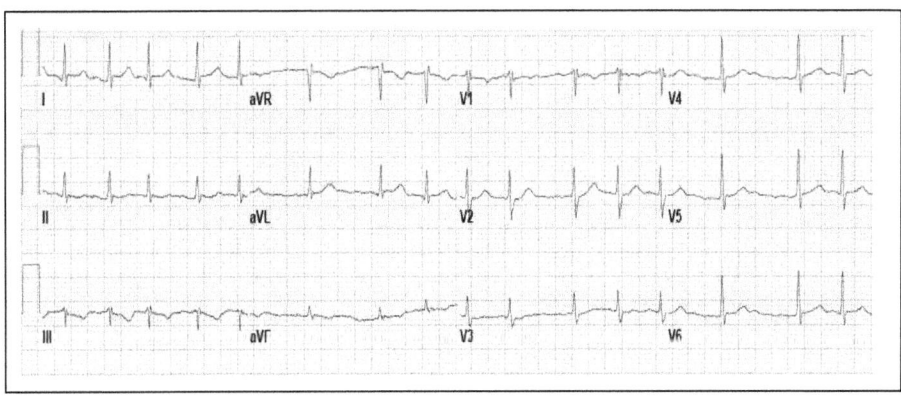

EKG 9

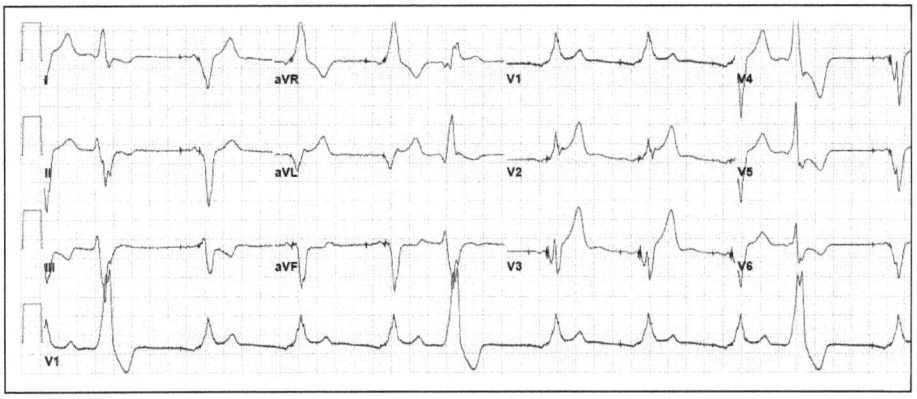

CLINICAL EKG INTERPRETATION

EKG 10

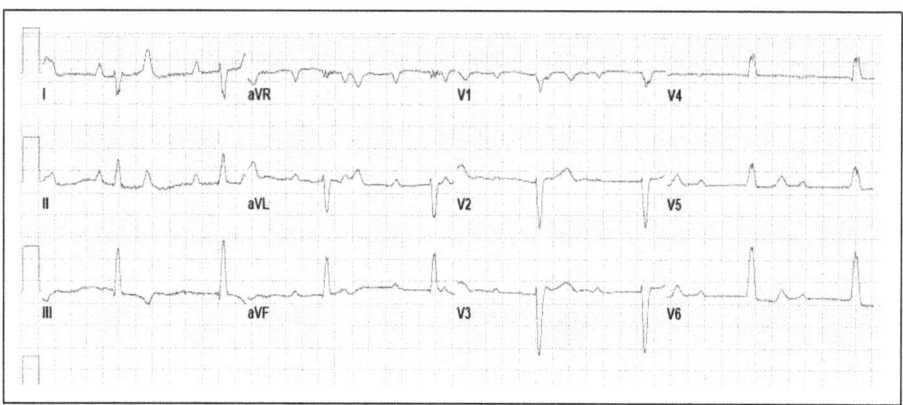

EKG 11

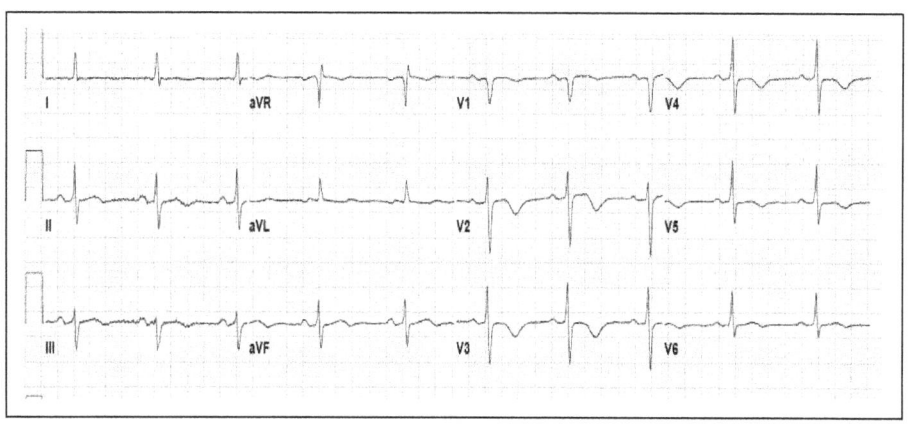

EKG 12

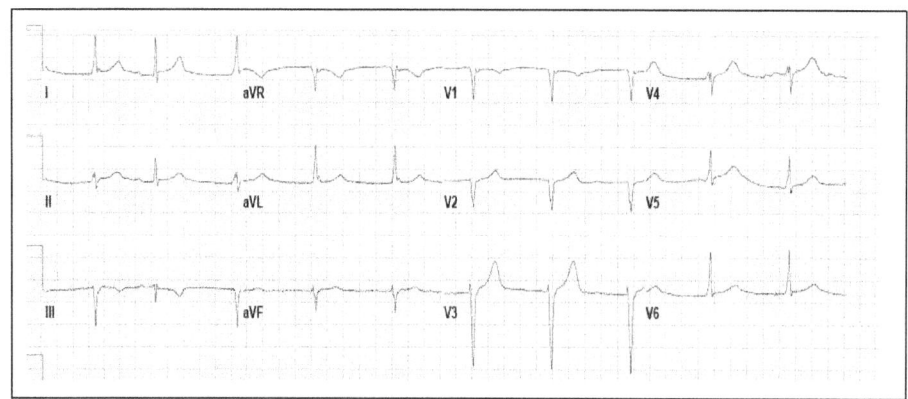

EKG INTERPRETATIONS QUIZ 1-50

EKG 13

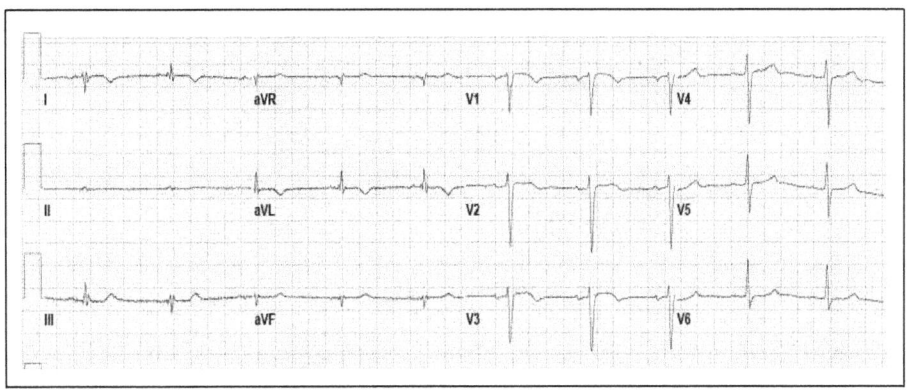

EKG 14

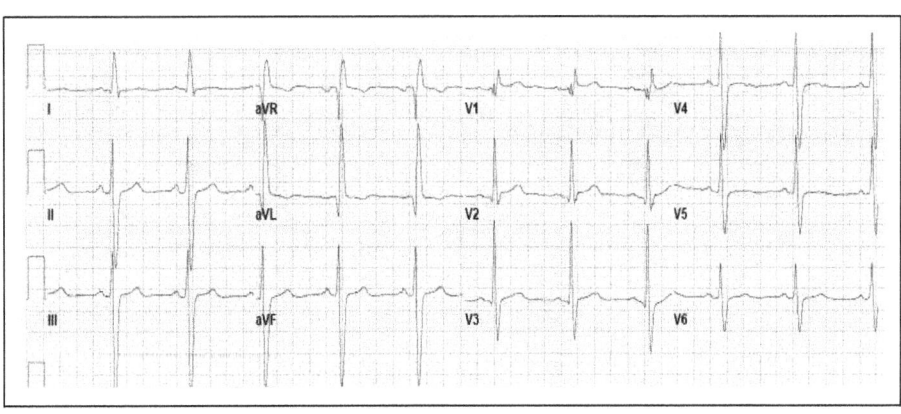

EKG 15

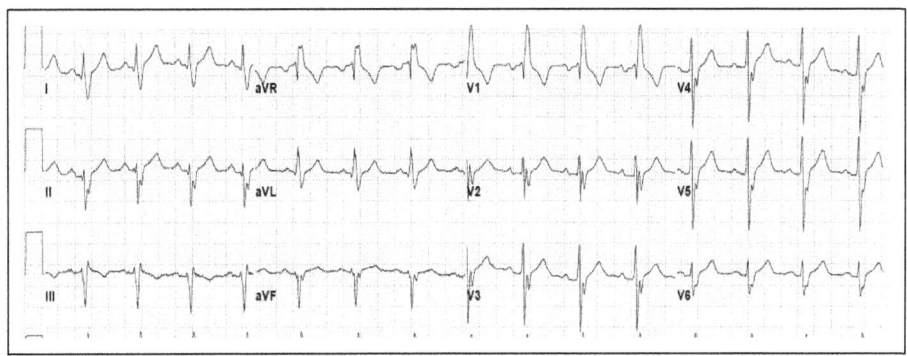

CLINICAL EKG INTERPRETATION

EKG 16

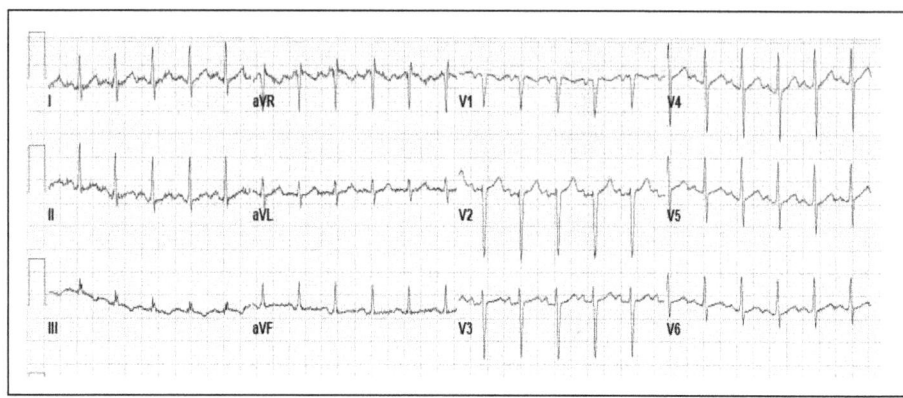

EKG 17

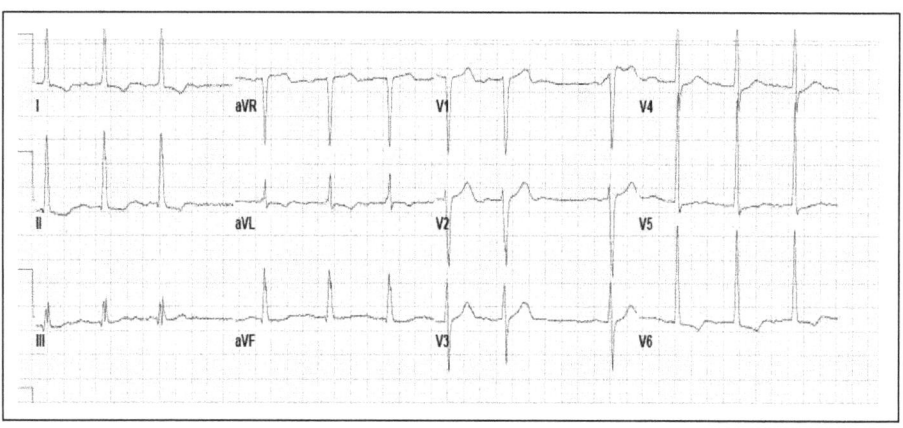

EKG 18

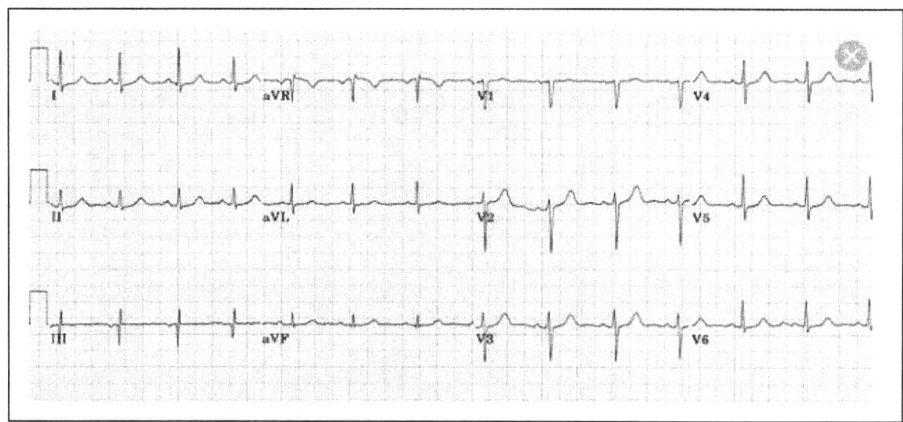

EKG INTERPRETATIONS QUIZ 1-50

EKG 19

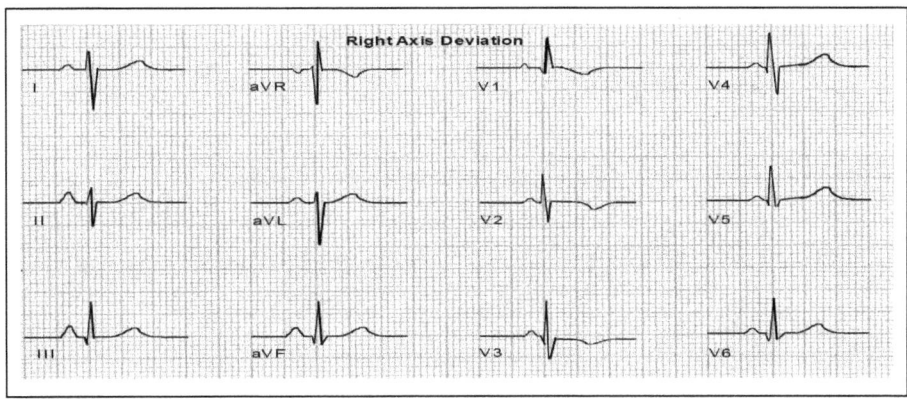

EKG 20

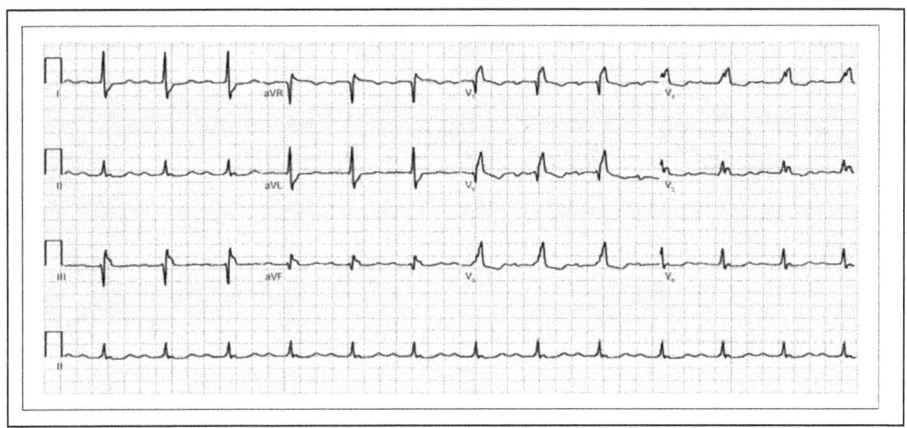

EKG 21

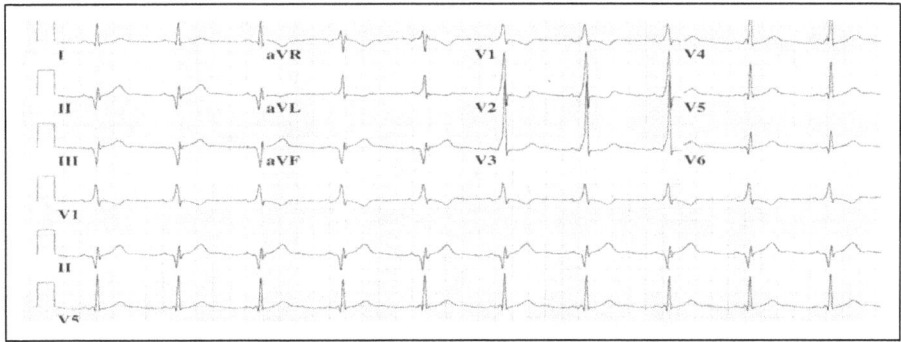

CLINICAL EKG INTERPRETATION

EKG 22

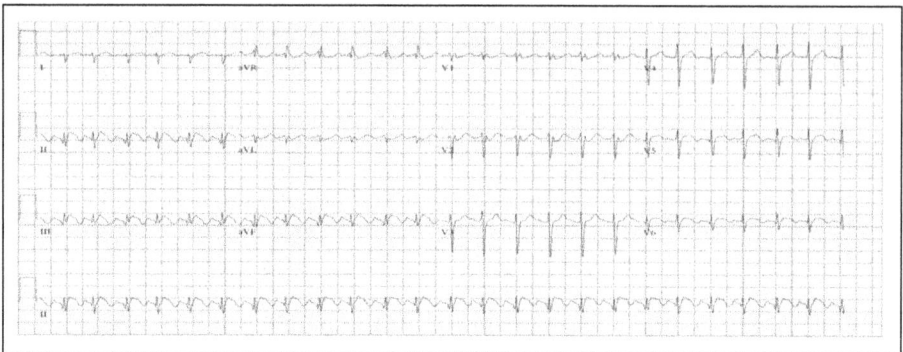

EKG 23

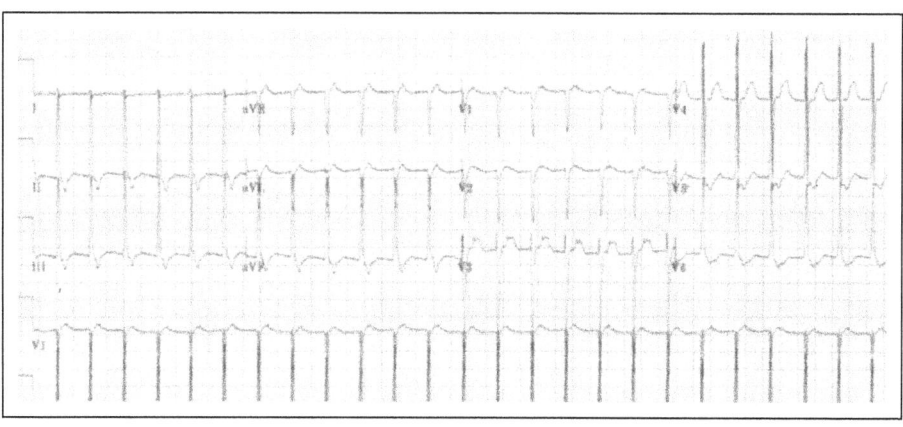

EKG 24

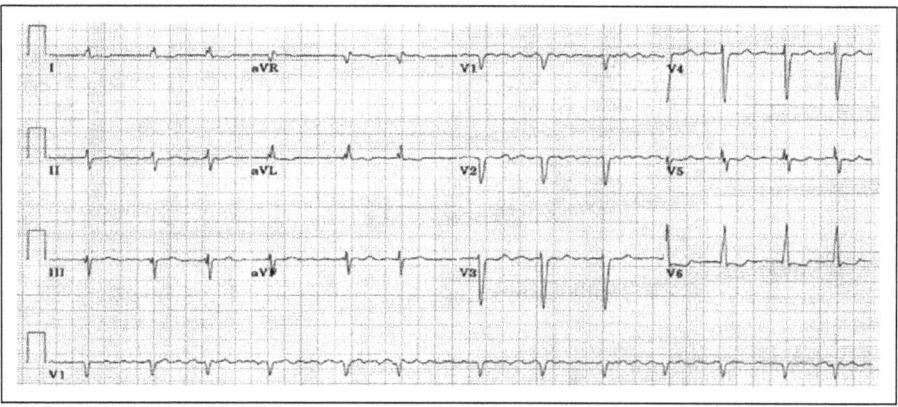

EKG INTERPRETATIONS QUIZ 1-50

EKG 25

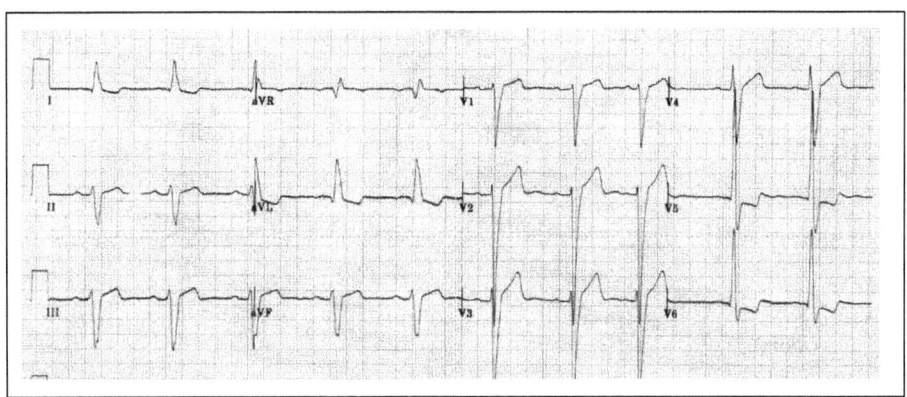

EKG 26

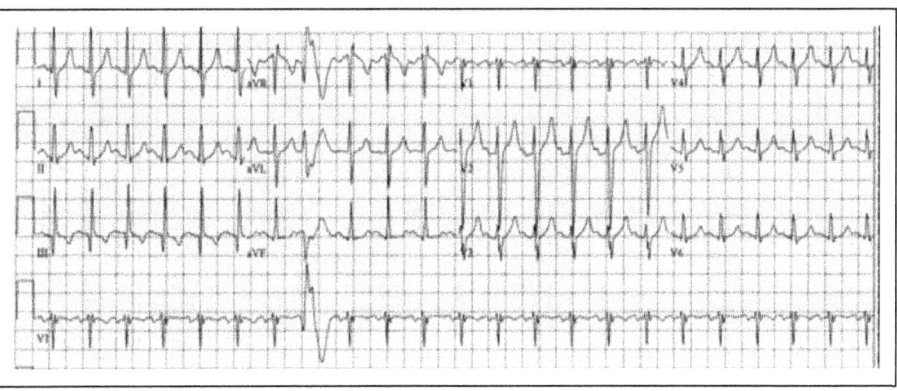

EKG 27

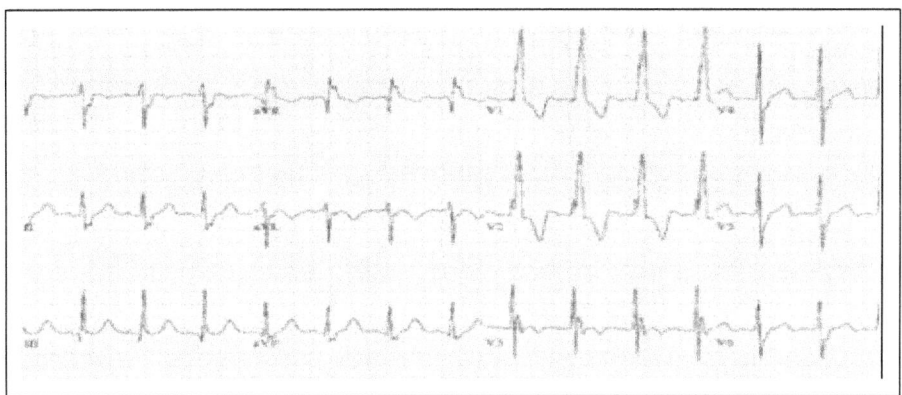

CLINICAL EKG INTERPRETATION

EKG 28

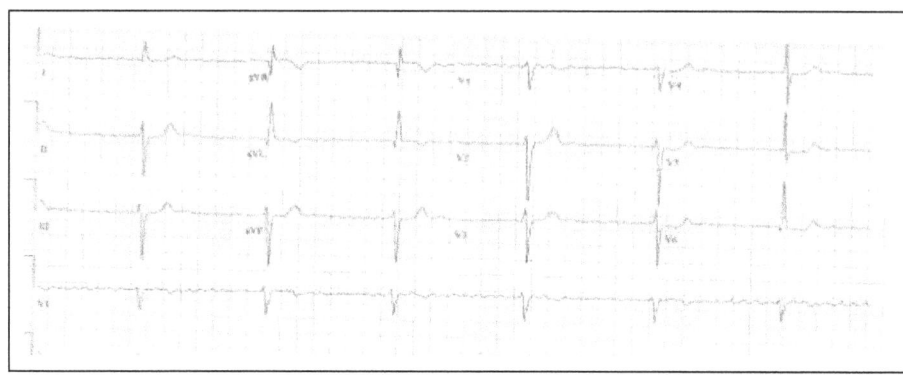

EKG 29

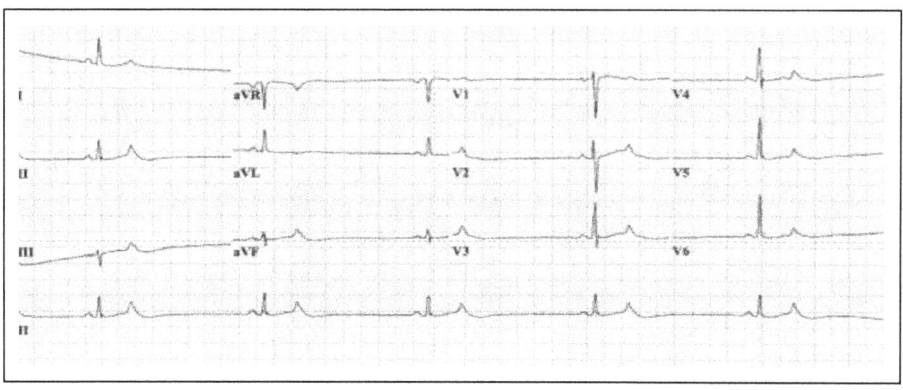

EKG 30

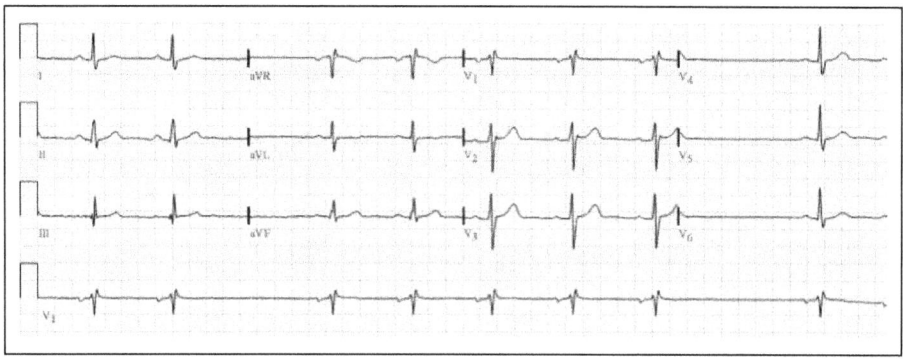

EKG INTERPRETATIONS QUIZ 1-50

EKG 31

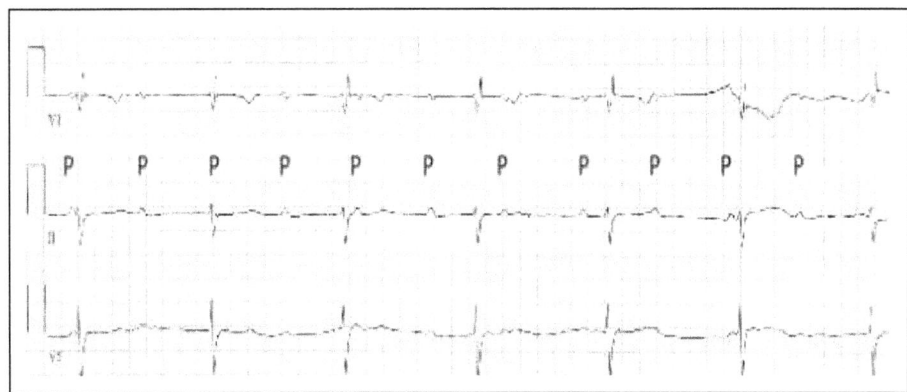

EKG 32

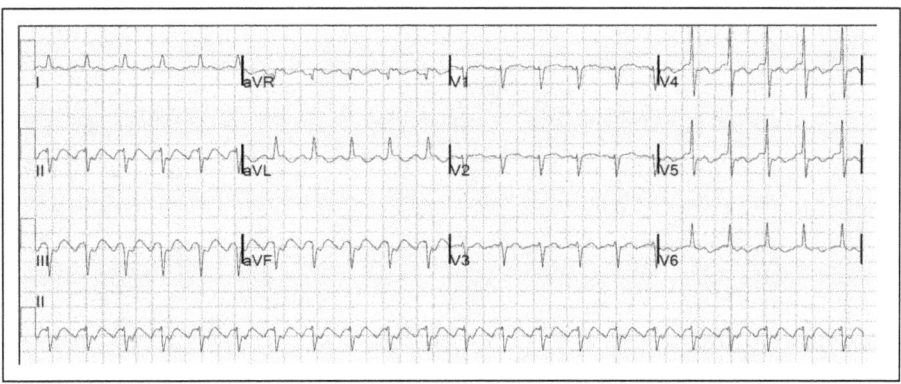

EKG 33

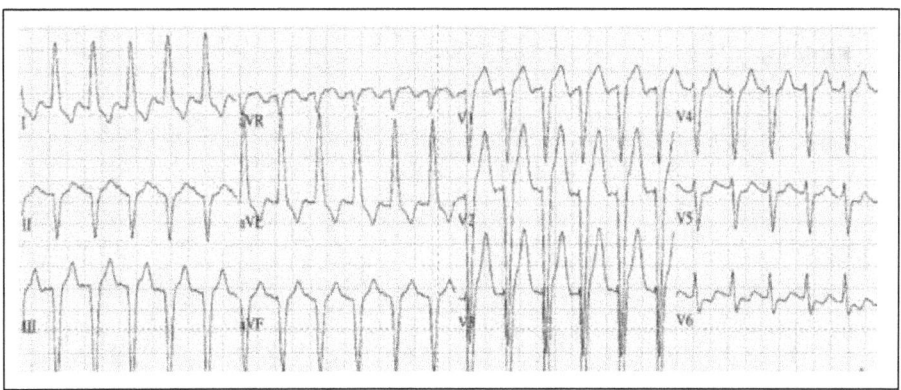

CLINICAL EKG INTERPRETATION

EKG 34

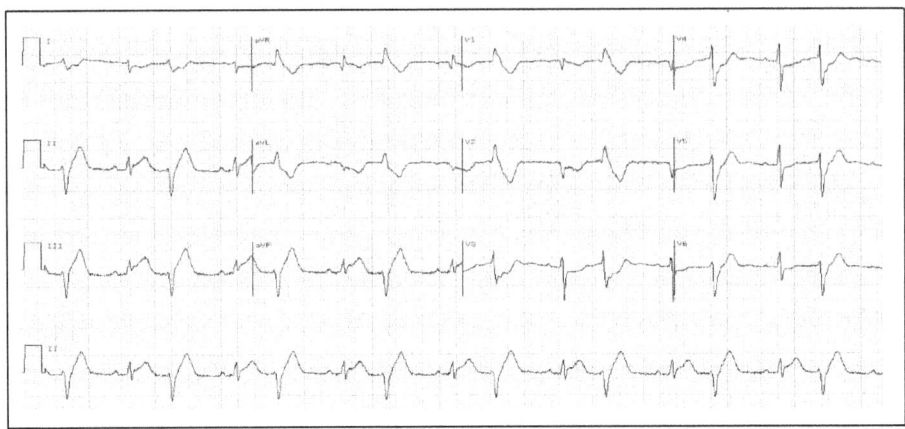

EKG 35

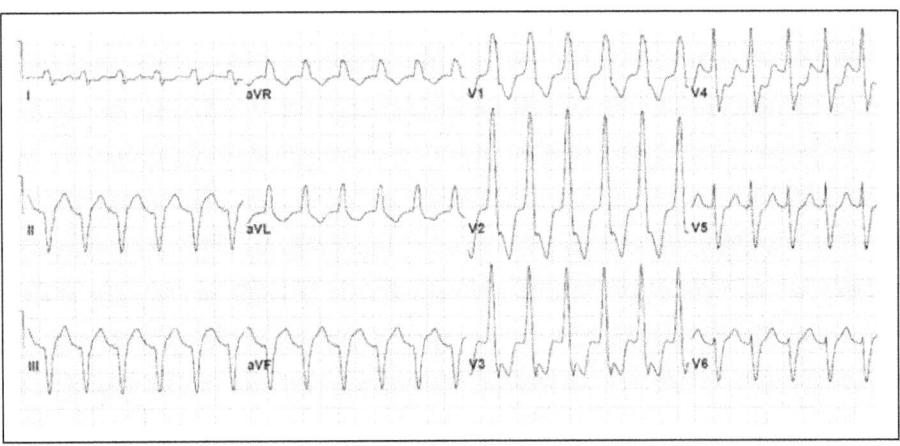

EKG 36

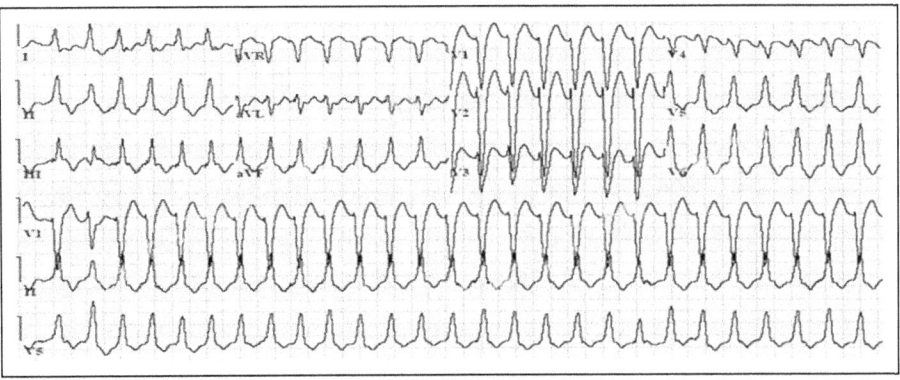

EKG INTERPRETATIONS QUIZ 1-50

EKG 37

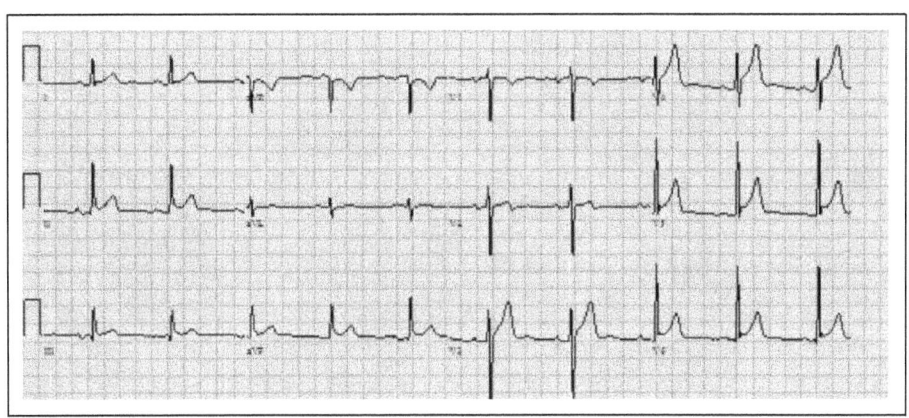

EKG 38

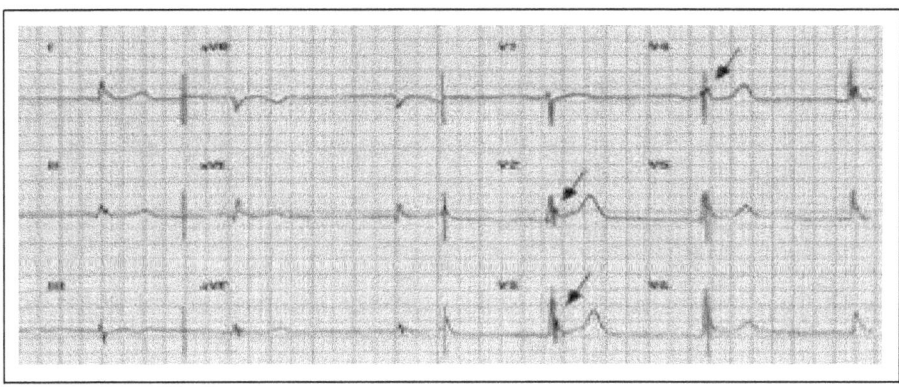

EKG 39

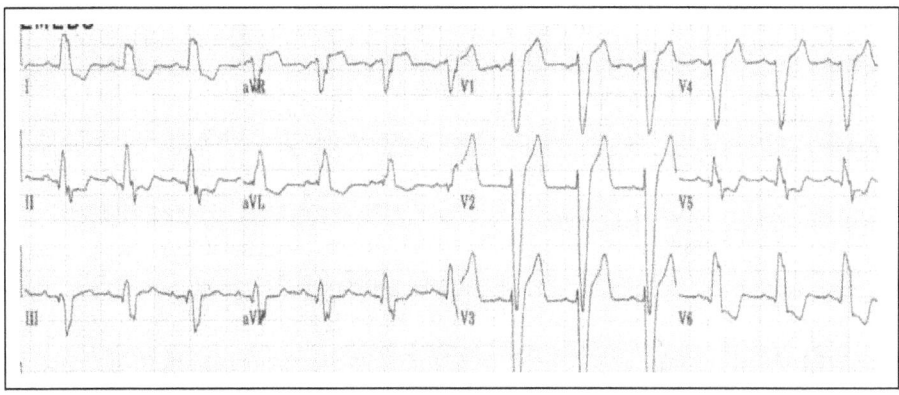

CLINICAL EKG INTERPRETATION

EKG 40

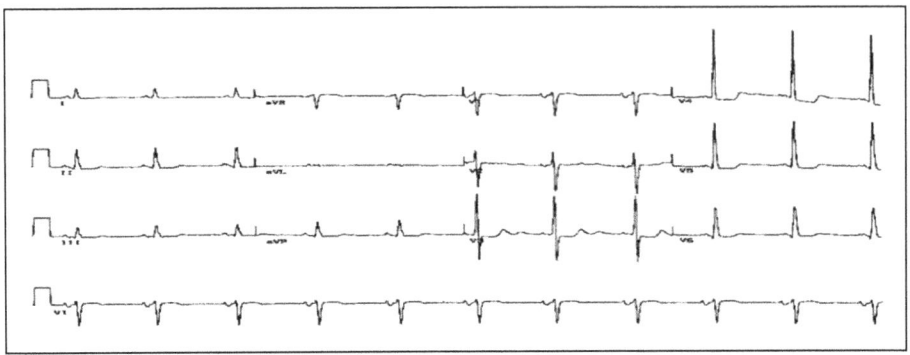

EKG 41

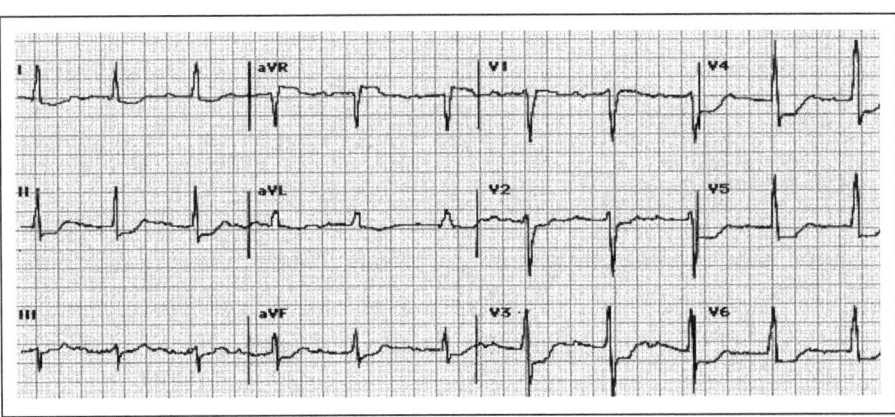

EKG 42

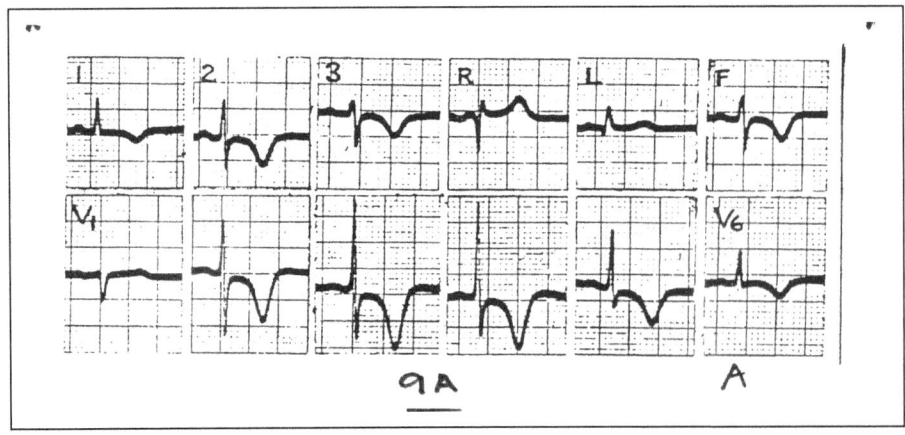

EKG INTERPRETATIONS QUIZ 1-50

EKG 43

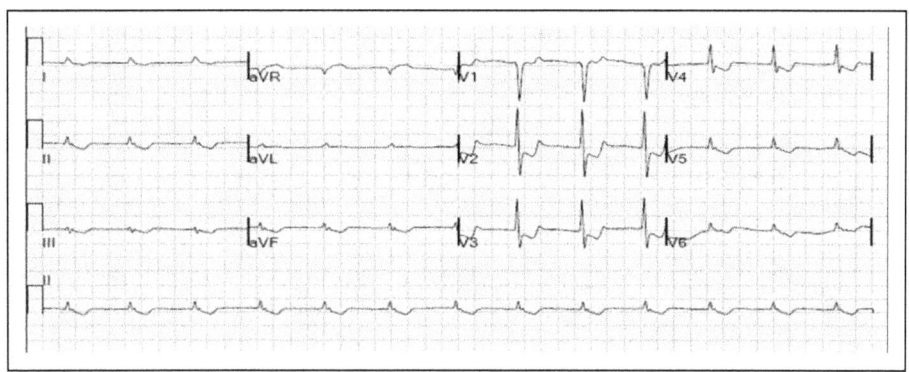

EKG 44

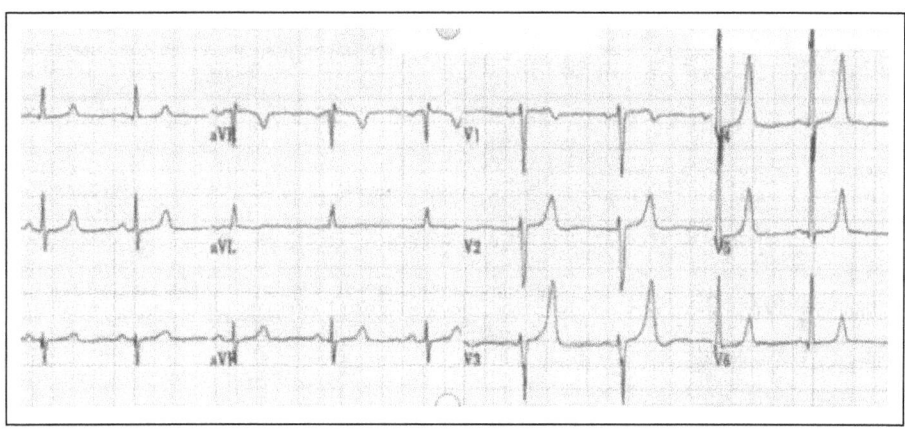

EKG 45

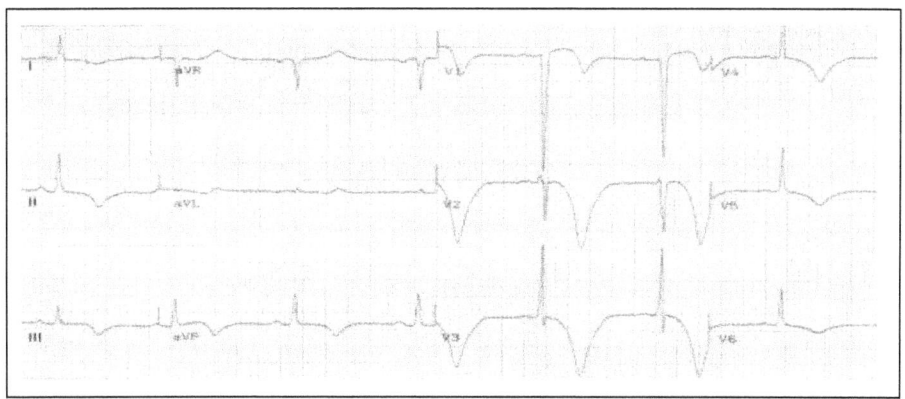

CLINICAL EKG INTERPRETATION

EKG 46

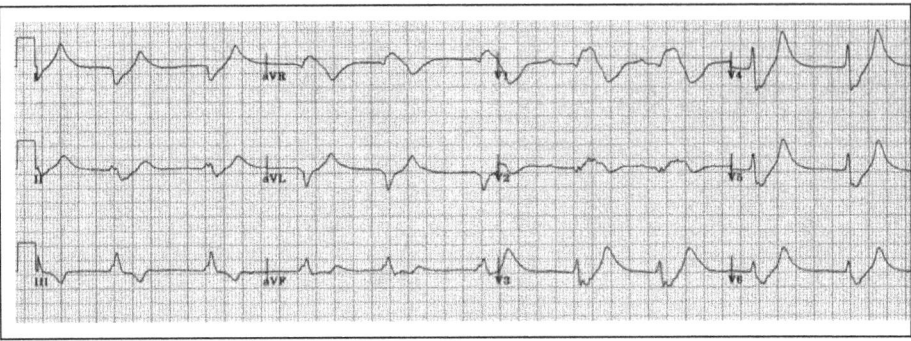

EKG 47

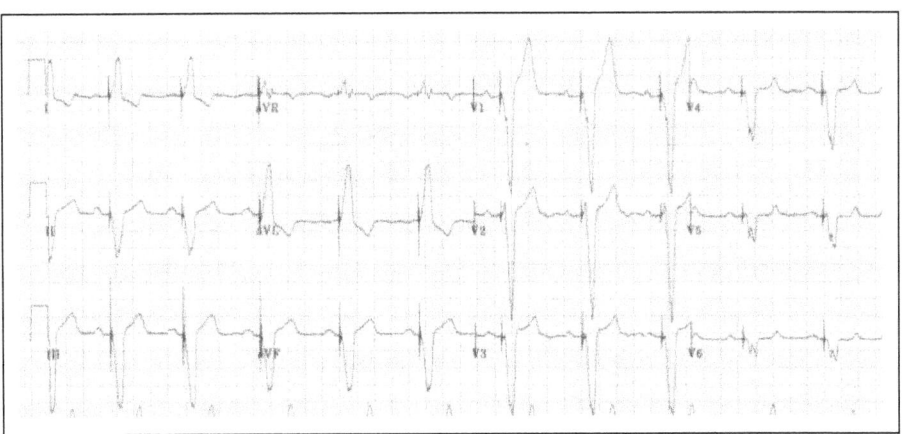

EKG 48

EKG INTERPRETATIONS QUIZ 1-50

EKG 49

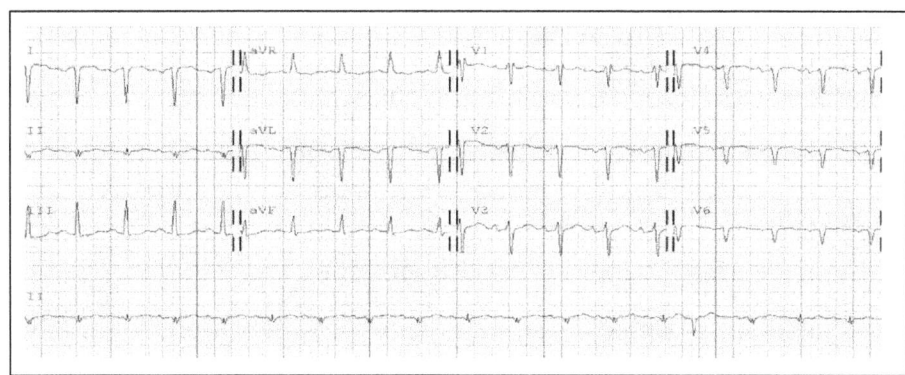

EKG 50

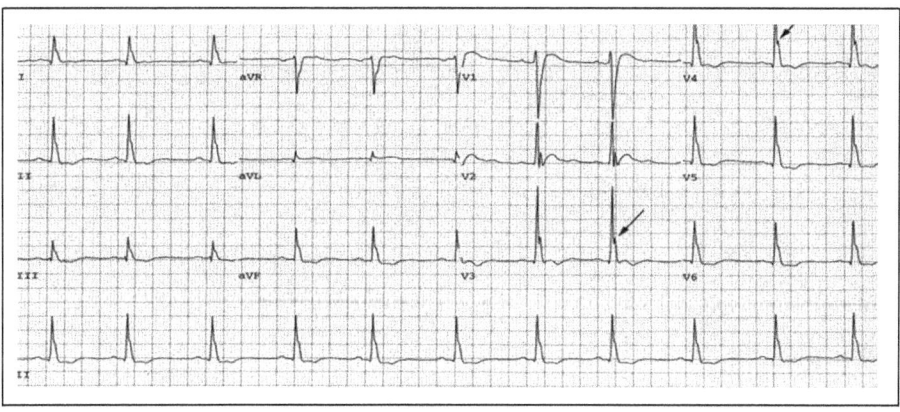

EKG 51

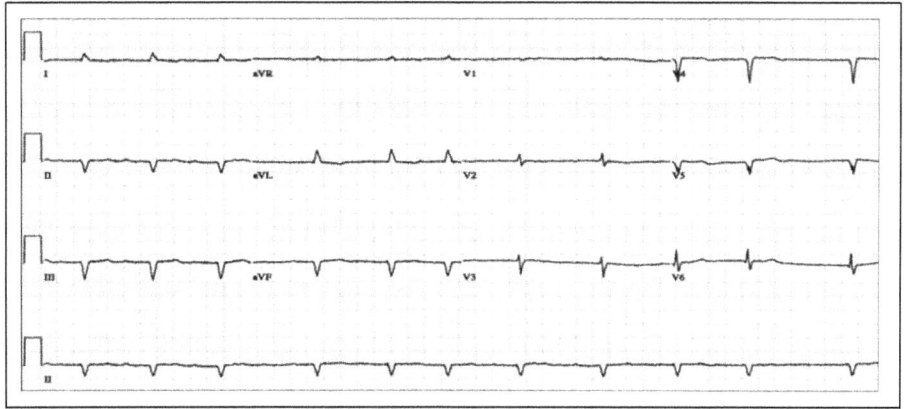

CLINICAL EKG INTERPRETATION

EKG Quiz Answers:

EKG 1. Sinus rhythm. There are hyperacute ST elevations noted in leads I, aVL, and V2 to V6. Notice the elevation of the J point along with straightening of the ST segment in the anterior chest leads. ST depression in leads III and aVF represents the reciprocal changes. You do not see reciprocal changes in pericarditis. There is an involvement of the high anterior wall which is generally supplied by the diagonal branch. And, there is an anterolateral involvement as show in V2 to V6 ST elevation. This points to an acute extensive anterolateral . There are also Q waves in V2 to V6. It takes at least 6 hours for Q waves to develop. Would you take this person to the catheterization lab since there is already development of the Q waves even if the chest pain is of 3-4 hour duration? Since this involves an extensive area of the left ventricle, an open LAD is far better than an occluded LAD to salvage any border zone ischemia. Yes, it would make sense to take this patient to the catheterization lab and open up a proximal totally occluded LAD if present. What do you think?

EKG 2. This is an interesting electrocardiogram. Sinus rhythm. Right axis deviation. Immediately you should think about the conditions that cause right axis deviation. Next, we see tall R waves in the V1, V2, V3, and V4. In fact, there are deep S waves in the lateral chest leads that suggest right ventricular hypertrophy. So far, we have RVH with RAD. Whenever you see right ventricular hypertrophy, you should also look for right atrial enlargement. The P waves look peaked in leads II, III, and aVF, suggestive of right atrial enlargement. These findings go hand in hand. There is a large negative P wave in V1 suggestive of left atrial enlargement. There are discordant ST-T changes in V1 to V5. A combination of RVH, RAD, RAE, and

EKG INTERPRETATIONS QUIZ 1-50

LAE should raise the possibility of mitral stenosis. It could also be due to pulmonary embolus; you would not see an LAE.

EKG 3. Your interpretation.

EKG 4. Appearances could be deceptive on purpose. At first glance, lead I may look like sinus bradycardia. Upon close observation you notice there is no correlation between the P wave and the QRS complexes. The PR intervals are not constant. The P waves come before and after the QRS complexes. In fact, if you closely look at the T waves and the TP segments, there appears to be another P wave! The atrial rate if 93 bpm, while the ventricular rate is 48 bpm. The QRS complex seems to be independent of the P waves. It is not a Wenckebach as there is no progressive PR prolongation. It is not 2nd-degree AV block as there are no constant PR intervals in the conducted beats. It is unlikely to be atrial bigeminy as the non-conducted P waves don't appear to be premature. The ventricular rhythm could be Junctional, with RBBB. There is AV dissociation. The most likely diagnosis is complete heart block with escape junctional rhythm with RBBB.

EKG 5. There is sinus rhythm with 1st-degree AV block. Hyperacute ST elevation is noted in leads II, III, and aVF, along with ST elevation in leads V5 and V6. This suggests the involvement of the inferolateral walls. If you are taking this patient to the catheterization lab, which artery is most likely involved? Remember that the lateral wall is generally supplied by the circumflex marginal branches. And, in 15% of the cases, the circumflex artery also supplies the inferior wall. The other option would be the RCA, which generally supply the inferior wall but not the lateral wall. Occasionally, the RAC may supply the apex of the left ventricles and when that is involved we might see changes in V3 and V4. Here we see reciprocal changes in V1 to V3. If I was in Las Vegas I would bet on the circumflex branch as it involves the inferolateral wall of the left ventricle.

EKG 6. Sinus rhythm. The most obvious picture is one of a wide QRS complex. The PR interval is at the upper limit of normal (200 ms). There is left atrial enlargement as the negative deflection in V1 covers more than one small box. Leads I, aVL, and V5 and v6 have wide QRS complexes. There is a left bundle branch block. In addition, there is a slight left axis deviation as the S wave in lead II is slightly greater than the R wave. There are also discordant ST-T changes in the lateral chest leads (another point on board exams). Also, note the J point elevation in V1, V2, V3, and V4 with ST elevation, which is a normal finding in a patient with LBBB. The QRS duration is 160 ms.

EKG 7. Sinus rhythm at a rate of 80 bpm. Left atrial enlargement. Pacemaker spikes. Wide QRS following the spikes. The QRD complexes are positive in leads I, aVL, V1, and V2. There is atrial sensing and ventricular pacing. There is also left atrial enlargement. The QRS duration is 120 ms.

EKG 8. There are no visible P waves. The RR intervals are irregularly irregular. There is an incomplete RBBB. There are nonspecific T wave changes. Terminal S waves related RBBB are noted in the anterolateral leads. Less than 1 mm ST elevation in leads I, aVL, and V4 to V6. Atrial fibrillation with a variable ventricular response.

EKG 9. It is a paced rhythm. There is atrial pacing and capture. There is ventricular pacing and capture. In addition, you see premature ventricular complexes. The pacemaker rate is 60 bpm. The QRS complex is 160 ms. The fact that both the atria and the ventricles are being paced suggests far advanced disease involving the sinus node and the conduction system.

EKG 10. Sinus rhythm. RBBB. LAD. LAHB. Left atrial enlargement. Poor R wave progression in the lateral chest leads may be related to lead placement. Nonspecific T wave changes in inferolateral leads.

EKG 11. Sinus arrhythmia. Symmetrical T wave inversions in the inferior and anterolateral chest leads. This is suggestive of ventricular ischemia involving more the one territory. There is also QT prolongation. Conditions that prolong QT interval would include hypocalcemia, antidepressants, and some antiarrhythmic drugs.

EKG 12. It appears to be junctional rhythm at a rate of 60 bpm with a retrograde P wave seen in aVL and V1. One sinus beat seen in leads I, II, and III. No other P waves are noted. Since there is one conducted sinus beat, it cannot be complete heart block. It would qualify as a high-grade AV block. The difference may be more academic than clinical. There is a disease involving the sinus node and the AV node. Unless this rhythm is related to drugs such as digitalis, beta blockers, or calcium channel blockers, based on the symptoms this patient may be a candidate for a pacemaker. Any type of 48-hour monitoring might shed more light on the degree of conduction problems and atrial activity, which might help determine the type of pacemaker that might be suitable for this patient.

EKG 13. Sinus bradycardia. There are T wave inversions involving leads I, aVL, and V1 to V3, suggestive of ischemia involving the high anterior and anteroseptal regions. Low voltage in limb leads. Left atrial enlargement.

CLINICAL EKG INTERPRETATION

EKG 14. Sinus rhythm. Left axis deviation. RBBB. Nonspecific T wave changes in leads I, aVL, and V4 to V6. Lack of natural R wave progression across the chest leads may be due to lead misplacement.

EKG 15. Sinus rhythm. RBBB. LAD. LAHB. Terminal slurred S waves noted in multiple leads.

EKG 16. SVT loss of R waves anteriorly. ST- T changes.

EKG 17 Sinus rhythm. Wenckebach type I. Voltage criteria for LVH. ST-T changes.

EKG 18. NSR Normal.

EKG 19. RAD P wave, RVH. Tall R waves in V1, V2. Discordant ST-T changes in V1 and V2.

EKG 20. Sinus rhythm. Old ASMI, RBBB. Discordant ST-T changes in V1 and V2. Nonspecific ST-T changes in V4, V5, and V6.

EKG:21. Sinus rhythm. WPW syndrome with delta waves. Type A WPW.

EKG 22. Atrial flutter with 2:1 conduction. Notice the flutteR waves in leads II, III, and aVF

EKG 23. SVT. Retrograde P waves. Voltage criteria for LVH. Downsloping ST depression in the lateral leads.

EKG 24. Atrial Fib with adequate VR. Low QRS voltage in limb leads and chest leads. Loss of R waves anteriorly. Generalized nonspecific ST-T changes.

EKG INTERPRETATIONS QUIZ 1-50

EKG 25. Sinus rhythm. Left axis deviation. LVH with strain pattern. Notice 2 to 3 mm upsloping ST elevation in V1, V2, and V3, which are common findings in LVH and also in LBBB.

EKG 26. Sinus tachycardia. S1, Q3, and T3. The combination of findings suggestive of acute pulmonary embolus. It can be seen in any situation where there is acute right ventricular strain. In addition, there is an rSr'' in V1.

EKG 27. Sinus rhythm with extreme right axis deviation. RBBB with a QRS complex of >120 ms. There are also RS complexes all the way to V6, suggestive of RVH with strain.

EKG 27. Sinus rhythm with extreme right axis deviation. RBBB, RVH with strain.

EKG 28. Atrial Fib. Whenever you see regular narrow QRS rhythm, think of junctional rhythm nonspecific ST-T changes.

EKG 29. At first glance, it looks like bradycardia. If you pay attention to the T waves, there may be a hidden P wave which is premature. That makes this rhythm sinus with atrial bigeminy and pause.

EKG 30. Sinus rhythm with constant PP intervals. There are dropped P waves. Second-degree AV block Type II.

EKG 31. Sinus rhythm. Third-degree AV block. None of the P waves are conducted. Narrow QRS suggest the impulse can be from the junction or the common bundle.

EKG 32. Atrial flutter with 2:1 conduction. The sawtooth appearance of flutteR waves in the inferior leads. There is ST elevation in aVL along with downsloping ST segments in the lateral chest leads.

33. Wide QRS tachycardia. SVT with LBBB and ST-T changes related to LBBB. LAD. Some ST depression in the lateral chest leads may also suggest ischemia.

EKG 34. Sinus rhythm. Acute IMI. Ventricular bigeminy, reciprocal changes in leads 1 and aVL and nonspecific ST-T changes laterally.

EKG 35. Ventricular tachycardia at 150 bpm. The tachycardia has an RBBB pattern, suggestive of left ventricular origin. The QEX complex is 160 ms. Significant ST-T changes noted in the anterior leads.

EKG 36. Ventricular tachycardia at a rate of 165 bpm. The tachycardia has an LBBB pattern, suggesting its origin might be from the right side. In addition, there are two beats that have a different morphology that may suggest fusion beats. There is a suggestion of a retrograde P in leads I and aVR but they are not consistent.

EKG 37. Sinus rhythm. There are ST elevations in multiple leads. The ST segment is concave upward, unlike in an acute MI in which they are straight up or convex upward. In pericarditis, it is associated with symptoms and may improve with time. This is an example of early repolarization seen in young individuals.

EKG 38. Sinus bradycardia. First-degree AV block. Low QRS voltage. Osborne waves in V2, V3, and V4. Low amplitude T waves. Prolonged QT interval. A sign of slowing of the metabolism. This is an example of hypothermia. Some similar features may be seen in severe hypothyroidism even though not Osborne waves.

EKG 39. Sinus rhythm. Left bundle branch pattern. QRS duration >120 ms. Wide QRS in leads I, aVL, and the lateral chest leads. Discordant ST-T changes in the anterolateral chest leads. Notice the marked ST elevation in V1, V2, and V3, simulating an acute MI which is a normal finding. There is a suggestion of a left atrial enlargement with a negative deflection of the P wave in V1, occupying more than 1 small box.

EKG 40. Sinus rhythm. Left atrial enlargement. Voltage criteria for LVH. Nonspecific ST-T changes. These are not the typical discordant ST-T changes we notice with LVH. There is horizontal ST depression in V3, V4, and V5 but it is not clear about the depth. If it is more than 1 mm, it may suggest subendocardial ischemia or infarction.

EKG 41. Sinus rhythm. There is horizontal ST depression noted in leads II, III, aVF, V3, V4, V5, and V6. The ST depression is more than 3-4 mm. This is an example of subendocardial ischemia. If this is associated with chest pain and positive cardiac enzymes, it would be called subendocardial infarction. Thus, these patients are at an increased risk for subsequent cardiac events in the following three-month period and need a more thorough evaluation for inducible ischemia after the acute event settles down. There is also a first-degree AV block.

EKG 42. This is an example of deeply inverted T waves seen in the inferior and anterolateral chest leads. These T wave changes represent ventricular ischemia, which in this case appears to be global ischemia. If the same EKG changes are associated with chest pain and positive cardiac enzymes, it may represent non-Q MI.

EKG 43. Sinus rhythm. Low QRS voltage in the chest leads. The absence of P waves raises the question of accelerated junctional rhythm. Tall R waves and ST depression noted in V2, V3, and V6, which suggest posterior myocardial infarction. There are also ST-T changes noted in the infer-lateral leads, suggestive of strain pattern. Notice the biphasic T waves in the anterior leads.

EKG 44. Sinus rhythm. Tall peaked T waves in the anterolateral chest leads. These changes are seen in patients with hyperkalemia. There is increased voltage criteria for LVH. This may go along with a patient with hypertension and renal failure or those on potassium-sparing diuretics. So, an EKG tells a lot about a patient's cardiovascular and metabolic states.

EKG 45. Sinus bradycardia with giant negative T waves in the inferior and anterolateral chest leads. There is a prolongation of the QT interval. This type of change is typical in patients with acute cerebrovascular accidents.

EKG 46. Sinus rhythm with very wide QRS complexes. First-degree AV block. Loss of R waves across the EKG. ST depression and tall T waves. Hyperkalemia.

EKG 47. Pacemaker rhythm. Atrial sensing. Ventricular pacing. Rate 63 bpm. LBBB pattern suggests right ventricular pacing. The significant ST elevation may be present in paced beats, LBBB, and in patients with LVH. This is not a sign of acute myocardial ischemia or infarction.

CLINICAL EKG INTERPRETATION

EKG 48. Paced rhythm. Two pacemaker spikes are seen, suggesting atrial pacing and ventricular pacing. This is a dual chamber-pacing. There is an LBBB pattern in leads I, aVL, and V6. Note the left axis deviation. Since there is atrial capture, we can assume there is no atrial fib or flutter. However, there seems to be advanced changes in the conduction system since the ventricles are also paced.

EKG 49. Sinus rhythm. Inverted P, QRS, and T waves in leads I and aVL. Right axis deviation. Incomplete RBBB. Poor R wave progression across the left chest leads. Positive QRS complex in aVR. Nonspecific ST-T changes. All these findings should raise the suspicion of Dextrocardia. You can confirm that by right-sided chest, reversing the right and left arm leads. On a chest x-ray you will see the heart located on the right side of the chest.

EKG 50. Sinus rhythm. Rate 66 bpm. Notice the notch in the downstroke of the R waves. These are Osborn waves. There is also shortening of the QT interval. There is an ST depression in the lateral chest leads. Tall R waves in V2 and V3. These findings are consistent with hypercalcemia.

EKG 51. Sinus rhythm. Prolonged PR interval. Low QRS voltage (<5 mm in the limb leads and <10 mm in the chest leads). Left axis deviation. Nonspecific ST-T changes. Consider hypothyroidism, larger pericardial effusion, COPD, cardiomyopathy, and infiltrative cardiomyopathy.

The V1 usually has a negative T wave. However, in an inferior MI, if we see a positive T wave it may suggest right ventricular ischemia or infarction as V1 also represents the right ventricle. When we see these changes, we should consider proximal RCA occlusion leading to inferior myocardial infarction with a possible right ventricular infarction. Patients' right ventricular involvement may present with hypotension. Patients may need fluids and vasopressors for several days before we can stabilize them.

References

Recommended readings

- *The Only EKG Book You'll Ever Need*—Malcolm S. Thaler
- *Rapid Interpretation of EKGs*—Dale Dubin, M.D.
- Up to Date blog at wordpress.com
- ekgcasestudies.com
- healio.com
- lifeinthefastlane.com
- learntheheart.com
- https://meds.queensu.ca/central/assets/modules/tsecg/acute_right_ventricular_mi.html
- http://clevelandclinic.flywheelsites.com/cardio/?gclid=EAIaIQobChMIk-rup-Kz3wIVA77ACh1fKwGCEAAYASAAEgJdI_D_BwE

CLINICAL EKG INTERPRETATION

NIK'S COMEDY CLUB:

One day, I was getting ready to do a heart catheterization on a patient. The nurses were taking a little longer to get him ready. I walked up to him and said, "Mr. John, you've been waiting for this test for a long time, haven't you?"

"Yes, Dr. Nik, 72 years! Don't you think that's a long time to be waiting for this one test?"

"I see what you mean," I said.

"Have you done this before?"

"No, you are my first patient."

"What?"

"I, meant today!"

"You better get moving. If you are not ready in 5 minutes, I'm going to put you on the table and start the procedure myself."

ACLS QUIZ:

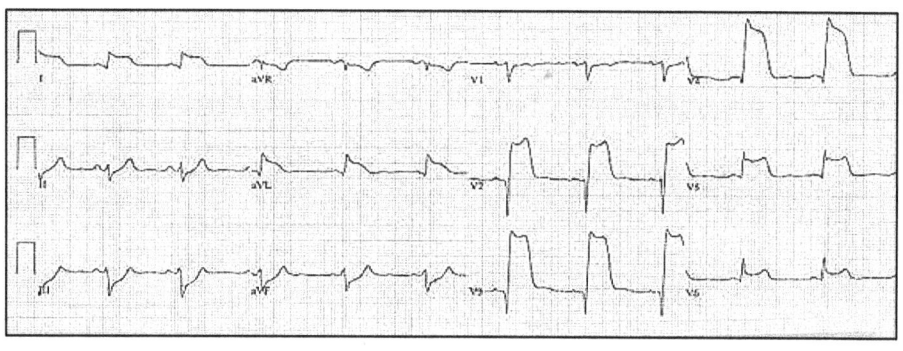

Concerned? _____

EKG INTERPRETATIONS QUIZ 1-50

Author: NIK NIKAM, MD, MHA

Dr. Nik Nikam has practiced cardiology in Houston and Sugar Land, Texas for over 38 years.

He had vast exposure to the medical field at the world-famous Texas Medical Center for over three decades. His public speaking skills and his interactions with a community of diverse people have created an everlasting reservoir of knowledge and experience.

He uses his experience in explaining the interpretation of the electrocardiogram from a clinical perspective and to create a visual image of the heart in the patient's body. He explains how the heart reflects the electrocardiographic changes and how these changes may reflect the patient's overall prognosis

Dr. Nik has made hundreds of presentations on Heart-Healthy Lifestyle. He has published over 100 articles in many local newspapers in Houston and across the US.

He is a Distinguished Toastmaster, speaker, writer, auctioneer, and a talk show host. His YouTube channel, "NIK NIKAM NETWORK - NNN," has more than 140 videos covering important cardiology topics, including ACLS protocols.

He loves to deliver an engaging educational presentation sprinkled with a unique sense of humor.

For speaking engagements, you can contact Dr. Nik Nikam at:

NIK NIKAM, MD, MHA
NNN MEDIA
3130 GRANTS BLVD #17034
SUGAR LAND, TX 77496
281-745-4161
drniknikam@gmail.com

CLINICAL EKG INTERPRETATION

YOUTUBE: NIK NIKAM

Please visit our YouTube channel, "NIK NIKAM," and Subscribe to it.

It has more than 150 presentations under "Cardiology Lecture Series," play list, including a comprehensive coverage of the cardiology section of the Internal Medicine Board Examination's cardiology section, the ACLS protocols, and ACLS EKG interpretations.

In fact, our presentation on ACLS EKG interpretation has been watched by more than 250,000 people from all across the globe.

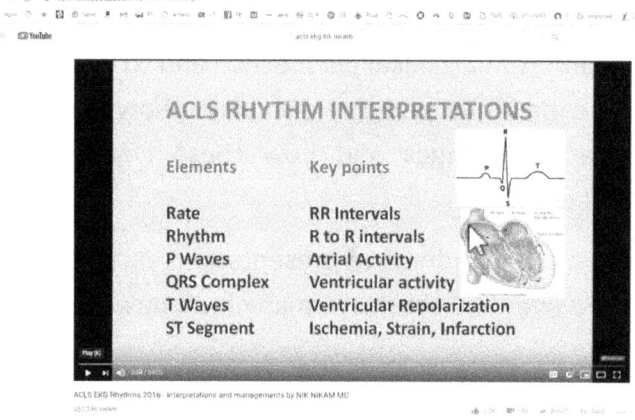

Let's Keep in Touch

As we continue to provide basic, clinical, patient focused, EKG interpretations that can help you at besides, we invite your input, tracings, and suggestions for the next edition so we can surely provide the readers on maximum return for their time and effort.

Also, please take a moment to comment on Amazon website about your impressions on the book and how we can improve it in the future.

EKG INTERPRETATIONS QUIZ 1-50

The End

CLINICAL EKG INTERPRETATION

www.ingramcontent.com/pod-product-compliance
Lightning Source LLC
Chambersburg PA
CBHW081453040426
42446CB00016B/3231